MEDICAL ASSISTANT
Urinary, Blood, Lymphatic, and Immune Systems and Laboratory Procedures
Module E

MEDICAL ASSISTANT

Urinary, Blood, Lymphatic, and Immune Systems and Laboratory Procedures
Module E

Material Selected from:

Mastering Healthcare Terminology
Second Edition
by
Betsy J. Shiland, MS, RHIA, CPHQ, CTR

Saunders Textbook of Medical Assisting
(textbook and workbook)
by
Diane M. Klieger, RN, MBA, CMA

Medical Transcription: Techniques and Procedures
Sixth Edition
by
Marcy O. Diehl, BVE, CMA-A, CMT, FAAMT

SAUNDERS

ELSEVIER

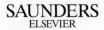

SAUNDERS
ELSEVIER

11830 Westline Industrial Drive
St. Louis, Missouri 63146

Notice

Knowledge and best practice in this field are constantly changing. As new research and
experience broaden our knowledge, changes in practice, treatment and drug therapy may
become necessary or appropriate. Readers are advised to check the most current
information provided (i) on procedures featured or (ii) by the manufacturer of each
product to be administered, to verify the recommended dose or formula, the method and
duration of administration, and contraindications. It is the responsibility of practitioners,
relying on their own experience and knowledge of the patient, to make diagnoses, to
determine dosages and the best treatment for each individual patient, and to take all
appropriate safety precautions. To the fullest extent of the law, neither the Publisher nor
the Authors assume any liability for any injury and/or damage to persons or property
arising out of or related to any use of the material contained in this book.

The Publisher

ISBN: 978-1-4377-0344-3

Printed in the United States of America

Last digit is the print number: 9 8 7 6 5

ACKNOWLEDGMENTS

Thank you to our advisory board members and the CCi Medical Assisting Program community for your dedication, teamwork, and support over the years.

This textbook has been designed for your success. Each feature has been chosen to help you learn medical assisting quickly and effectively. Colorful boxes, tables, and illustrations will visually spark your interest, add to your knowledge, and aid in your retention of the material. Most chapters end with a review that asks you to apply the terms and concepts you have learned.

USE ALL THE FEATURES IN THE CHAPTER

Key Terms

The key terms list provides you with a quick overview of the terms you will encounter as you work your way through the chapter. You can also use this page to help you review for tests.

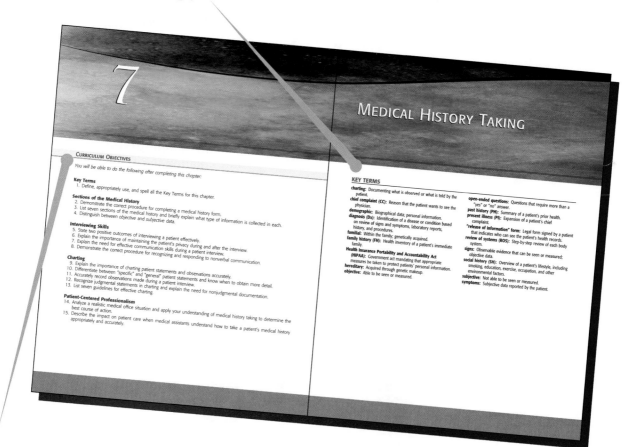

Objectives

Each objective is a goal for you. You should refer to these objectives before you study the chapter to see what your goals are and then again at the end of the chapter to see if you have accomplished them.

Exercises

Some chapters have exercises located after passages of information. Make sure you do these exercises to help you retain your new knowledge. Your instructor can check your work.

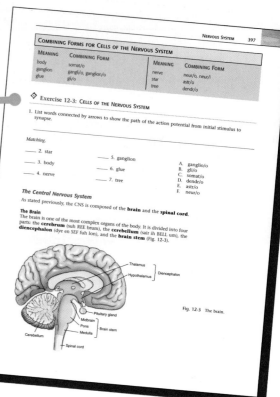

Procedures

Many chapters will contain illustrated step-by-step procedures showing you how to perform administrative and clinical procedures. Rationales for most steps explain why the step is important, and icons let you know which standard precautions to follow:

 Handwashing

 Gloving

 Personal Protective Equipment

 Biohazardous Waste Disposal

 Sharps Disposal

Plus, sample documentation shows you how to chart clinical procedures.

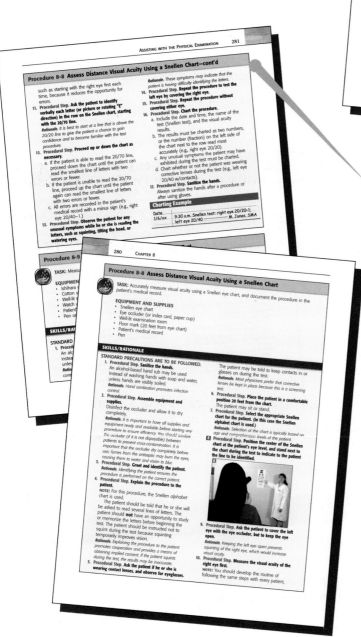

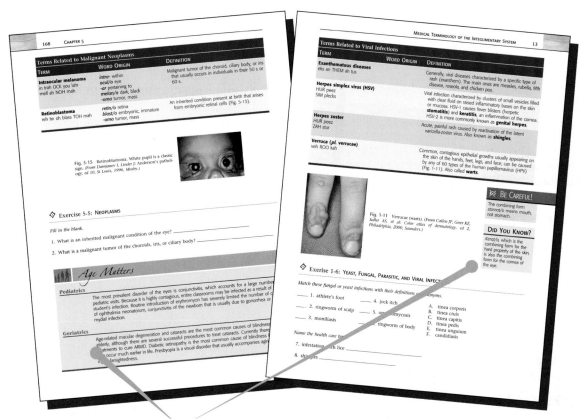

Special Information Boxes

Special information boxes that offer interesting facts or cautions are scattered throughout each chapter.

- *Did You Know?* boxes highlight the fascinating, sometimes strange history that underlies the origins of health care terms.
- *Be Careful!* boxes point out common pitfalls that you might experience when health care terms and word parts are spelled similarly but have different meanings.
- *Age Matters* boxes highlight important concepts and terminology for both pediatric and geriatric patients.

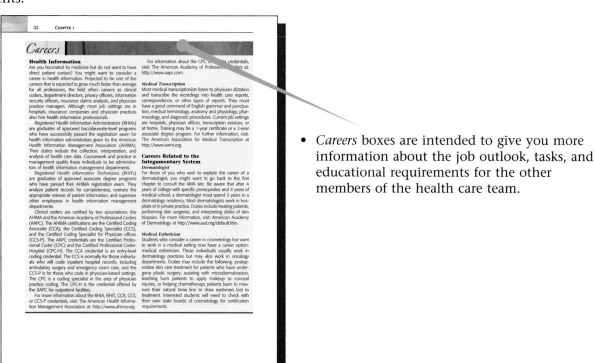

- *Careers* boxes are intended to give you more information about the job outlook, tasks, and educational requirements for the other members of the health care team.

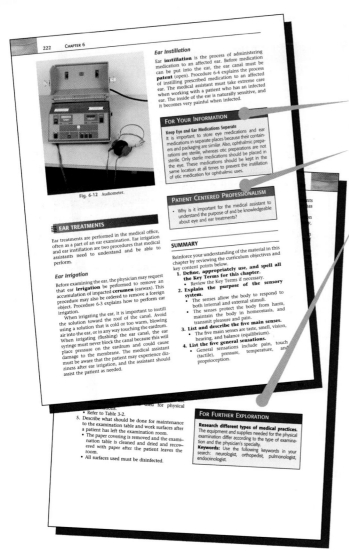

- *For Your Information* boxes provide interesting informational "tid-bits" on topics related to the subject at hand.
- *Patient-Centered Professionalism* boxes prompt you to think about the patient's perspective and encourage empathy.
- *For Further Exploration* boxes suggest topics for further Internet research to expand your comprehension of concepts and inspire you to "learn beyond the text."

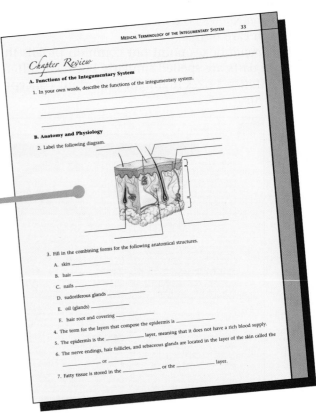

Chapter Review

A variety of exercises, including reviews of chapter terminology, theory, and critical-thinking, are included at the end of each chapter to help you test your knowledge. Most chapter reviews also include case studies to give you the opportunity to apply your recently gained knowledge to real-life situations. Your instructor can check your work on the chapter review section.

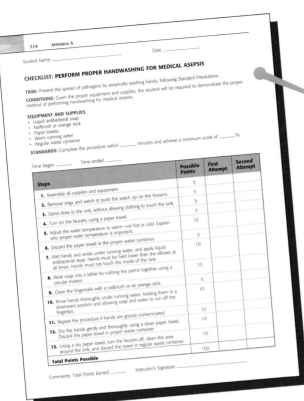

514   APPENDIX A

Student Name _____   Date _____

CHECKLIST: PERFORM PROPER HANDWASHING FOR MEDICAL ASEPSIS

TASK: Prevent the spread of pathogens by aseptically washing hands, following Standard Precautions.

CONDITIONS: Given the proper equipment and supplies, the student will be required to demonstrate the proper method of performing handwashing for medical asepsis.

EQUIPMENT AND SUPPLIES
- Liquid antibacterial soap
- Nailbrush or orange stick
- Paper towels
- Warm running water
- Regular waste container

STANDARDS: Complete the procedure within _____ minutes and achieve a minimum score of _____%.

Time began _____   Time ended _____

Steps	Possible Points	First Attempt	Second Attempt
1. Assemble all supplies and equipment.	5		
2. Remove rings and watch or push the watch up on the forearm.	5		
3. Stand close to the sink, without allowing clothing to touch the sink.	5		
4. Turn on the faucets, using a paper towel.	5		
5. Adjust the water temperature to warm—not hot or cold. Explain why proper water temperature is important.	10		
6. Discard the paper towel in the proper waste container.	5		
7. Wet hands and wrists under running water, and apply liquid antibacterial soap. Hands must be held lower than the elbows at all times. Hands must not touch the inside of the sink.	10		
8. Work soap into a lather by rubbing the palms together using a circular motion.	10		
9. Clean the fingernails with a nailbrush or an orange stick.	5		
10. Rinse hands thoroughly under running water, holding them in a downward position and allowing soap and water to run off the fingertips.	10		
11. Repeat the procedure if hands are grossly contaminated.	10		
12. Dry the hands gently and thoroughly using a clean paper towel. Discard the paper towel in proper waste container.	10		
13. Using a dry paper towel, turn the faucets off, clean the area around the sink, and discard the towel in regular waste container.	10		
Total Points Possible	100		

Comments: Total Points Earned _____   Instructor's Signature _____

Appendixes

Appendixes include competency checklists. They are organized into two groups. There are Core Competency Checklists for core skills, such as taking vital signs, giving injections, and assigning insurance codes, that you will be practicing in every module. The Core Competency Checklists are followed by the Procedure Competency Checklists, which are unique to the topics you are learning in this module. Each group of checklists has a Grade Sheet to summarize your performance scores when demonstrating your competencies to your instructor.

CONTENTS

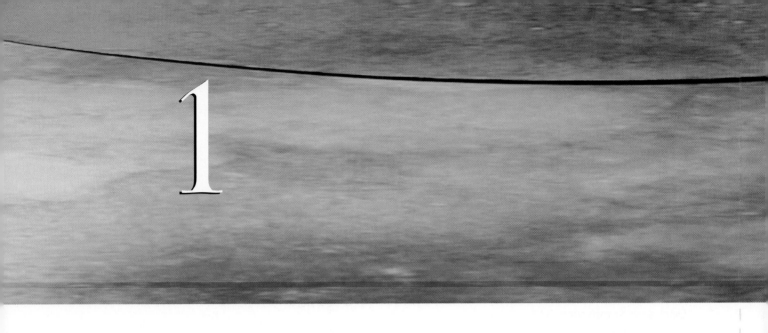

1

OBJECTIVES

You will be able to do the following after completing this chapter:

Key Terms
1. Define, appropriately use, and spell all the Key Terms for this chapter.

Laboratory Regulations and Safety
2. Explain the purpose of the Clinical Laboratory Improvement Amendments of 1988 (CLIA 88).
3. List three factors that determine whether a medical office will perform and process a specimen.
4. Briefly describe three CLIA-waived urine tests, six CLIA-waived blood tests, and seven CLIA-waived tests of other types.
5. Differentiate between quality assurance (QA) and quality control (QC) and briefly explain how each is accomplished in the medical office.
6. Demonstrate the correct procedure for using methods of quality control.
7. Explain the need for safety precautions in the medical office laboratory and how they protect both staff and patients.

Basic Laboratory Equipment
8. Identify the parts of a compound microscope, and explain its proper use and maintenance.
9. Demonstrate the procedure for successfully focusing a microscope from lower to higher power.
10. Explain the purpose and proper use of a centrifuge.

Laboratory Tests
11. List six categories of laboratory tests and briefly explain the purpose of each.
12. Explain the importance of effective patient preparation before laboratory tests are performed.
13. Explain the importance of completing a laboratory request form accurately.
14. Demonstrate the procedure for accurately completing a laboratory request form.
15. List three methods of specimen collection, and explain the need for collecting specimens accurately.
16. Demonstrate the procedure for accurately collecting a specimen for transport to an outside laboratory.
17. Explain the purpose of a laboratory report and why it must be accurate and transmitted to the physician in a timely manner.
18. Demonstrate the correct procedure for screening and following up on patient test results.

Culture Collection
19. Demonstrate the correct procedure for collecting an uncontaminated throat specimen to test for group A beta-hemolytic streptococci.

INTRODUCTION TO THE PHYSICIAN OFFICE LABORATORY

Urine Collection

20. Explain the purpose of a urinalysis and the need for avoiding sources of contamination and for processing urine specimens in the required time.
21. List four instructions the medical assistant should give to a patient who is to collect a random urine specimen and bring it to the medical office.
22. Demonstrate the correct procedure for obtaining a urine specimen from an infant using a pediatric urine collector.
23. Demonstrate the correct procedure for providing patient instructions on collecting a midstream clean-catch urine specimen to ensure validity of test results.
24. Demonstrate the correct procedure for providing patient instructions on collecting a 24-hour urine specimen to ensure validity of test results.
25. Explain the special considerations for handling drug screenings and specimens that may be used as evidence in a court of law.

Blood Collection

26. List methods of collecting blood and give the three factors that determine which method will be used.
27. Explain the purpose of a lancet in capillary blood collection.
28. Briefly describe five types of containers that can be used to collect capillary blood specimens.
29. Demonstrate the correct procedure for obtaining a capillary blood specimen acceptable for testing using the index or middle finger.
30. List four acceptable sites for performing venipuncture and the two factors in selecting the site.
31. State two reasons for failed venipuncture draws.
32. List the order of draw for the evacuated-tube (Vacutainer) system recommended by the Clinical and Laboratory Standards Institute (CLSI).
33. Demonstrate the correct procedure for obtaining a venous blood specimen acceptable for testing using the evacuated-tube system.
34. Demonstrate the correct procedure for obtaining a venous blood specimen acceptable for testing using the syringe method.
35. Demonstrate the correct procedure for obtaining a venous blood specimen acceptable for testing using the butterfly method.
36. Demonstrate the correct procedure for successfully separating serum from a blood specimen and transferring the serum from the collection tube to a transfer tube.

Stool Collection

37. Explain the considerations for collecting stool specimens.

Sputum Collection

38. Explain the considerations for collecting sputum specimens.

Patient-Centered Professionalism

39. Analyze a realistic medical office situation and apply your understanding of the purpose and use of the physician office laboratory to determine the best course of action.
40. Describe the impact on patient care when medical assistants have a solid understanding of the processes and procedures used to collect specimens for testing in the medical office.

KEY TERMS

24-hour urine specimen Collection of urine over a 24-hour period to test kidney function, checking for high levels of creatinine, uric acid, hormones, electrolytes, and medication.

arm (microscope) Part of the microscope that is held when moving the equipment; connects the objective and ocular lenses to the base.

bacteremia Bacteria in the blood; sepsis.

bacteriuria Bacteria in the urine.

base (microscope) Bottom part of the microscope that contains the light source.

binocular Having two eyepieces or ocular lenses.

blood bank Organization that conducts studies for ABO blood grouping and Rh typing.

blood culture Sterile blood specimen drawn for use with a special medium to diagnose specific infectious diseases.

butterfly method Blood collection method using a winged infusion set.

capillary puncture Skin puncture to obtain a capillary blood sample.

capillary collection tube Small tube used to collect capillary blood.

Centers for Medicare and Medicaid Services (CMS) Federal agency that oversees financial regulations of Medicare and Medicaid.

centrifuge Laboratory equipment that separates solids or semisolids from liquids by forced gravity.

certificate of provider-performed microscopy (PPM) procedures Certificate that allows a physician in the office laboratory to conduct both low-complexity and moderate-complexity tests.

certificate of waiver Certificate that allows a physician office laboratory to perform low-complexity testing.

chain of custody Process by which evidence is handled.

chain of evidence Collection routine for a specimen used as evidence.

chemistry Tests run on serum or other body fluids to identify specific chemicals and drugs.

Clinical Laboratory Improvement Amendments of 1988 (CLIA 88) Legislation enacted to ensure the quality of laboratory results by setting performance standards.

coagulation studies Studies that evaluate the clotting process of blood.

coarse focus adjustment knob Part of the microscope used to lower the stage for rapid focusing; used only with low-power objective.

compound Having two sets of lenses on a microscope.

condenser Mechanism located between the stage and light source on a microscope that condenses the light for vision.

control samples Samples used for testing in which the values are known.

counterbalanced Balanced on both sides.

crossmatching Process of identifying blood compatibility by determining proteins on the red blood cells of the donor and recipient.

cultures Growth of microorganisms in special media used to provide nutrition to the microbes.

drug screening Urine or blood collection to determine the presence or absence of specific substances.

engineering controls Devices that promote safety in the laboratory.

evacuated tube Blood collection tube in which the internal atmosphere is a vacuum allowing blood to flow into the tube.

evacuation blood collection system System that includes a holder, double-ended sterile needle, color-coded stopper, and vacuum blood tube.

eyepiece Part of the microscope through which the viewer looks to see an object; magnifies the visual field by 10 times.

filter paper Special paper used to pass a liquid through or to collect a blood specimen.

fine focus adjustment knob Part of the microscope used for precise focusing of a specimen on a slide; used with both high power and oil immersion.

first morning specimen Urine specimen taken when the patient first awakens; most concentrated specimen.

forensics Collection of evidence (e.g., specimen) in a methodical manner for use in a court of law.

glass slide Flat piece of glass used to hold a specimen for microscopic examination.

glucose tolerance test (GTT) Test in which urine and blood are collected at specified intervals after a special glucose solution is ingested; measures the body's ability to absorb glucose. Also called an oral glucose tolerance test (OGTT).

hematology Tests that assess the formed elements of blood, including red blood cells, white blood cells, and platelets.

heparin Natural substance that prevents clotting; a vacuum tube additive that prevents the clotting of blood in the tube.

iris diaphragm Mechanism just below the microscope stage that adjusts the amount of light that enters the field of vision; connected to the condenser.

laboratory requisition Laboratory form showing the identification of a specimen and the laboratory test to be performed.

lancet Sterile needle-like piece of metal used to puncture the skin to collect a capillary blood specimen.

lens Piece of glass with refracting capabilities.

light source Part of the microscope located in the base that allows for a better view of the specimen.

mechanical stage control knobs Parts of the microscope that move a slide right to left or front to back.

microbiology Tests performed to study microorganisms.

microcontainer Small tubes for blood collection.

microhematocrit centrifuge Machine used to process a blood sample for a hematocrit reading by separating cells from plasma.

microscope Optical instrument used in a laboratory setting to view an organism too small to be seen with the naked eye.

midstream clean-catch urine specimen Urine specimen that requires a strict cleaning procedure and collection during the middle of voiding.

monocular Having only one eyepiece.

multisample needle Needle that can be used to take multiple blood samples because it has a retractable sleeve on one end of a double-ended needle; used with vacuum tubes.

nosepiece Part of the microscope that holds the objectives.

objectives Common name for objective lenses of a microscope that magnify by different powers or strengths.

objective lens Lens within the objective of the microscope that magnifies a specimen by a certain power.

ocular lens Eyepiece; magnifies the field by 10 times.

oil-immersion lens Microscope lens that uses a special oil to allow magnification of 100 times the size of the specimen.

order of draw Order or manner in which blood collection tubes are to be drawn.

personal protective equipment (PPE) Protective clothing worn by all health care workers exposed to body fluids and blood, as required by CDC Standard Precautions to minimize exposure.

phlebotomy Process of drawing blood from a vein; venipuncture.

physician office laboratory (POL) Laboratory within the medical office setting.

pipette Narrow tube used for transferring liquids by suction.

pipetting Taking a small sample from a larger sample using a pipette.

plasma Liquid portion of the blood.

postprandial specimen Urine or blood specimen taken after a meal.

quality assurance (QA) Process designed to monitor and evaluate the quality and accuracy of test results.

quality control (QC) Process that provides for accuracy of laboratory tests performed by using a known value for a precheck.

quantity not sufficient (QNS) Insufficient amount of a specimen for performing the desired test.

random urine specimen Urine specimen collected at any time.

rapid screening test Test used to detect disease using various methods; can be used to detect group A beta hemolytic streptococci.

reagents Solutions used when testing specimens in the laboratory.

serology Tests that study the body's immune response by detecting antibodies in the serum.

serum Liquid portion of blood after blood cells and clotting elements form a clot; used for testing chemicals found in blood.

single-sample needle Double-ended blood collection needle without a retractable sleeve.

solutes Materials suspended in liquid that are not dissolvable.

sputum Lung secretions produced by the bronchi.

stage Part of the microscope that holds the slide.

Standard Precautions Guidelines established by the CDC to reduce the spread of infection.

stool Feces; end product of the digestive system expelled from the rectum.

swab-transport media system Device used to keep a swab with a specimen moist until it can be processed for testing.

syringe method Blood collection method using a syringe and sterile needle.

timed specimen Urine or blood specimen collected at specified intervals for a set time.

urinalysis Analysis of urine to include physical, chemical, and microscopic properties.

Vacutainer Blood collection tube with a colored stopper; used with the evacuation blood collection system.

vacuum tube Blood collection tube with a vacuum; evacuated tube.

venipuncture Puncture of a vein to obtain a venous blood sample.

winged infusion set Blood collection needle set with "wings" to aid in guiding the needle.

What Would You Do?

Read the following scenario and keep it in mind as you learn about the physician office laboratory (POL).

The full-time laboratory technician at Dr. Macinto's office is on sick leave for a week. Dr. Macinto asks Sherri, a medical assistant, to fill in for the sick technician. Sherri has just been hired from another office, where she was trained by the physician. She has not done laboratory tests and has not prepared patients for laboratory work.

On the first day, Dr. Macinto asks Sherri to collect a midstream urine sample on a patient for a culture and sensitivity and to send some of the urine to an outside laboratory for a drug screen. Sherri hands the urine collection container to the patient without any instructions and allows the patient to go to the bathroom alone to collect the specimen. When the specimen is collected, Sherri leaves the drug screen on the counter to await the arrival of the laboratory courier for transport to the outside laboratory. Neither Sherri nor the courier signs for the specimen. Furthermore, the laboratory form is not complete, and no documentation was made of the collection of the specimen.

Mrs. Gorchetzki, a postmastectomy patient, is seen next. Dr. Macinto has ordered a fasting blood sugar and a fasting blood chemistry test. Without talking to Mrs. Gorchetzki about the preparation she has made for the test, Sherri gathers the supplies for the testing. Mrs. Gorchetzki mentions that she had bacon and eggs for breakfast. Sherri draws the blood sugar using a capillary puncture. Sherri performs the testing before doing quality control for the day. When the specimen is drawn for the blood chemistry, the laboratory request form asks for serum. Sherri starts the process of drawing the venipuncture specimen from the side of the mastectomy in a heparinized tube. Mrs. Gorchetzki tries to tell Sherri to collect the specimen from the other arm because it is easier to draw blood from that arm, but Sherri does not listen.

When Sherri places the specimen in the centrifuge, she spins only one tube. She pipettes off the liquid and sends it to the laboratory. As it turns out, the liquid sent to the laboratory is plasma, but the laboratory had requested serum.

What things would you have done differently in this situation?

One of the many duties of the medical assistant is to collect, prepare for transport, and process different types of specimens. Medical laboratories perform chemical, physical, and microscopic tests on blood, urine, and other body fluids. A medical laboratory's function is to collect and test specimens provided by the patient. The physician analyzes test results to assess the patient's general health, diagnose, and form a treatment plan as needed. A medical laboratory can be located in a variety of settings, including the physician office laboratory (POL), hospital, and outside (independent) reference laboratory. This chapter focuses on the POL.

When a specimen is collected and transported, the medical assistant must understand the importance of following federal and state protocols. Adherence to guidelines helps ensure the accuracy and usefulness of the results. In addition to understanding the laboratory regulations and safety guidelines, medical assistants must also be familiar with basic laboratory equipment; the process of carrying out laboratory tests; culture, urine, and blood collection; stool and sputum collection; and the range of normal test results.

LABORATORY REGULATIONS AND SAFETY

Not all medical offices have a **physician office laboratory (POL).** Offices that do have a POL are regulated by government standards. Medical offices that do not have a POL are still required to take proper procedural steps in obtaining, labeling, and preparing any specimens to be sent to outside laboratories. Strict adherence to CLIA and OSHA regulations is required.

CLIA Performance Standards

In 1988 the Federal Health Care Financing Administration (HCFA), now called the **Centers for Medicare and Medicaid Services (CMS),** developed the **Clinical Laboratory Improvement Amendments of 1988 (CLIA 88).** These regulations set minimum performance standards in the laboratory and mandated quality assurance and quality control standards. This act divided laboratory tests into three levels of complexity and established standards for personnel qualifications and quality control for testing at each of the three levels. The three levels are high complexity, moderate complexity, and waived tests (referred to as "CLIA-waived" tests). The more complex the test, the more training the laboratory personnel performing the test must have.

Whether a medical office performs and processes the specimen will depend on the type of practice, cost-effectiveness for performing the test "on site," and the level of complexity as defined by CLIA 88.

Laboratory Regulations

Medical laboratories are regulated by both state and federal agencies. CLIA 88 is monitored through CMS, the Centers for Disease Control and Prevention (CDC), and the Occupational Safety and Health Administration (OSHA). CMS issues the certificate, and CDC and OSHA monitor compliance. The state health department is responsible for making certain

their regulations meet or exceed the federal regulations. The amount of regulation to which a POL is subjected depends on the complexity of tests performed at the medical office.

CLIA-Waived Tests

Tests in the "waived" category are not held to the same personnel educational requirements as the other tests, but waived tests are still held to the same quality control and quality assurance standards. Waived tests do not require personnel to have specific training because the procedures are considered simple tests that can be performed with only a small amount of complexity. Table 1-1 lists typical CLIA-waived tests, which are discussed further in Chapter 2.

Moderate-Complexity Tests

A medical assistant with additional training in laboratory testing may qualify to perform some tests in the moderate-complexity range. Moderate-

---

TABLE 1-1   Typical CLIA-Waived Tests

Waived Tests	Use
Urine	
Dipstick or tablet reagent: nonautomated tests for bilirubin, glucose, hemoglobin, ketones, leukocytes, nitrite, pH, protein, specific gravity, and urobilinogen	Screening of urine to monitor or diagnose various diseases (e.g., diabetes) and asses condition of kidneys and urinary tract
Urine pregnancy test (visual color comparison test)	Diagnosis of pregnancy
Urine chemistry analyzer	Screening of urine to detect abnormal values
Blood	
Erythrocyte sedimentation rate (ESR) (nonautomated)	Screening for inflammatory activity
Hemoglobin test: copper sulfate (nonautomated)	Monitors hemoglobin level in blood
Spun microhematocrit, blood count	Screening for anemia
Blood glucose level by monitoring device approved by FDA for home use	Monitors blood glucose level
Hemoglobin test by analytical instrument providing direct readout	Monitors hemoglobin level in blood; measures concentration of hemoglobin A_{1c} in blood, indicating glucose levels over a 3-month period
Hematocrit	Screening for anemia
Other	
Serum cholesterol and HDL	Total cholesterol monitoring
Prothrombin time	Evaluates anticoagulant effect
Ovulation tests (visual color)	Detection of ovulation
Fecal and gastric occult blood	Detection of blood in feces or presence of blood in gastric contents
Tests for *Helicobacter pylori*	Detects antibodies specific for *H. pylori*
Streptococcus	Detects group A beta-hemolytic streptococci
Saliva alcohol tests	Detects alcohol in saliva

FDA, Food and Drug Administration; *HDL*, high-density lipoprotein.

complexity testing involves proficiency testing, test management, quality control, quality assurance, and specialized training. These tests require that the medical assistant follow a certain protocol when performing each test.

High-Complexity Tests

High-complexity tests require high levels of training and are not performed in the POL. They include cytology (Pap smear) and blood typing and cross-matching. Each state has its own regulations for laboratory personnel, and individual states' regulations may be more stringent than CLIA 88, which requires a facility to be appropriately certified for each test performed.

Certificates

A **certificate of waiver** is issued to a physician office laboratory qualified to perform only low-complexity tests.

A **certificate of provider-performed microscopy (PPM) procedures** is issued to a POL qualified to perform moderate-complexity and waived (low-complexity) tests and microscopic procedures. A medical assistant with additional training can perform moderate-complexity tests in the laboratory under the direct supervision of a medical technologist, medical laboratory technician, or physician (e.g., hematology and chemistry done with automated analyzers).

Quality Assurance

A **quality assurance (QA)** program for laboratory testing is designed to monitor and evaluate the quality and accuracy of the test results. It requires the medical office to ensure the reliability of test results by establishing a comprehensive set of written policies and procedures for performing the test and for patient education related to the testing. The facility must develop detailed instructions for specimen collection that include labeling, preservation, and transportation of specimens, as well as specific guidelines for training new personnel. A plan for the continuing education of employees and a program for the maintenance of equipment must also be included.

Quality Control

Quality control (QC) is a process that provides the medical assistant (or POL) the means to ensure that test results are accurate. This requires the following actions:

- Using **control samples** for each new batch of reagents or new supply of test kits daily.
- Using unexpired (fresh) **reagents** (Box 1-1).

BOX 1-1   Use of a Control Sample for Quality Control

1. A control sample having a known value is provided by the manufacturer.
2. This control sample is run as if it were a patient sample. This tests the technique of the operator, reagent effectiveness, and accuracy of the equipment.
3. The reagent is used to produce a chemical reaction. This chemical reaction provides a value.
4. This value is compared to a value range provided by the manufacturer.
5. Not all control samples use a reagent. For example, the Hemocue Photometer uses a control cuvette to check the machine's calibration. Each control cuvette has an assigned value (e.g., 12.1). Every morning before the machine is used, the control cuvette is placed into the machine, and the registered value must match the assigned control value. Manufacturers will identify acceptable deviations (e.g., ±0.3 g/dL). Any reading not within the acceptable range means the machine must not be used until it has been serviced.

- Conducting daily instrument calibration. All instruments must be calibrated according to the manufacturer's recommendations. This ensures that each patient's sample is measured under the same conditions.
- Properly documenting the samples and test results. Proper documentation should be used for every test. Document when a new test kit or reagent is tested. Include the date, time, expected results, actual results, and corrective action taken if results were not within known values.
- Performing preventive maintenance of equipment. Maintenance guidelines are provided with each piece of equipment. A regular schedule for routine maintenance should be established and documented by the user to maintain proper functioning of each piece of laboratory equipment.

Procedure 1-1 outlines the process of using methods of quality control.

Laboratory Safety

Attention to safety in the POL protects both the patient and the medical assistant. The ultimate goal of the medical assistant is to provide for quality patient care. Quality patient care depends on following safety guidelines established by government

Procedure 1-1 Use Methods of Quality Control

TASK: Practice quality control procedures in the medical laboratory to ensure accuracy of test results through detection and elimination of errors.

EQUIPMENT AND SUPPLIES
- Quality control logbook
- Quality control samples (as provided in CLIA-waived prepackaged test kits)
- CLIA-waived prepackaged test kit
- Patient sample
- Copy of CLIA 88 guidelines
- Copy of state regulations and guidelines
- Patient's medical record

SKILLS/RATIONALE

NOTE: For this procedure, a CLIA-waived human chorionic gonadotropin (hCG) pregnancy test is performed.

STANDARD PRECAUTIONS ARE TO BE FOLLOWED.

1. **Procedural Step. Sanitize the hands.**
   An alcohol-based hand rub may be used instead of washing hands with soap and water, unless hands are visibly soiled.
   Rationale. Hand sanitization promotes infection control.

2. **Procedural Step. Assemble equipment and supplies.**
   Obtain the quality control (QC) sample provided in a CLIA-waived prepackaged test kit.
   NOTE: Specially prepared QC samples are included with each CLIA-waived test kit. Manufacturer's directions must be followed and the QC samples tested along with patient samples. Each QC sample will specify how often the test must be performed to maintain the integrity of the test results. For example, a positive and a negative QC sample must be run each time that a patient sample pregnancy test is performed.
   Rationale. It is important to have all supplies and equipment ready and available before starting any procedure to ensure efficiency.

3. **Procedural Step. Check the expiration date on the prepackaged test kit and on each QC specimen.**
   Rationale. Outdated test kits and QC samples will cause inaccurate test results.

4. **Procedural Step. Obtain the specimen from the patient, and identify the specimen as belonging to the patient.**

Rationale. Identifying that the specimen belongs to the patient ensures that the procedure is performed on the correct patient.

5. **Procedural Step. Perform testing of the specimen following the specific protocols outlined for the sample by the manufacturer.**

6. **Procedural Step. Perform quality control testing as outlined by the manufacturer's protocols for the specimen being tested.**

7. **Procedural Step. Determine the results for both the patient's specimen and the QC sample.**
   Compare the test results with the standard reference values provided with the prepackaged CLIA-waived test kit.

8. **Procedural Step. Document the results in the QC logbook and the patient's medical record.**
   Rationale. When patient records are audited, the physician's office must be able to provide proof that a QC sample was completed for any CLIA-waived procedure that has been documented in a patient's medical record, as required by CLIA guidelines.

9. **Procedural Step. Sanitize the hands.**
   Always sanitize the hands after every procedure or after using gloves.

Charting Example

Date	
8/2/xx	9:10 a.m. Pregnancy test performed on first morning urine specimen brought from home. Appropriate QC and patient tests performed. QC results documented in QC log. Negative test results for pregnancy. ———————— L. Negle, CMA (AAMA)

BOX 1-2   OSHA Guidelines for Laboratory Safety*

Physical Hazards
If improperly used, any piece of laboratory equipment or its surroundings could promote hazardous work conditions. Proper training is therefore required.

Electricity
All equipment must be grounded according to established guidelines. Overloaded electrical circuits, frayed electrical cords, and use of extension cords must be avoided.

Fire
Fire extinguishers of the correct type to handle electrical or chemical fires must be present. All flammable chemicals must be stored in a fireproof cabinet.

Equipment
Laboratory equipment must be used according to the manufacturer's guidelines (e.g., autoclave, centrifuge).

Chemical Hazards
Many chemical agents are used in the laboratory setting. If used improperly, chemicals can cause injury from toxic gas or can be caustic to skin.

Labeling
All chemicals must be identified with a label that contains hazard information, including name of the chemical, warnings, and name and manufacturer of the product.

Material Safety Data Sheet (MSDS)
An MSDS must be available for every potentially hazardous chemical in the laboratory (e.g., alcohol, bleach). The MSDS identifies the chemical, protective clothing needed when handling, which body systems could be affected by exposure to the chemical, and the first-aid or medical treatment required. MSDSs must be available in all medical offices. An MSDS should come with each chemical product when ordered and should be stored in a yellow notebook in the work area (Fig. 1-1).

Storage
Proper storage of flammable liquids and caustic chemicals is required.

*The employer must systematically evaluate the workplace and POL for any hazardous situation that could harm an employee.

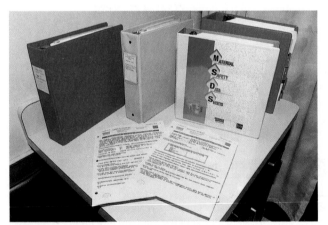

Fig. 1-1 Laboratory MSDS notebook. *(From Stepp CA, Woods MA: Laboratory procedures for medical office personnel, Philadelphia, 1998, Saunders.)*

agencies (e.g., OSHA) that provide a safe working environment for employees. In turn, if the work setting is safe, the patient will benefit.

Review the information about the **Standard Precautions** developed by CDC and enforced by OSHA, including information on the Bloodborne Pathogens Standard and its requirements concerning exposure control plans, **engineering controls, personal protective equipment (PPE),** exposure incidents, and the "right to know" law. Box 1-2 lists other OSHA safety guidelines for the POL. Box 1-3 lists general safety guidelines for the POL.

PATIENT-CENTERED PROFESSIONALISM

- Why must the medical assistant be aware of laboratory regulations and safety precautions in the POL?

BASIC LABORATORY EQUIPMENT

Because medical assistants perform several laboratory tests using technical equipment and supplies, they must be familiar with basic laboratory equipment. Medical assistants may be asked to order supplies, use automated equipment to process tests (e.g., Hemocue for hemoglobin, glucometer for glucose levels), maintain the equipment, and perform many tasks related to the care and maintenance of the equipment. As when using administrative office equipment, it is important to follow the manufacturer's instructions when performing tests with laboratory equipment.

The microscope and centrifuge are two basic pieces of equipment found in most POLs. Other automated pieces are advanced equipment (e.g., blood and urine analyzers) and may require additional training to operate. These types of equipment are fully computerized, and some automatically print out the test results.

BOX 1-3 General Guidelines for Laboratory Safety

1. No shoes with open toes or heels.
2. Laboratory coats or protective outerwear must be worn while in the laboratory and removed when leaving the area.
3. Broken glass and sharps must be disposed in a sharps container.
4. Long hair must be pulled back to prevent contamination and injury.
5. All work surfaces must be cleaned before and after procedures.
6. Hands must be sanitized before and after laboratory procedures.
7. Personal protective equipment (PPE) must be worn when a "splash" or aerosol contamination could occur.

Microscope

The **microscope** is one of the most important and frequently used pieces of equipment in the POL. The microscope magnifies objects too small to be seen with the naked eye. It is used when examining urine sediment, evaluating blood smears, performing cell counts, and identifying microorganisms.

Medical assistants who work in a facility with a POL may be required to use a microscope. Therefore it is necessary to be familiar with its parts and their function, be capable of operating it properly, and be able to maintain it.

Parts of a Microscope

Fig. 1-2 shows the microscope and its various parts. Microscopes are either **monocular** (having one eyepiece, or **lens**) or **binocular** (**compound,** or having two eyepieces, or two sets of lenses). The parts of a microscope are mounted in a stand, which consists of an **arm** and a **base.** The stand supports the magnification system (objectives), accessories

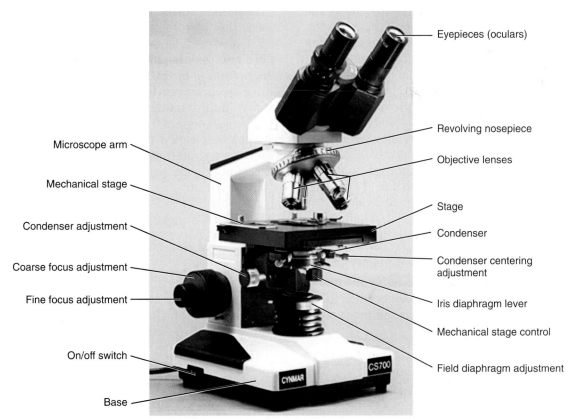

Fig. 1-2 Parts of a binocular microscope. *(Courtesy CARLSAN, Carlinville, Ill.)*

TABLE 1-2	Total Magnification = Ocular Lens × Objective Power		
Ocular Lens	**Objective Power**	**Total Magnification**
10	4× (lowest power)	40×
10	10× (low power)	100×
10	40× (high power)	400×
10	100× (oil immersion)	1000×

needed to operate it, and the stage, which holds the slide. The light or illumination source is situated in the base.

Operating the Microscope

To operate the microscope properly, the medical assistant needs to understand how magnification occurs, how the stage is used, how the light source functions, and how to focus the microscope.

MAGNIFICATION

The compound microscope is the type most often used in the POL. It uses two sets of lenses to magnify an object. The first lens set is located in the **eyepiece,** or **ocular lens,** and the second lens set is the **objective lens,** commonly referred to as the **objectives.** The objectives are the set closest to the object being viewed. These two sets of lenses work together to magnify the specimen.

Magnification found in the ocular lens is 10 times (10×) the actual size of the object. Table 1-2 shows the total magnification. Most microscopes have three or four objectives: 4×, 10×, 40×, and 100× (oil immersion). The objectives are attached to the revolving **nosepiece.** Only one objective is used at a time. The lowest power is the shortest objective, and this is used first to scan the visual field and then focus on an object. To attain greater detail, the viewer advances to the next objective. The longest objective is the **oil-immersion lens** (100×), which allows for the most detail. This objective refracts light when a drop of immersion oil is placed between the lens and the specimen. Oil also allow the objective to move or slide without breakage. Differential of cells and Gram stain for bacteria are most often analyzed using this objective.

STAGE

The **stage** is a platform that holds the slide for viewing and extends from the arm of the microscope. A hole located in the center of the stage allows light rays to enter from the light source (located below the stage) and reach the specimen. Movable clips are used to hold the slide securely on the stage. The **mechanical stage control knobs** allow the slide to be moved from right to left or front to back.

Take extra care when placing the slide on the stage. Ease the slide gently between the clips, without releasing them too quickly, to avoid breaking the slide.

LIGHT SOURCE

The **light source** is usually located in the base of the microscope. Light passes upward to the specimen. The objective lens and the ocular lens of the eyepiece allow the viewer to have a magnified or enlarged image of the specimen. The **condenser** and the **iris diaphragm** are located between the stage and the light source, so the amount of light reaching the objective can be adjusted and controlled.

FOCUSING

Above the base, located on each side of the microscope, are the focusing knobs. The **coarse focus adjustment knob** (large knob) is used to bring the specimen into focus when the lower power objective is used. Once focused, the nosepiece can be rotated to increase the magnification by using higher power objectives. The **fine focus adjustment knob** is then used to bring the specimen into sharper focus. Procedure 1-2 describes how to focus the microscope from lower to higher power.

Care and Maintenance

To maintain optimal working order, microscopes must be properly maintained. They should have yearly maintenance performed by the manufacturer or a service representative. The microscope should be cleaned before and after each use. The following should be done to prevent damage to the microscope during cleaning, storage, and transportation:

- Clean all nonglass surfaces using a soft cloth.
- Use lens paper to clean all lenses. Wipe the ocular lens first, then the objectives. The oil-immersion objective should be cleaned last.
- Place the microscope in a protective covering or in a cabinet for storage.
- When transporting the microscope, firmly hold the arm of the microscope with one hand and support the base with the other.
- Clean the oil-immersion lens with xylene or a special lens cleaner.

The microscope usually requires only minimal care to operate properly. Securing the microscope

Procedure 1-2 Focus the Microscope

TASK: Focus the microscope on a prepared slide from low power to high power.

EQUIPMENT AND SUPPLIES
- Microscope with cover
- Lens paper
- Lens cleaner
- Specimen slide
- Soft cloth
- Tissue or gauze

SKILLS/RATIONALE

STANDARD PRECAUTIONS ARE TO BE FOLLOWED.

1. **Procedural Step. Sanitize the hands.**
   An alcohol-based hand rub may be used instead of washing hands with soap and water, unless hands are visibly soiled.
   Rationale. Hand sanitization promotes infection control.

2. **Procedural Step. Assemble equipment and supplies and verify the order.**
   Rationale. It is important to have all supplies and equipment ready and available before starting any procedure to ensure efficiency.

3. **Procedural Step. Clean the ocular and objective lenses of the microscope with lens paper and lens cleaner.**

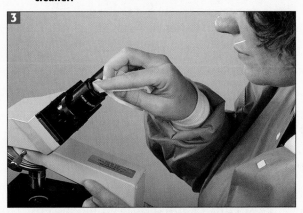

4. **Procedural Step. Turn on the light source, and adjust the ocular lenses to fit your eye span.**

5. **Procedural Step. Rotate the nosepiece to the scanning objective (4×) or to the low-power objective (10×) if the scanning objective is not attached to your microscope.**
   Make sure the objective clicks securely into place.

6. **Procedural Step. Place the slide on the stage and secure in the slide clip.**
   The specimen side should be up.

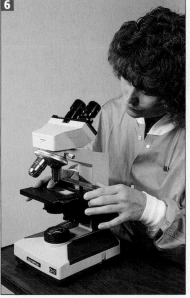

7. **Procedural Step. Adjust the coarse focus adjustment knob.**
   Viewing from the side, position the low-power objective until it almost touches the slide, either by raising the stage or by lowering the objective.
   Rationale. It is important to view from the side to prevent the objective from touching the slide.

8. **Procedural Step. Open the diaphragm to allow in the maximum amount of light.**

9. **Procedural Step. Focus the specimen.**
   Look through the ocular lens(es), and slowly turn the coarse focus adjustment knob to move the objective away from the specimen.

10. **Procedural Step. Further focus the specimen into finest detail by using the fine focus adjustment knob.**

11. **Procedural Step. Adjust the diaphragm and condenser to regulate and adjust the amount of**

Continued

Procedure 1-2 Focus the Microscope—cont'd

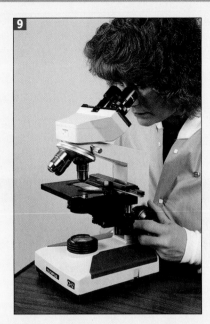

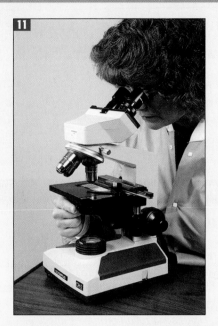

light focused on the specimen to obtain the sharpest image.

12. **Procedural Step. Rotate the nosepiece.**
Rotate the nosepiece to the low-power objective if the scanning objective was initially used, or to the high-power objective if the low-power objective was initially used. Click securely into place. The specimen should still be in coarse focus. Using the fine focus adjustment knob, bring the specimen back into fine focus.

13. **Procedural Step. Examine the specimen by scanning the slide using the stage controls to move it in four directions.**

14. **Procedural Step. Examine the specimen as required for the procedure or test, and report the results.**

15. **Procedural Step. On completing your examination of the specimen, once again lower the stage or raise the objective, turn off the light, and remove the slide from the stage.**

16. **Procedural Step. Clean the stage with lens paper or gauze.**

17. **Procedural Step. Clean the objectives and ocular(s) with dry lens paper.**

18. **Procedural Step. Once clean, cover the microscope with a dust cover and return it to storage.**

19. **Procedural Step. Sanitize the hands.**
Always sanitize the hands after every procedure or after using gloves.

Photos from Bonewit-West K: *Clinical procedures for medical assistants*, ed 6, Philadelphia, 2004, Saunders.

---

when transporting it (holding the arm and supporting the base), placing it gently on work surfaces, and cleaning it after use help to avoid costly repairs.

Centrifuge

A **centrifuge** is a piece of laboratory equipment used to separate solid (or semisolid) material from a liquid by forced gravity. As the contents of the centrifuge tube are spun at a high speed, the solid or semisolid materials separate from the liquid portion and settle to the bottom of the tube. The centrifuge can separate **solutes** (materials suspended in a liquid) from urine and can separate **serum** or **plasma** from blood cells. This separation allows each part of the specimen to be studied.

Two types of centrifuge are typically used in the POL. A regular centrifuge uses large or small tubes to separate urine or blood components (Fig. 1-3, *A*). The **microhematocrit centrifuge** processes blood in a capillary tube (Fig. 1-3, *B*). Some centrifuges have both components in one machine.

Using the Centrifuge

Tubes placed in the centrifuge must always be **counterbalanced** (Fig. 1-4). The area directly

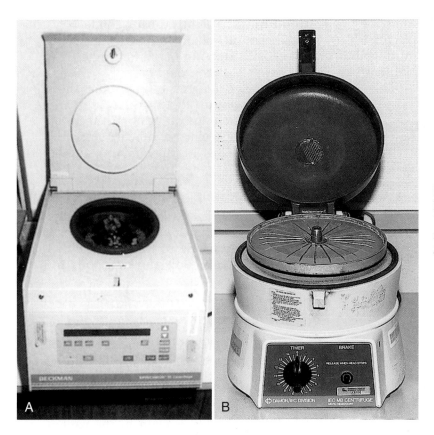

Fig. 1-3 **A,** Regular centrifuge. **B,** Micro-hematocrit centrifuge. *(From Stepp CA, Woods MA:* Laboratory procedures for medical office personnel, *Philadelphia, 1998, Saunders.)*

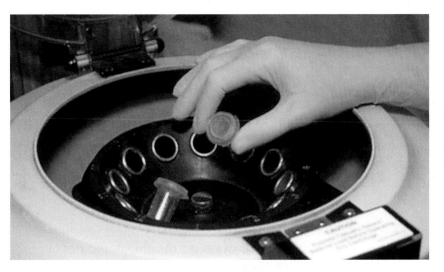

Fig. 1-4 Placing specimen tubes in a centrifuge. *(From Zakus SM:* Clinical skills for medical assistants, *ed 4, St Louis, 2001, Mosby.)*

opposite the specimen tube must contain a tube of equal size and shape and must have an equal amount of fluid. Tubes with water are often used for this purpose when there are an unequal number of tubes to be centrifuged.

Centrifuges have a flat or domed safety cover. This cover must be closed before turning on the machine. This prevents glass and fluids from spraying into the air (aerosol droplet contamination). Some centrifuges have an additional safety feature

that prevents the machine from working unless the cover is closed. A timer is set to process the specimen according to the manufacturer's instructions. A safety feature on most centrifuges is a safety lock that prevents the lid from being lifted during the spin cycle.

Centrifuge Tubes

Tubes used for centrifuging can have a cone-shaped or rounded bottom. The tubes can be made of glass or plastic and are disposable (glass tubes must be disposed of in a sharps container). Before placing a tube in the test tube compartment of the centrifuge, a rubber cushion should be placed in the bottom of the tube holder to minimize breakage.

PATIENT-CENTERED PROFESSIONALISM

- Why must the medical assistant understand the proper use and storage of laboratory equipment?

LABORATORY TESTS

Laboratory tests can be divided into several categories. Although the medical assistant will not perform some of these tests, it is important to be aware of their purpose in the POL. Categories and types of tests performed include the following:

- **Chemistry.** Chemistry test procedures are performed on a patient's serum (the liquid portion of the blood after a clot has formed and is then separated from the formed elements), plasma (from unclotted blood), urine, spinal fluid, and other body fluids. The tests are conducted to check for specific levels of chemicals, such as glucose, cholesterol, electrolytes (e.g., sodium, potassium), proteins, and drugs.
- **Hematology.** Hematology tests assess the formed elements of whole blood. This includes actual counting of the number of white cells (leukocytes), red cells (erythrocytes), and platelets in a blood sample. The cell shape, size, and level of maturity are also observed.
- **Coagulation studies** evaluate the clotting process of a patient's blood. These studies are often performed by the hematology department. Coagulation studies are performed to evaluate anticoagulant therapy and the blood's ability to clot.
- **Microbiology.** Microbiology tests are performed to study bacteria, fungi, viruses, and parasites found in body fluids. These tests aid in the identification of microorganisms and determination of their antibiotic sensitivity.
- **Serology.** Serology tests are performed to study the body's immune responses by detecting the antibodies in the serum. Serology includes testing for pregnancy, infectious mononucleosis, human immunodeficiency virus (HIV) infection, hepatitis, and some sexually transmitted diseases (STDs).

- **Blood bank.** The blood bank conducts studies for ABO blood groupings, Rh typing, and **crossmatching** blood for surgical patients.
- **Urinalysis.** Urinalysis testing studies the physical, chemical, and microscopic structure of urine. Tests are done on urine to screen for infection, drugs, glucose, human chorionic gonadotropin (hCG for pregnancy), and other chemicals.

In addition to understanding the various types of testing, the medical assistant must understand the process of conducting laboratory tests, including patient preparation, use of the laboratory request form, specimen collection and transport, and the resulting laboratory reports.

Patient Preparation

The results of laboratory tests are only as good as the integrity (correctness) of the specimen collected. For example, if an ordered test required the patient to fast and this did not occur, the accuracy of the test would be in question. It is the medical assistant's responsibility to explain to the patient any special requirements, such as fasting or withholding medications, before collection of the needed specimen, and to schedule the testing early enough that the patient can carry them out in time. Verbal and written instructions should be given to patients in a manner they understand.

- *Fasting* requires the patient to refrain from eating and drinking (except water in some cases) to prevent the results from being altered by certain foods and excess water or fluid. Fasting usually starts after midnight, but can begin at 9 a.m. for some tests, such as cholesterol testing. The specimen is collected in the early morning so that the patient can resume daily activities.
- *Medications* can sometimes interfere with test results. For example, insulin should not be taken until after the fasting blood specimen has been drawn to assess glucose tolerance. The physician will determine which medications the patient can take before testing.

A preprinted instruction sheet explaining the test to be done and its preparation is an ideal tool to help the patient be compliant. The medical assistant needs to make certain the patient understands the importance of preparing for the test properly. Allow the patient time to ask questions, and provide any specific details as needed.

Lab Services

IMPORTANT
Patient instructions
and map on back

PHYSICIAN ORDERS

Patient _____ _____ _____ D.O.B. _____ M ☐ Patient
                    Last Name   First   M.I.   F ☐ SS# ___ - ___ - ___

Address _____ City _____ Zip _____ Phone # _____

Physician _____
          ATTACH COPY OF INSURANCE CARD

Date & Time of Collection: _____
Drawing Facility: _____

Diagnosis/ICD-9 Code _____
                    (Additional codes on reverse)

☐ ROUTINE   ☐ PHONE RESULTS TO: # _____
☐ ASAP   ☐ FAX RESULTS TO: # _____
☐ STAT   ☐ COPY TO: _____

☐ 789.00 Abdominal Pain   ☐ 414.9 Coronary Artery Disease (CAD)   ☐ 244.9 Hypothyroidism
☐ 285.9 Anemia (NOS)   ☐ 250.0 DM (diabetes mellitus)   ☐ 272.4 Hyperlipidemia
                           ☐ 780.7 Fatigue/Malaise   ☐ 401.9 Hypertension
                           ☐ 272.0 Hypercholesterolemia   ☐ 485.9 URI (upper respiratory infection)

HEMATOLOGY
☐ 1021 CBC, Automated Diff (incl. Platelet Ct.)
☐ 1023 Hemoglobin/Hematocrit
☐ 1020 Hemogram
☐ 1025 Platelet Count
☐ 1150 Pro Time Diagnostic
☐ 1151 Pro Time, Therapeutic
☐ 1155 PTT
☐ 1315 Reticulocyte Count
☐ 1310 Sed Rate/Westergren

URINE
☐ 1059 Urinalysis
☐ 1082 Urinalysis w/Culture if indicated
   Urine-24 Hr _____ Spot _____
   Ht. _____ Wt. _____
☐ 3033 Creatinine
☐ 3036 Creatinine Clearance (also requires blood)
☐ 3398 Protein
☐ 3096 Sodium/Potassium
☐ Microalbumin 24 Hr _____ Spot _____

SEROLOGY
☐ 8020 ANA (Antinuclear Antibody)
☐ 8040 Mono Spot
☐ 3494 Rheumatoid Factor
☐ 8010 RPR
☐ 5365 Rubella

CHEMISTRY
☐ 5550 Alpha Fetoprotein, Prenatal
☐ 3000 Amylase
☐ 3153 B12/Folate
☐ 3156 Beta HCG, Quantitative
☐ 3321 Bilirubin, Total
☐ 3324 Bilirubin, Total/Direct
☐ 3009 BUN
☐ 3159 CEA
☐ 3348 Cholesterol
☐ 3030 Creatinine, Serum
☐ 3509 Digoxin (recommend 12 hrs., after dose)
☐ 3515 Dilantin
☐ 3168 Ferritin
☐ 3193 FSH
☐ 3066 ▼ Glucose, Fasting
☐ 3061 Glucose, 1° Post 50 g Glucola
☐ 3075 ▼ Glucose, 2° Post Glucola
☐ 3060 Glucose, 2° Post Prandial (meal)
☐ 3049 ▼ Glucose Tolerance Oral GTT
☐ 3047 ▼ Glucose Tolerance Gestational GTT
☐ 3650 Hemoglobin, A1C

CHEMISTRY
☐ 5232 HBsAg
☐ 3175 HIV (Consent required)
☐ 3581 Iron & Iron Binding Capacity
☐ 3195 LH
☐ 3590 Magnesium
☐ 3527 Phenobarbital
☐ 3095 Potassium
☐ 3689 Pregnancy Test, Serum (HCG, qual)
☐ 3653 Pregnancy Test, Urine
☐ 3197 Prolactin
☐ 3199 PSA
☐ 3339 SGOT/AST
☐ 3342 SGPT/ALT
☐ 3093 Sodium/Potassium, Serum
☐ 3510 Tegretol
☐ 3551 Theophylline
☐ 3333 Uric Acid

MICROBIOLOGY
☐ 7240 Culture, AFB
☐ 7200 Culture, Blood x _____
☐   Draw Interval _____
☐ 7280 Culture, Fungus
☐   Culture, Routine
☐ 7005 Culture, Stool
☐ 7010 Culture, Throat
☐ 7000 Culture, Urine
☐ 7300 Gram Stain
☐ 7355 Occult Blood x _____
☐ 7365 Ova & Parasites x _____
☐ 7400 Smear & Suspension
       (Includes Gram Stain/Wet Mount)
☐ 7060 Rapid Strep A Screen (Negs confir by cult)
☐ 7065 Rapid Strep A Screen only
☐ 7030 Beta Strep Culture
☐ 5207 GC by DNA Probe
☐ 5130 Chlamydia by DNA Probe
☐ 5555 Chlamydia/GC by DNA Probe
☐ 7375 Wright Stain, Stool

Additional Tests _____

PANELS & PROFILES

☐ X 3309 CHEM 12
   Albumin, Alkaline Phosphatase,
   BUN, Calcium, Cholesterol, Glucose,
   LDH, Phosphorus, AST, Total
   Bilirubin, Total Protein, Uric Acid

☐ ▼ 3315 CHEM 20
   Chem 12, Electrolyte Panel,
   Creatinine, Iron, Gamma GT, ALT,
   Triglycerides

☐ ▼ 3357 CARDIAC RISK PANEL
   Cholesterol, HDL, LDL, Risk Factors,
   VLDL Triglycerides

☐ X 3042 CRITICAL CARE PANEL
   BUN, Chloride, CO2, Glucose,
   Potassium, Sodium

☐ 3046 ELECTROLYTE PANEL
   Chloride, CO2, Potassium, Sodium

☐ ▼ 3399 EXECUTIVE PANEL
   Chem 20, Iron, Cardiac Risk Panel,
   CBC, RPR, Thyroid Cascade

☐ 5242 HEPATITIS PANEL, ACUTE
   HAVIgMAb, HBsAg, HBsAb, HBcAb, HCVAb

☐ ▼ 3355 LIPID MONITORING PANEL
   Cholesterol, Triglycerides, HDL, LDL, VLDL,
   ALT, AST

☐ 3312 LIVER PANEL
   Alkaline Phospatase, AST, Total Bilirubin,
   Gamma GT, Total Protein, Albumin, ALT

☐ X 3083 METABOLIC STATUS PANEL
   BUN, Osmolality (calculated), Chloride, CO2
   Creatinine, Glucose, Potassium, Sodium,
   BUN/Creatinine, Ratio, Anion Gap

☐ X 3376 PANEL B
   Chem 12, CBC, Electrolyte Panel

☐ ▼ 3382 PANEL D
   Chem 20, CBC, Thyroid Cascade

☐ X 3388 PANEL F
   Chem 12, CBC, Electrolyte Panel,
   Thyroid Cascade

☐ ▼ 3391 PANEL G
   Chem 20, Cardiac Risk Panel, CBC,
   Thyroid Cascade

☐ ▼ 3393 PANEL H
   Chem 20, CBC, Cardiac Risk Panel
   Rheumatoid Factor, Thyroid Cascade

☐ ▼ 3397 PANEL J
   Chem 20, Cardiac Risk Panel

☐ 5351 PRENATAL PANEL
   Antibody Screen ABO/Rh, CBC
   Rubella, HBsAg, RPR
   ☐ 1059 with Urinalysis, Routine
   ☐ 1082 with Urinalysis w/Culture
          if indicated

☐ X 3102 RENAL PANEL
   Metabolic Status Panel, Calcium,
   Phosphorus

☐ 3188 THYROID CASCADE
   TSH, Reflex Testing

▼ - patient **required** to fast
    for 12-14 hours

X - patient recommended to
    fast 12-14 hours

LAB USE ONLY   INIT _____
☐ SST   ☐ PLASMA
☐ PURPLE   ☐ SERUM
☐ YELLOW   ☐ SWAB
☐ BLUE   ☐ SLIDES
☐ GREEN   ☐ DNA PROBE
☐ GREY   ☐ B. CULT BTLS
☐ URINE
☐ BLACK
☐ OTHER: _____
REC'V. SPECIMEN: ☐ FROZEN
☐ AMBIENT ☐ ON ICE

Special Instructions/Pertinent Clinical Information _____

Physician's Signature _____   Date _____
These orders may be FAXed to: 449-5288   7060-500 (7/96)

LAB

Fig. 1-5 Laboratory requisition form. *(From Young AP, Kennedy DB: Kinn's the medical assistant, ed 9, Philadelphia, 2003, Saunders.)*

Laboratory Request Form

For laboratory tests to be processed correctly, a **laboratory requisition** must be completed correctly (Fig. 1-5). When incorrect paperwork accompanies a specimen to an outside laboratory, the test could be delayed or not performed at all, or the wrong test could be completed, or the test could be documented for the wrong patient. Patients do not like to come back for another specimen collection, and the physician does not expect a delay in testing, which in turn delays making a diagnosis and determining treatment plans. An incorrect form also suggests that the staff is unprofessional or incompetent. All outside laboratories have a requisition or request form; it may vary in style and format, but the information required is similar.

Procedure 1-3 explains the process of completing a laboratory requisition. Box 1-4 lists the necessary documentation for charting the transport of specimens to an outside laboratory. The completed requisition is attached to the specimen before transport. The laboratory requisition provides laboratory personnel with the physician's requested tests. Incomplete information delays the results and thus delays patient treatment.

Specimen Collection

Quality control measures should always be maintained during the collection process. The three different methods of specimen collection are as follows:

Procedure 1-3 Complete a Laboratory Requisition Form

TASK: Accurately complete a laboratory requisition form for specimen testing.

EQUIPMENT AND SUPPLIES
- Physician's written order for laboratory tests
- Laboratory requisition form
- Patient's medical record
- Pen

SKILLS/RATIONALE

STANDARD PRECAUTIONS ARE TO BE FOLLOWED.

1. **Procedural Step. Obtain the patient's medical record, and confirm the physician's orders for laboratory test(s).**
   Rationale. Only tests that are ordered by the physician should be requested; confirming the order in the patient's record ensures accuracy.

2. **Procedural Step. Obtain the laboratory requisition form for the laboratory where the test will be performed.**
   Rationale. Requisition forms are typically provided by the laboratory; the physician's office may use several laboratories, and it is important that the correct form and laboratory be used.

3. **Procedural Step. Complete the section of the requisition requiring the physician's name and address.**
   Rationale. If this section is left blank, the laboratory will not know where to send the test results, causing a delay in diagnosis and treatment for the patient.

4. **Procedural Step. Complete the patient's demographic information.**
   Some laboratory references require knowing a patient's age and gender.
   Rationale. Completing the patient demographic section ensures that the test results are reported for the correct patient.

5. **Procedural Step. Complete the section of the requisition requiring the patient's insurance and billing information.**
   Rationale. If this section is not completed, the physician and the laboratory may not receive a timely payment for services rendered.

6. **Procedural Step. Complete the desired laboratory test(s) information.**
   Indicate the ordered laboratory test(s) on the requisition. Include the type of specimen collected and the source of the specimen. All boxes must be clearly marked.
   Most laboratory requisition forms list all the tests that the laboratory routinely performs. Each

test will have a box to check (or a bubble to fill in) or an area to circle to indicate which test is being ordered. A blank area toward the bottom of the form is usually provided to order tests not listed on the form.
   Rationale. It is important to indicate the specimen source, since many tests can be performed on several types of specimens (e.g., hCG pregnancy tests can be performed on urine and blood).

7. **Procedural Step. Complete the section of the requisition requiring date and time of specimen collection.**
   Rationale. Many laboratory tests are time sensitive, and the specimens must be processed within the time frame for the test results to be accurate.

8. **Procedural Step. Enter the patient's diagnosis on the requisition as required.**
   It may be necessary to code symptoms until the laboratory test rules in or rules out a diagnosis (e.g., nausea and vomiting; after test results, diagnosis becomes pregnancy).
   Rationale. Laboratory testing is performed to confirm or rule out a diagnosis. Diagnosis is required for billing the insurance company.

9. **Procedural Step. Enter the type and amount of medication the patient is taking.**
   Rationale. Some medications interfere with the accuracy of the test results.

10. **Procedural Step. Complete the patient authorization to release, and assign the benefits portion as applicable.**
    Rationale. This section must be completed in order for the laboratory to bill the patient's insurance company and release the test results to the physician's office.

11. **Procedural Step. Attach the laboratory requisition securely to the specimen before sending it to the laboratory.**
    Rationale. When specimens arrive at the laboratory without a requisition securely attached, the specimen is considered invalid, and the ordered tests will not

Procedure 1-3　Complete a Laboratory Requisition Form—cont'd

be performed, requiring the specimen to be recollected and reprocessed.

12. **Procedural Step. Document in the patient's medical record and in the laboratory logbook that a specimen was sent for testing.**
List type of specimen, special preparation that the patient may have performed, date, time, patient's name, where the specimen was sent, when the results are due to be returned (if known), and your initials.
Rationale. *This step is important for follow-up.*

Charting Example

Date	
7/7/xx	9:20 a.m. Urine 20 mL, clean-catch container, Vacutainer tube sent to Mullins Lab for urinalysis and C&S. Picked up at 10:05 a.m. ——————— L. Williams, RMA

Charting Example

Date	
8/4/xx	9:00 a.m. Pt. presents to office fasting since 9:00 p.m. 8-3-xx. Blood sample drawn and spun for serum. Sent to Woodland Park Lab for Lipid Panel. Pt. tolerated procedure well. Juice and crackers provided after blood collection. Pt. instructed to schedule appt. in 5-7 days for test results. ——————— L. Williams, RMA

BOX 1-4　## Documentation when Charting for Transport of a Specimen to an Outside Laboratory

1. Date
2. Time
3. Name of specimen being sent
4. Name of laboratory to which the specimen is sent
5. Test to be completed
6. Proper signature and credential
7. Diagnosis code at time of examination
8. Name and patient demographics, including insurance information

1. The specimen is collected and tested at the medical office.
2. The specimen is collected at the medical office, but it is transferred to an outside medical laboratory.
3. A physician with a written order refers the patient to an outside laboratory, where specimen collection and testing take place.

Regardless of the method, the medical assistant is responsible for making certain the patient has received proper preparation instructions for the test to be done. For continued patient consideration, the medical assistant should ensure that the laboratory requisition is completed properly, then follow through to make certain the laboratory report is provided to the physician for analysis in a timely manner. If the report does not arrive in a timely manner, the medical assistant should follow up with the laboratory.

Specimen Containers

Before a laboratory test result can reflect the patient's true health status, the collection technique must be correct. Use of proper specimen containers is necessary to avoid contamination or deterioration of the specimen. Some specimens may require specific additives or preservatives to be added if the specimen will be sent to an outside laboratory or if it will involve a 24-hour urine collection. Remember, if you are not sure about the right test container for collection or proper times, call your laboratory personnel for clarification. They would rather answer questions before than after the test.

Timing

Proper collection times of a specimen are necessary to make the test values reliable, as follows:

- Glucose tolerance test (GTT) specimens must be carefully timed over a specified period to represent a patient's blood glucose level accurately.
- Most urine specimens need to be collected as the first specimen of the day because they provide more information about the patient's kidney function because of the concentration of the urine.

Transport

Outside laboratory testing requires the specimen be collected and taken to, or picked up by, the testing laboratory. Each laboratory service will supply the physician's office with transporting containers, special directions (if applicable) for obtaining the specimens and the amount needed, storage until picked up, and instructions for transporting the specimens. Most laboratory services have carriers trained to handle and deliver the specimens properly and on a timely basis. Outside laboratories have scheduled pickups, so when scheduling patients for specimen collection, remember to take this into consideration. Procedure 1-4 provides instructions on proper collection techniques for specimens sent to an outside laboratory.

Laboratory Reports

The function of the laboratory report form is to provide the physician with the results of the laboratory test(s) performed. It contains necessary information to assist the physician with a diagnosis (Fig. 1-6). Typical information for an outside laboratory includes the following:

1. Laboratory demographics (name, address, telephone number)
2. Ordering physician's name, phone number, and address
3. Patient's information (name, insurance, diagnosis, age, gender)
4. Date and time the laboratory received the specimen
5. Date and time results were reported to the physician's office
6. Tests to be performed
7. Normal range or reference values for each test performed
8. Results of the tests performed

Most laboratory test results are meaningless unless standard values are available to compare the results. Because many factors can affect a person's results, such as gender, age, and race, a normal range is provided for each test. These values represent the range for the general population. Note that each laboratory's range may vary because of the equipment and reagents used to perform the tests. Therefore all tests should be compared to the range of the laboratory performing the test.

The medical assistant may be required to review the laboratory reports when received, immediately notifying the physician of abnormal findings. The physician must review and initial all laboratory reports before they are filed in the patient's medical record. If the patient does have an abnormal test result, the physician may want to see the patient. Laboratory reports can be mailed, delivered by the outside laboratory, or transmitted via the Internet, fax, or telephone. If receiving laboratory reports over the telephone, the medical assistant should repeat results recorded to verify correctness, obtain the identity of the phone reporter, and sign his or her initials to the report. Telephoned results should be followed by a hard copy or electronic copy.

Accuracy in recording results is important to avoid a misunderstanding and a possible misdiagnosis. A misdiagnosis could generate a lawsuit for misfeasance, so it is imperative to be accurate when documenting test results. Procedure 1-5 outlines the process of screening and following up on patient test results.

PATIENT-CENTERED PROFESSIONALISM

- What professional components must a medical assistant have to make certain the patient is properly prepared, the correct collection method is used, and the specimen is transported to the laboratory within the proper time frame?

CULTURE COLLECTION

Cultures of a specific body area can be collected using a sterile polyester (Dacron) swab. Because delays in processing cannot be anticipated, a **swab-transport media system** should be used. Swabs in a transport media should be processed within 24 hours.

Wound

When wound cultures are collected, one or two sterile Dacron swabs should be used with transport media to ensure an adequate specimen has been collected (Fig. 1-7). If the wound is deep, an *anaerobic* culture kit (which detects bacteria not needing oxygen to survive) may also be used to check for the presence of gangrene or other anaerobic bacteria.

Throat

A throat culture is collected by using a sterile Dacron swab. The posterior pharyngeal and tonsillar areas are swabbed to perform a **rapid screening test** to detect the presence of group A beta-hemolytic streptococci. Touching the tongue and the inside of the cheeks and teeth must be avoided to prevent the

Procedure 1-4 **Collect a Specimen for Transport to an Outside Laboratory**

TASK: Properly collect a specimen to be sent to an outside laboratory.

EQUIPMENT AND SUPPLIES
- Nonsterile disposable gloves
- Personal protective equipment (PPE)
- Specimen and container
- Laboratory request form
- Pen
- Patient's medical record
- Laboratory logbook
- Biohazardous waste container

SKILLS/RATIONALE

STANDARD PRECAUTIONS ARE TO BE FOLLOWED.

1. **Procedural Step. Provide the patient with any advance preparation or special instructions.**
   Such preparation may involve the following:
   a. Diet modification
   b. Fasting
   c. Medication restrictions
   d. Collection of specimen at home
      Explain the instructions thoroughly, and provide the patient with written instructions to take home as a reference. If specimen collection is to be done in the physician's office, notify the patient of the time to report to the medical office.
   Rationale. The patient must prepare properly in order to provide a quality specimen that will lead to accurate test results. The patient should not have to return to the office to have another specimen collected.

2. **Procedural Step. Review the requirements in the laboratory directory for the collection and handling of the specimen ordered by the physician.**
   These instructions may include the following:
   a. Materials required for collection
   b. Type of specimen to be collected
   c. Amount of specimen required for laboratory analysis
   d. Procedure to follow as the specimen is collected
   e. Proper handling and storage of the specimen after collection
      Telephone the laboratory with any questions regarding the collection or handling of the specimen to ensure specimen quality.
   Outside laboratories will provide a reference

manual detailing their specimen collection requirements.
Rationale. Reviewing the requirements beforehand prevents errors in collection and handling of the specimen and ensures quality that is acceptable for an accurate test.

3. **Procedural Step. Complete the laboratory requisition form (Procedure 1-3).**
   If the tests results are needed by the physician as soon as possible, mark "STAT" on the request in bold letters.
   Rationale. The completed form provides the laboratory with the information necessary to perform the tests accurately.

4. **Procedural Step. Sanitize the hands.**
   An alcohol-based hand rub may be used instead of washing hands with soap and water, unless hands are visibly soiled.
   Rationale. Hand sanitization promotes infection control.

5. **Procedural Step. Assemble equipment and supplies.**
   Be sure to use the appropriate specimen container required by the outside laboratory. Inspect the container to make sure it is not broken, chipped, or cracked. If the specimen is to be collected in a sterile container, make certain the packaging material has not been broken.
   Rationale. It is important to have all supplies and equipment ready and available before starting any procedure to ensure efficiency. The appropriate specimen container must be used to ensure the collection of the proper type of specimen required by the laboratory. Damaged specimen containers are unsuitable for collection and should be discarded.

Continued

Procedure 1-4 Collect a Specimen for Transport to an Outside Laboratory—cont'd

6. **Procedural Step. Greet and identify the patient, and escort the patient to the examination room.**
   If the patient was required to prepare for the test, determine whether the patient has prepared properly. Specimen collection is often an anxiety-producing experience for the patient, and reassurance should be offered to help reduce apprehension.
   Rationale. Identifying the patient ensures the specimen is collected from the correct patient.

7. **Procedural Step. Collect the specimen.**
   Use the following guidelines in specimen collection:
   a. Follow the OSHA standard (apply gloves or PPE as necessary).
   b. Collect the specimen using proper technique.
   c. Collect the proper type and amount of the specimen required for the test.
   d. Process the specimen further as required by the outside laboratory (e.g., separating serum from whole blood).
   e. Place the lid tightly on the specimen container.
   f. Dispose of any materials used in the specimen collection in the appropriate waste container.
   Rationale. Proper collection of a specimen provides the laboratory with an acceptable sample for testing.

8. **Procedural Step. Clearly label the tubes and specimen containers.**
   Include the patient's name, date, physician's name, your initials, and any other information required by the laboratory, such as the source of the specimen.
   NOTE: Quality assurance procedures require labeling of blood specimen tubes *after* collection to ensure tubes have been drawn on the correct patient.
   Rationale. Properly labeled tubes and specimen containers prevent a mix-up of specimens.

9. **Procedural Step. Record information about the collection in the patient's medical record and the laboratory logbook.**
   Include the date and time of the collection, type and source of the specimen, laboratory tests ordered by the physician, and information indicating its transport to the outside laboratory, including the date the specimen will be sent.

10. **Procedural Step. Properly handle and store (if necessary) the specimen, according to the laboratory's specifications.**
    Rationale. The specimen must be handled and stored properly to maintain the integrity of the specimen.

11. **Procedural Step. Prepare the specimen for transport to the outside laboratory.**
    Be sure to include the completed laboratory request with the specimen, and double-check to make sure the name on the laboratory request and the specimen label is the same.

12. **Procedural Step. Remove gloves and sanitize the hands.**
    Always sanitize the hands after every procedure or after using gloves.

13. **Procedural Step. When the laboratory report is returned to the physician's office, review the test results.**
    a. Compare each test result with the normal range provided by the laboratory. If the test results are grossly abnormal, notify the physician immediately.
    b. Attach the laboratory report to the patient's record, and submit it to the physician for review.
    c. Once the physician has reviewed and initialed the report, file the report in the patient's medical record and document on the flow chart as per office protocol.

Charting Example

Date	
3/10/xx	8:00 a.m. Venous blood specimen collected for lipid profile from Ⓡ arm. Pt. was in a fasting state. Transported to Medical Laboratory Corp. on 3/10/xx. ———————————— E. Daly, CMA (AAMA)

PHYSICIANS CLINICAL LABORATORY, INC.

1925 E Oregon Avenue, Our Town, US 65432   FINAL
(800)000-0000
Ronald B. Woodman M.D., Medical Director

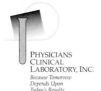

PHYSICIANS
CLINICAL
LABORATORY, INC.
*Because Tomorrow
Depends Upon
Today's Results*

32497
To:UNITED HLTH CENTER—HEALTH FAIRE
   1925 Oregon Ave.
   Our Town, US 65432

Patient : DOE, JOHN
Med Rec# : 004-81-8408
DOB/Sex : 06/18/70 25 YRS MALE
Acc #   : 5226481140   Non-Fasting
Spec Coll: 08/12/XX   Loc: CV01
Spec Rec : 08/14/XX
Req Phys : UNITED HLTH CENTER - HEAL

LOCATION	TEST	RESULTS		REFERENCE RANGE	UNITS
Loc		WITHIN RANGE	OUT OF RANGE		

— — — — — — — — — — CHEMISTRY — — — — — — — — — — — —

		WITHIN RANGE	OUT OF RANGE	REFERENCE RANGE	UNITS
C	Chemistry Panel				
	Glucose	94		70-110	mg/dL
	Sodium	138		135-145	mmol/L
	Potassium	4.6		3.5-5.1	mmol/L
	Chloride	100		98-110	mmol/L
	BUN	18		7-22	mg/dL
	Creatinine	1.2		0.5-1.5	mg/dL
	BUN/Creat Ratio	15		8-24	Ratio
	Uric Acid	7.1		3.5-7.2	mg/dL
	Bili, Total	0.7		0.2-1.2	mg/dL
	GGT		55 H	11-51	IU/L
	AST (SGOT)	16		0-40	IU/L
	ALT (SGPT)	24		0-45	IU/L
	LD	146		100-210	IU/L
	Alkaline Phos	67		31-102	IU/L
	Calcium	10.0		8.6-10.1	mg/dL
	Phosphorus	3.5		2.5-4.6	mg/dL
	Total Protein	7.4		6.0-8.0	g/dL
	Albumin	4.9		3.5-5.0	g/dL
	Globulin	2.5		1.5-4.0	g/dL
	A/G Ratio	2.0			
	Iron	126		65-175	ug/dL
	Cholesterol		239 H	0-200	mg/dL
	Triglyceride	115		10-140	mg/dL
C	HDL	51		30-85	mg/dL
C	CHOL + LDL Group				
	CHOL/HDL Ratio	4.7			mg/dL

			Male	Female
	1/2 Average Risk		3.4	3.3
	Average Risk		5.0	4.4
	2x Average Risk		10.0	7.0
	3x Average Risk		24.0	11.0

	LDL		165 H	0-130	mg/dL

Printed: 08/15/XX 8:02AM

Fig. 1-6   A test result form showing normal ranges and results. *(From Stepp CA, Woods MA: Laboratory procedures for medical office personnel, Philadelphia, 1998, Saunders.)*

Procedure 1-5 Screen and Follow Up on Patient Test Results

TASK: Follow up with a patient who has abnormal test results.

EQUIPMENT AND SUPPLIES
- Laboratory test results
- Tickler file (3 × 5 cards or computer software program) or laboratory log of patient results
- Follow-up reminder cards
- Pen
- Patient's medical record

SKILLS/RATIONALE

STANDARD PRECAUTIONS ARE TO BE FOLLOWED.

NOTE: Follow office policy and procedures for contacting a patient with abnormal test results. Some physicians prefer to personally contact patients with abnormal results. Some test results should not be provided to the patient over the telephone, and the physician will require the patient to make an appointment and come to the office.

1. **Procedural Step. When the laboratory report is returned to the physician's office, review the test results.**
   Compare each test result with the normal range provided by the laboratory. Identify and highlight results outside the normal range. The laboratory will provide the reference ranges and may indicate on the report any results that fall outside the normal range. If abnormal results

   are not indicated by the laboratory, you should indicate them before submitting to the physician for review according to office protocol.

2. **Procedural Step. Attach the laboratory report to the patient's medical record, and submit it to the physician for review.**
   After reviewing and initialing the report, the physician will determine what follow-up should occur.

3. **Procedural Step. If the physician requests that you schedule the patient for a follow-up appointment, determine the most appropriate method of contact.**
   Remember to follow HIPAA guidelines.

4. **Procedural Step. Contact the patient and schedule an appointment.**
   NOTE: Do not discuss test results with a patient unless the physician has given you permission to do so.

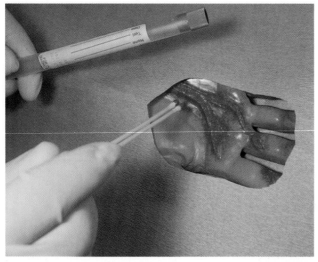

Fig. 1-7 Culturing of a wound. A swab is used to collect the specimen, which is then placed in the holder that contains transport media to preserve the culture. *(From Chester GA:* Modern medical assisting, *Philadelphia, 1998, Saunders.)*

gathering of extraneous microorganisms. Immediately after the specimen is taken, the swab must be placed in the sterile collection tube containing the holding media. Procedure 1-6 outlines the process of throat culture collection.

PATIENT-CENTERED PROFESSIONALISM

- What collection criteria must be met for obtaining a swab culture?

≋ URINE COLLECTION

The collection of a urine specimen from a patient is one of the most frequently performed procedures by a medical assistant. The process is simple, and the information provided about the patient's urinary system and body function is invaluable. A urinalysis can detect diseases of the kidney, other diseased

Procedure 1-6 Collect a Specimen for CLIA-Waived Throat Culture and Rapid Strep Test

TASKS: Collect an uncontaminated throat specimen to test for group A beta-hemolytic streptococci. Perform a rapid strep test.

EQUIPMENT AND SUPPLIES
- Nonsterile disposable gloves
- Facemask
- Sterile polyester (Dacron) swab
- Culture transport system
- Test tube rack
- Tongue depressor
- Gooseneck lamp
- Timer
- Biohazardous waste container
- Patient's medical record

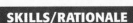

SKILLS/RATIONALE

STANDARD PRECAUTIONS ARE TO BE FOLLOWED.

Specimen Collection for Throat Culture

1. **Procedural Step. Sanitize the hands.**
   An alcohol-based hand rub may be used instead of washing hands with soap and water, unless hands are visibly soiled.
   Rationale. Hand sanitization promotes infection control.

2. **Procedural Step. Assemble equipment and supplies and verify the order.**
   Rationale. It is important to have all supplies and equipment ready and available before starting any procedure to ensure efficiency.

3. **Procedural Step. Obtain the patient's medical record.**

4. **Procedural Step. Greet and identify the patient, and escort the patient to the examination room.**
   Rationale. Identifying the patient ensures the procedure is performed on the correct patient.

5. **Procedural Step. Instruct the patient to have a seat on the end of the examination table, and explain the procedure to the patient.**
   Rationale. Explaining the procedure to the patient promotes cooperation and provides a means of obtaining implied consent.

6. **Procedural Step. Visually inspect the patient's throat.**
   If the patient is chewing gum or eating, ask the patient to dispose of the gum or food. Provide the patient with a tissue and throw the item in the waste container.
   Adjust lighting, such as a gooseneck lamp, as necessary to obtain proper visualization of the throat.

Rationale. Visualization of the throat must be unobstructed to obtain an uncontaminated specimen.

7. **Procedural Step. Apply gloves and facemask.**

8. **Procedural Step. Prepare the culture transport system.**
   Peel open the wrapper containing the culture transport system. Stand the tube in the test tube rack.
   Rationale. The culture transport system will be used to send a specimen to the laboratory for confirmation of rapid strep test results.

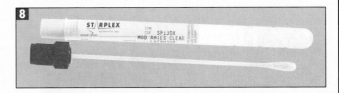

9. **Procedural Step. Prepare the polyester (Dacron) swab.**
   Open the sterile Dacron swab by peeling apart the paper wrapper halfway, leaving the tip of the swab inside the wrapper.
   Rationale. The Dacron swab will be used for collection of a specimen for the rapid strep test.

10. **Procedural Step. Remove the culture transport system swab from the peel-apart package, being careful not to contaminate it by touching the tip to anything.**
    Hold the swab in your dominant hand.

11. **Procedural Step. Remove the Dacron swab from the paper wrapper, again being careful not to contaminate it by touching the tip.**

Continued

Procedure 1-6 Collect a Specimen for CLIA-Waived Throat Culture and Rapid Strep Test—cont'd

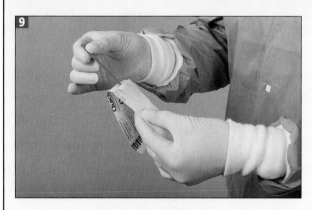

12. **Procedural Step. Place both swabs in your right hand with the tips close together, almost like one swab.**
    The tips of the swabs may touch without becoming contaminated because both are sterile.
13. **Procedural Step. Ask the patient to tilt the head back and open the mouth wide.**
14. **Procedural Step. Use a tongue depressor to hold down the tongue.**
    Rationale. Using a tongue depressor to hold down the tongue provides visualization and access to the back of the throat.
15. **Procedural Step. Carefully insert the swabs into the patient's mouth without touching the inside of the mouth, tongue, or teeth.**
    Rationale. Touching the swabs to the inside of the patient's mouth, tongue, or teeth may contaminate the specimen, providing inaccurate test results.

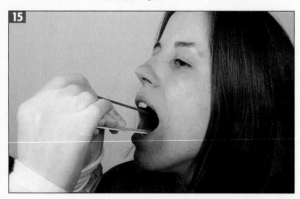

16. **Procedural Step. Ask the patient to say "Ahh ..."**
    Rationale. This reduces the tendency to gag.
17. **Procedural Step. Firmly swab the back of the throat (posterior pharynx) with a figure-eight motion between the tonsillar areas.**
    Make sure to touch any reddened areas, white patches, or areas where you see pus. Rotate the swabs to make sure each swab contacts as

much of the tonsillar area as possible. To minimize gagging, swab quickly and firmly but without excess pressure.
    Rationale. The rotating motion is used to deposit as much of the material as possible onto the swabs. Most patients gag slightly, but excessive pressure on the back of the throat or moving the swab very slowly in the figure-eight pattern will increase discomfort for the patient.
18. **Procedural Step. Continue to hold down the tongue with the depressor, and carefully remove the swabs from the patient's mouth without touching the tongue, teeth, or inside of the cheeks.**
19. **Procedural Step. Discard the tongue depressor in a biohazardous waste container.**
20. **Procedural Step. Remove and discard the cap from the tube, and place the swab from the transport system firmly into the bottom of the tube so that it is dampened with the transport medium, and secure tightly. Return the Dacron swab to the original wrapper.**
    Avoid contamination of the swabs with anything from the environment. Some swab-transport systems require breaking an ampule after inserting the swab back into the collection device to release the transport medium.
21. **Procedural Step. Label the transport tube and swab with the patient's name.**
    Never label until the specimen has been collected.
    If the transport tube is sent to the laboratory for confirmation, the label and a test requisition form must be completed.
22. **Procedural Step. Once the specimens have been returned to their individual packaging, remove personal protective equipment (PPE) and sanitize the hands.**
    Always sanitize the hands after every procedure or after using gloves.

Rapid Strep Test (QuickVue)
NOTE: There are several manufacturers of rapid strep tests. Follow the manufacturer's directions for testing. Directions below are specific to the QuickVue strep test but are relatively standard.
1. **Procedural Step. Sanitize the hands.**
    Sanitize the hands if you are not completing the strep test immediately after obtaining the specimen. An alcohol-based hand rub may be used instead of washing hands with soap and water, unless hands are visibly soiled.

Procedure 1-6 Collect a Specimen for CLIA-Waived Throat Culture and Rapid Strep Test—cont'd

Rationale. Hand sanitization promotes infection control.

2. **Procedural Step. Apply PPE (if not already applied).**

3. **Procedural Step. Assemble equipment and supplies.**

   Obtain three of everything because a positive and a negative control must be run in addition to the patient's sample. Positive and negative controls must be run whenever a new kit is opened. The manufacturer supplies swabs that have been impregnated with different types of streptococcal bacteria. These swabs are treated the same as the patient swab. If they react as expected, this shows that the test has been performed correctly and everything is working properly. Before patient results can be reported, quality control data must be satisfactory.

4. **Procedural Step. Unwrap each of the three cassettes that are wrapped in foil pouches.**

5. **Procedural Step. Record the lot number and expiration date of the kit on the logsheets.**

   Rationale. Control and patient results are recorded after testing has been completed. The laboratory director reviews all logsheets.

6. **Procedural Step. Label each cassette for the controls and patient.**

7. **Procedural Step. Insert the swab into the swab chamber of the cassette.**

   The shaft will rest in a little notch in the back. **NOTE:** There are two important things to remember:

   a. Recheck the swab and cassette labels to make sure the correct swab goes into the correct cassette.

   b. Make sure the swab is inserted *completely* into the swab chamber so that the shaft rests in the notch on the back. When the extraction solution is added, it must cover the swab.

8. **Procedural Step. Make sure there is a glass ampule inside and that the solution is not green, then squeeze the bottle to break the ampule.**

9. **Procedural Step. Shake the bottle vigorously five times to mix the solution from inside the ampule with the solution outside it.**

   The extraction solution should turn green.

10. **Procedural Step. Add the extraction solution.**

    Fill the swab chamber to the rim with the extraction solution. If you are counting drops, it should take about 10 drops. Set a timer for 5 minutes, and don't move the cassette during that time.

11. **Procedural Step. Examine the results window at the end of 5 minutes.**

    Each cassette should have a blue line at the "C" mark. This is the internal control and is a measure of quality assurance. If there is no blue line at the "C" mark, the results are invalid and the test must be repeated with a new specimen, a new cassette, and fresh extraction solution. The negative internal quality assurance is reflected as a clear background behind the lines in the results window and indicates that nothing interfered with the test.

    Rationale. Quality assurance is the procedural control confirming that the reaction between specimen and solutions took place as expected. For this system, the appearance of a blue line at the "C" mark is an internal positive quality assurance, which indicates that the extraction solution was prepared correctly and that it migrated through the chamber adequately.

12. **Procedural Step. Check for positive or negative test results.**

    Any pink or purple line next to the "T" mark means the test is positive. No line next to the "T" mark means the test is negative.

13. **Procedural Step. Sanitize the hands.**

    Always sanitize the hands after every procedure or after using gloves.

14. **Procedural Step. Record the known controls on the quality control logsheet.**

15. **Procedural Step. Record the results from the patient's cassette, including the internal quality assurance.**

16. **Procedural Step. Document the test results.**

Charting Example

Date	
7/12/xx	11:15 a.m. Throat specimen collected from tonsillar area. QuickVue rapid strep test neg. Sent specimen to Medical Lab Corp. for confirmation test. ———————————— L. Patton, CMA (AAMA)

Photos from Bonewit-West K: *Clinical procedures for medical assistants*, ed 6, Philadelphia, 2004, Saunders.

BOX 1-5 | Documentation when Charting Laboratory Procedures Done in the POL

1. Date
2. Time
3. Name of test performed
4. Results (using interpretation guide if provided by the manufacturer)
5. Patient reaction, if any
6. Proper signature and credential

---

states of body systems, and infections in the urinary tract. Proper collection of the specimen is imperative for the test results to be valid. Quality control practices require that all sources of contamination be avoided during the collection and while handling the specimen after the collection.

The medical assistant must process urine specimens within 1 hour of collection or refrigerate the specimen until processing can occur. Urine is an excellent culture medium, and any bacteria present in a urine specimen multiply rapidly at room temperature. Because one purpose of collecting a urine specimen is to screen for **bacteriuria** (bacteria in the urine) and, if necessary, to culture a urine specimen to identify the bacteria, timing is important. Box 1-5 provides information for charting laboratory procedures, such as urinalysis, done in the POL.

Medical assistants should be familiar with the various types of urine specimens that are collected; the collection of random, midstream clean-catch, 24-hour, timed, and specimens for drug-screening are covered in this chapter. Chapter 2 offers more information about performing urinalysis and analyzing urine specimens that have been collected.

Random Urine Specimen

A **random urine specimen** (collected any time during the day) is the type of urine most frequently collected from the patient. The ideal specimen is the **first morning specimen** because it is the most concentrated and has an acid pH, which preserves cells present. If the specimen is to be collected by the patient at home and then brought to the office for examination, it should be refrigerated until it can be transported. It should also be collected in a clean container or one provided by the office or laboratory. Instruct the patient not to touch the inside of the container if possible.

The medical assistant may be asked to collect an uncontaminated urine specimen from an infant. Special pediatric urine collection bags are available for obtaining this type of specimen. Procedure 1-7 outlines the steps in the process of collecting an uncontaminated urine specimen from an infant using a pediatric urine collector.

Midstream Clean-Catch Urine Specimen

A **midstream clean-catch urine specimen** requires the patient to follow a strict cleaning procedure. The medical assistant must explain to the patient the purpose for this type of specimen collection as well as the instructions for obtaining it. The patient should be told the importance of not touching the inside of the sterile container and for wiping off the genital (urethral) area from front to back with the antiseptic wipes provided before urinating. Use of antiseptic wipes reduces bacterial contamination of the specimen, and although the specimen is not sterile, it is considered less contaminated than a random specimen.

Patients are instructed to start urinating in the toilet, stop, continue to urinate to collect a specimen, and then finish urinating in the toilet. By not collecting the first urine voided, the antiseptic residual and external bacteria from the urethral area are removed. This process also reduces the risk of contamination from the perineal area, which may contain anal contaminants. This procedure is usually done in the physician's office; the patient should be provided with detailed instructions and illustrations for collection. Procedure 1-8 provides patient instructions for collecting a midstream clean-catch urine specimen to ensure the validity of the test results.

24-Hour Urine Specimen

A **24-hour urine specimen** tests for kidney function. The patient collects urine over a 24-hour period. The specimen may need to be kept cool in an ice chest or other type of refrigeration. Some collection containers have a preservative that can be added to the specimen to maintain quality. This test is used to check for high levels of creatinine, uric acid, hormones, electrolytes, and medications. The medical assistant instructs the patient in proper collection technique. It is important to remind the patient that the first specimen is *not* collected. Instead, it is discarded, but the time is recorded. All urine is collected in this container through the first specimen the next morning. The specimen is processed in an outside laboratory. Procedure 1-9 provides instructions on preparing the patient to obtain an accurate 24-hour urine specimen.

Procedure 1-7 Obtain a Urine Specimen from an Infant Using a Pediatric Urine Collector

TASK: Collect an uncontaminated urine specimen from an infant.

EQUIPMENT AND SUPPLIES
- Nonsterile disposable gloves
- Antiseptic wipes, or gauze squares and antiseptic solution
- Sterile water and sterile gauze squares
- Pediatric urine collector bag
- Sterile urine specimen container and label
- Biohazardous waste container
- Patient's medical record

SKILLS/RATIONALE

STANDARD PRECAUTIONS ARE TO BE FOLLOWED.

1. **Procedural Step. Sanitize the hands.**
   An alcohol-based hand rub may be used instead of washing hands with soap and water, unless hands are visibly soiled.
   Rationale. *Hand sanitization promotes infection control.*

2. **Procedural Step. Assemble equipment and supplies and verify the order.**
   Rationale. *It is important to have all supplies and equipment ready and available before starting any procedure to ensure efficiency.*

3. **Procedural Step. Obtain the patient's medical record.**

4. **Procedural Step. Greet the infant's parent or guardian and identify the patient, and escort them to the examination room.**
   Rationale. *Identifying the patient ensures the procedure is performed on the correct patient.*

5. **Procedural Step. Explain the procedure to the parent or guardian.**
   Rationale. *Explaining the procedure to the parent or guardian promotes cooperation and provides a means of obtaining implied consent.*

6. **Procedural Step. Apply gloves.**

7. **Procedural Step. Position the infant.**
   Place the child in a supine position on the examination table. Remove the diaper, and ask the parent or guardian to help spread the child's legs apart.
   Rationale. *Placing the child in this position with the parent or guardian helping to spread the legs apart provides access to the genitalia and enables thorough cleansing of the area and application of the urine collection bag.*

8. **Procedural Step. Cleanse the child's genitalia thoroughly.**
   Female infant: Using a separate antiseptic wipe for each side, cleanse the urinary meatus, wiping once from the pubis to the anus. Using a third wipe, cleanse directly over the urinary meatus. Rinse the area thoroughly with sterile water and sterile gauze squares, then wipe the area dry with a new sterile gauze square.

   Male infant: For uncircumcised males, retract the foreskin of the penis. Cleanse the area around the meatus and the urethral opening in the same manner used in the female patient. Use a separate antiseptic wipe for each area. Use a fresh antiseptic wipe to clean the scrotum. Rinse the area thoroughly with sterile water and sterile gauze squares, then wipe the area dry with a new sterile gauze square.
   Rationale. *To prevent contamination of the specimen, the urinary meatus and surrounding area must be free from contaminants, which could affect the test results. Care must be taken to wipe only in a front-to-back motion, and each antiseptic wipe should be used only once to prevent contamination from the anal area. The cleansing agent must be rinsed off to prevent it from entering the urine specimen, which could affect the accuracy of the test results. The area must be wiped dry to ensure an airtight adhesion of the collection bag to prevent leakage of urine.*

9. **Procedural Step. Prepare the urine collection bag.**
   Remove the urine collection bag from the peel-apart packaging, and remove the paper backing from the adhesive strip around the sponge ring of the bag, being careful not to touch the bag to any surface that could cause contamination.

Continued

Procedure 1-7 Obtain a Urine Specimen from an Infant Using a Pediatric Urine Collector—cont'd

10 **Procedural Step. Firmly attach the urine collection bag.**

Female infant: The round opening of the bag should be placed so that it covers the upper half of the external genitalia. The opening of the bag should be directly over the urinary meatus with the bag directed toward the patient's feet.

Male infant: The bag should be positioned so that the child's penis and scrotum are projected through the opening of the bag. The loose end of the bag should be directed toward the feet.

Rationale. The urine collection bag must be attached securely to prevent leakage.

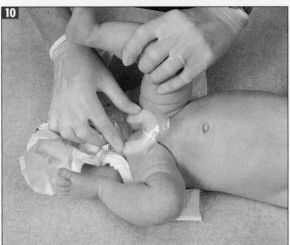

11. **Procedural Step. Loosely diaper the child and, having a parent or guardian remain with the child, check the urine collection bag every 15 minutes until a urine specimen is obtained.**

Rationale. The diaper helps hold the urine collection bag in place.

12. **Procedural Step. Remove gloves and sanitize the hands.**

Always sanitize the hands after every procedure or after using gloves.

13. **Procedural Step. When a sufficient volume of urine has been collected, apply new gloves and gently remove the urine collection bag.**

Rationale. Pulling the bag away from the child's skin too forcefully or too quickly may cause discomfort and irritation to the child's skin.

14. **Procedural Step. Clean the genital area and rediaper the child.**

15. **Procedural Step. Transfer the urine specimen into a sterile urine specimen container, and tightly secure the lid.**

Dispose of the collection bag in a biohazardous waste container.

16. **Procedural Step. Label the specimen container.**

Include the child's name, date, and time of collection, type of specimen, and the physician's name. Dispose of the collection bag in a biohazardous waste container.

17. **Procedural Step. Process the specimen based on the physician office laboratory protocol.**

Either test the urine specimen per the physician's orders or prepare it for transfer to an outside laboratory. If the specimen is to be sent to an outside laboratory, complete a laboratory requisition form and securely attach it to the specimen before transport. If the specimen cannot be tested or transferred immediately, refrigerate it.

Rationale. When a urine specimen cannot be tested immediately, a preservative must be added or the specimen must be refrigerated. When left sitting at room temperature, urine composition changes, such as a possible increase in bacteria and crystals.

18. **Procedural Step. Remove gloves and sanitize the hands.**

Always sanitize the hands after every procedure or after using gloves.

19. **Procedural Step. Document the procedure.**

Include the date, time of collection, and type of specimen. If the specimen is to be transported to an outside laboratory, document which tests were ordered and the name of the laboratory receiving the specimen.

Charting Example

Date	
1/24/xx	10:00 a.m. Urine specimen collected for culture and sensitivity. Picked up by Lab Center on 1/24/xx. ———————— ———————————— T. Moore, CMA (AAMA)

Photos from Bonewit-West K: *Clinical procedures for medical assistants*, ed 6, Philadelphia, 2004, Saunders.

Procedure 1-8   Instruct a Patient in Collection of a Midstream Clean-Catch Urine Specimen

TASK: Instruct a patient in the correct method for obtaining a midstream clean-catch urine specimen.

EQUIPMENT AND SUPPLIES
- Midstream urine collection kit

or
- Sterile specimen container
- Three antiseptic towelettes

SKILLS/RATIONALE

STANDARD PRECAUTIONS ARE TO BE FOLLOWED.

1. **Procedural Step. Sanitize the hands.**
   An alcohol-based hand rub may be used instead of washing hands with soap and water, unless hands are visibly soiled.
   Rationale. Hand sanitization promotes infection control.

2. **Procedural Step. Assemble equipment and supplies and verify the order.**
   Rationale. It is important to have all supplies and equipment ready and available before starting any procedure to ensure efficiency.

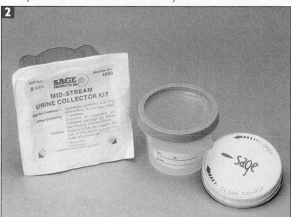

3. **Procedural Step. Greet and identify the patient, and escort the patient to the examination room.**
   Rationale. Identifying the patient ensures the procedure is performed on the correct patient.

4. **Procedural Step. Explain the procedure to the patient.**
   Rationale. Explaining the procedure to the patient promotes cooperation and provides a means of obtaining implied consent.

5. **Procedural Step. Label the container with the patient's name and clinic identification number.**

6. **Procedural Step. Instruct the patient to wash and dry his or her hands.**

7. **Procedural Step. Instruct the patient to loosen the top of the collection container, being careful not to touch the inside of the container.**
   Rationale. The container is sterile. Touching the inside of the container will cause contamination and possibly produce inaccurate test results.

8. **Procedural Step. Provide the patient with written and verbal instructions.**
   Female Patient
   a. Remove undergarments and sit on the toilet.
   b. Expose the urinary opening by spreading the folds of skin (labia) apart with one hand.
   c. While holding the labia apart with one hand, use the other hand to cleanse the area around the opening by wiping each side once from front to back with a separate antiseptic wipe. The third wipe should be used to wipe directly across the opening from front to back.
      Rationale. The microorganisms from the genital area must be removed by cleansing with an antiseptic solution. Cleansing from front to back prevents microorganisms from the surrounding perineal and anal region from being drawn into the area that is clean.
   d. Continue to hold the labia apart until the specimen has been collected.
   e. Begin collection by voiding a small amount of urine into the toilet.
      Rationale. Voiding a small amount flushes microorganisms out of the distal urethra.
   f. Instruct the patient to collect enough urine to fill the sterile container ²/₃ full, being careful not to touch the inside of the container.
      Rationale. Touching the inside of the container will contaminate it with microorganisms that normally reside on the skin.

Continued

Procedure 1-8   Instruct a Patient in Collection of a Midstream Clean-Catch Urine Specimen—cont'd

g. Void the remaining urine into the toilet.

h. Wipe the area dry with a tissue.

i. Replace the sterile lid onto the container. Do not touch the inside of the lid.
   Rationale. Touching the inside of the lid may introduce contaminants into the urine specimen.

j. Wipe the outside of the cup as needed, and leave the container on the counter, deliver it through the pass-through window into the lab, or hand it to the medical assistant, depending on office policy.

k. Discard the wipes, the kit, and everything else from the kit in a waste receptacle.

l. Wash hands with soap and water. Return to the examination room.

Male Patient

a. Expose the head of the penis. If the foreskin is in place, it should be retracted and held back until after the specimen has been collected.

b. Cleanse the area around the urethral opening by wiping each side once from top to bottom with a separate antiseptic wipe. The third wipe should be used to wipe directly across the opening from top to bottom. Cleansing from top to bottom prevents microorganisms

from the surrounding region from being drawn into the area that is clean.

c. Begin collection by voiding a small amount of urine into the toilet.
   Rationale. Voiding a small amount flushes microorganisms out of the distal urethra.

d. Instruct the patient to then collect 1 ounce of urine by voiding into the sterile container (approximately $^2/_3$ full), being careful not to touch the inside of the container.
   Rationale. Touching the inside of the container will contaminate it with microorganisms that normally reside on the skin.

e. Void the remaining urine into the toilet.

f. Replace the sterile lid onto the container. Do not touch the inside of the lid.
   Rationale. Touching the inside of the lid may introduce contaminants into the urine specimen.

g. Wipe the outside of the cup as needed, and leave the container on the counter, deliver it through the pass-through window into the lab, or hand it to the medical assistant, depending on office policy.

h. Discard the wipes, the kit, and everything else from the kit in a waste receptacle.

i. Wash the hands with soap and water, and return to the examination room.

Procedure 1-9 Instruct a Patient in the Collection of a 24-Hour Urine Specimen

TASKS: Instruct a patient in the correct method for obtaining a 24-hour urine specimen. Process the urine specimen.

EQUIPMENT AND SUPPLIES
- Large urine collection container
- Written instruction sheet
- Laboratory requisition
- Patient's medical record

SKILLS/RATIONALE

STANDARD PRECAUTIONS ARE TO BE FOLLOWED.
Collecting the Specimen
1. **Procedural Step. Sanitize the hands.**
   An alcohol-based hand rub may be used instead of washing hands with soap and water, unless hands are visibly soiled.

Rationale. Hand sanitization promotes infection control.

2. **Procedural Step. Assemble equipment and supplies and verify the order.**
   Rationale. It is important to have all supplies and equipment ready and available before starting any procedure to ensure efficiency.

Procedure 1-9 Instruct a Patient in the Collection of a 24-Hour Urine Specimen—cont'd

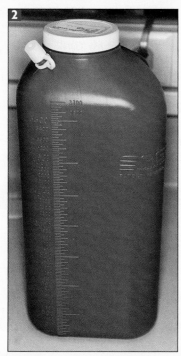

3. **Procedural Step. Greet and identify the patient, and escort the patient to the examination room.**

   Rationale. Identifying the patient ensures the procedure is performed on the correct patient.

4. **Procedural Step. Explain the procedure to the patient.**

   Instruct the patient to consume a normal amount of fluid for the duration of the procedure, except for the consumption of alcoholic beverages. Inform the patient there are no diet restrictions.

   Rationale. Explaining the procedure to the patient promotes cooperation and provides a means of obtaining implied consent. Intake of normal fluid amounts will provide more accurate information on the patient's normal output of urine.

5. **Procedural Step. Provide the patient with the collection container and written instructions.**

   Chart this information in the patient's medical record.

6. **Procedural Step. Provide verbal and written instructions to the patient for collection of the specimen.**

   a. On the first morning of the collection, empty the bladder as usual and note the time. Do not collect this first sample.

   b. Collect the next specimen either in a specified collection container (toilet hat) or

directly into the large, plastic collection container.

Some facilities will provide the patient with a "toilet hat" that can be placed over the toilet basin and under the seat, for ease of collection. The specimen is then transferred into the larger 24-hour collection container.

Rationale. The specified collection container must be large enough to accommodate the entire amount of the specimen because the goal is to collect all urine for a 24-hour period. If the patient forgets to collect a specimen or spills some of the urine, the collection must begin again the next morning.

c. Instruct the patient to replace the lid on the large collection container, and place the container in a refrigerator or cold ice chest. Some 24-hour urine collection containers are packaged with a urine preservative in the bottom of the collection container, so refrigeration of the specimen is not needed. If this is the case, instruct the patient not to remove the preservative. It must be left in the container.

Rationale. The specimen must be kept cold or a preservative must be added to slow down the growth of bacteria and decomposition of the urine.

d. Instruct the patient to repeat Steps b and c at each urination.

e. Inform the patient that the urine specimen must only be collected in the specified container and that all urine must be collected for the 24-hour period.

Rationale. If the patient collects the specimen in nonspecified containers, there is a risk of contamination of the specimen. There is also the risk that the container will not be large enough to contain the entire specimen. It is important that every drop be collected.

NOTE: If a 24-hour specimen collection has been ordered for a child, the parent or guardian must ensure that if the child wets the bed, the procedure is restarted the following morning.

f. On the second morning, the patient should wake at the same time as the first morning and collect this last specimen in the container.

Rationale. This provides an exact 24-hour specimen collection.

g. Instruct the patient to secure the lid on the collection container and return the specimen

Continued

Procedure 1-9 Instruct a Patient in the Collection of a 24-Hour Urine Specimen—cont'd

to the physician's office the same morning of the last specimen collection.

Processing the Specimen

7. **Procedural Step. When the patient returns the specimen, ask the patient whether he or she encountered any difficulties during the 24-hour collection process.**

   If problems were encountered that resulted in failure to collect the entire specimen, inform the patient that the procedure must be repeated starting the next morning. If this is the case, provide the patient with a second collection container, and review the collection process with the patient again. Pay particular attention to any areas that created difficulties during the first collection process.

   Rationale. *Because one component of the test requires measuring the quantity of urine, it must be stressed to the patient to follow the exact collection process and collect every specimen.*

8. **Procedural Step. Prepare the specimen for transport to the laboratory.**

Complete a laboratory requisition form, and label the specimen container. If the collection container does not already contain a preservative, one may be added to the specimen before transport to the laboratory. The laboratory will provide instructions if a preservative needs to be added.

9. **Procedural Step. Document the results.** Include the date and time, the type of specimen, and information on sending the specimen to the laboratory.

Charting Examples

Date	
1/26/xx	1300. Container and verbal/written instructions provided to patient for 24-hour urine specimen collection. ———————— S. Miller, CMA
1/28/xx	1000. 24-hour urine specimen sent to Medical Laboratory Corp. for creatinine clearance. ———— S. Miller, CMA (AAMA)

Timed Specimen

A **timed specimen** collection is when a specimen is collected at certain intervals. This type of specimen is often used to aid in the diagnosis of diabetes. A **glucose-tolerance test (GTT),** also called the oral glucose tolerance test (OGTT), requires the fasting patient to provide a urine and blood sample before ingesting a measured amount of glucose solution, then at timed intervals thereafter (½ hour, 1 hour, 2 hours, and 3 hours). Deviation from this schedule invalidates the test results.

A 2-hour **postprandial** (after meal) **specimen** is collected to assess glucose metabolism. A patient may be asked to fast, have a blood and urine sample taken, then eat a high-carbohydrate meal. Two hours after the meal, the patient provides blood and urine samples, which are screened for elevated glucose levels. Some physicians obtain only a postprandial specimen, without the fasting specimen.

Drug Screen

Special handling is required for specimens that may be used as evidence in a court of law. To be admissible, the collection, handling, processing, and testing of the specimen must maintain absolute quality and accuracy. A medical assistant may be involved in collecting a urine specimen for a **drug screening.** The **chain of custody** regulations describe how evidence—in this case the urine specimen—is to be collected and handled. These must be followed exactly to maintain the validity of the test results while protecting the donor's rights. The chain of custody provides strict guidelines for the collector of the specimen.

Forensic investigations are done in a methodical (step-by-step) manner and follow a **chain of evidence** (collection routine). The chain of evidence details each step and provides directions on handling every detail from beginning to end. Think of it as following a recipe: If you forget a step or an ingredient, the end result will not be very good. If the chain of evidence is not followed, the test results are suspect and are not usable in a court of law.

PATIENT-CENTERED PROFESSIONALISM

- Why must the medical assistant know the criteria for the different types of urine collection and the processing procedures?

≋ BLOOD COLLECTION

Two methods of collecting a blood specimen performed in a medical office are capillary puncture and venipuncture. The method selected depends on the test to be performed (e.g., point-of-care testing [POCT], hemoglobin, cholesterol) and the age and condition of the patient (e.g., infant, elderly adult with poor veins or weak veins).

Capillary puncture is a skin (dermal) puncture to obtain a capillary blood sample. When a small sample of blood is required (e.g., for a self-monitoring glucose test), the capillary puncture is the method of choice. Capillary puncture also is often the preferred choice for infants and elderly patients, because drawing blood by venipuncture in these age groups may be difficult and could cause damage to veins and surrounding tissue.

Venipuncture is a puncture of a vein to obtain a venous blood sample. A larger quantity of blood can be drawn with a venipuncture, and this is the method of choice when several tests are ordered, or a larger amount of blood is needed.

Capillary Puncture

The most common sites for the collection of a capillary puncture are the lateral sides of the ring and middle fingers, and the outer borders of the heel (medial and lateral plantar) for infants (Fig. 1-8). These sites are very vascular, and when punctured adequately, enough blood will be available to perform the ordered tests.

Poor collection techniques can alter the laboratory findings and therefore make the results useless.

- Avoid squeezing the area around the puncture site; this can also alter the results.
- To improve circulation before puncturing, the area can be warmed (e.g., moist heat, massaged or "milked," or warmed by having the patient wash his or her hands in warm water).
- Callused and scarred areas should be avoided because they are difficult to puncture.
- Areas that are edematous (swollen) or cyanotic (bluish) should also be avoided because blood obtained from these areas usually does not produce accurate test results.

Puncture Devices

A **lancet** is a small, sterile, needle-like piece of metal used to make a small puncture in the skin (dermis). Lancets are constructed to penetrate the skin at various depths depending on the type of patient (e.g., infant, child, adult). For example, a lancet for an infant usually has an incision depth of 1 mm, whereas a lancet for an adult is larger and provides a deeper incision. The depth of a lancet should never be 3 mm or greater because this can cause inflammation in the site or accidental contact with the bone. Care must be taken to maintain the sterility of the lancet to prevent the accidental introduction of microorganisms into the puncture site. Skin punctures require sterile technique because the skin is broken.

Lancets are disposable and can be manual (pushing the point of a lancet into the skin), retractable or spring-loaded (depressing a plunger to force the blade into the skin and then retract it), or a reusable semiautomatic device. An example of a reusable semiautomatic lancet device is the Glucolet II (Bayer Corporation). A disposable lancet is placed in a spring-loaded holder, and a release

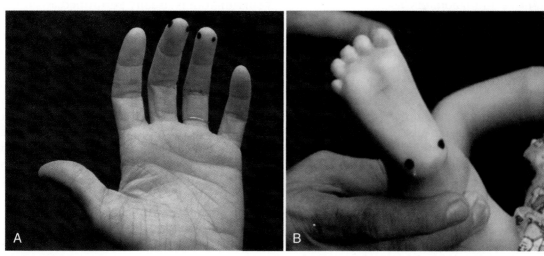

Fig. 1-8 Capillary puncture sites. **A**, Fingertips. **B**, Infant's heel. *(From Young AP, Kennedy DB: Kinn's the medical assistant, ed 9, Philadelphia, 2003, Saunders.)*

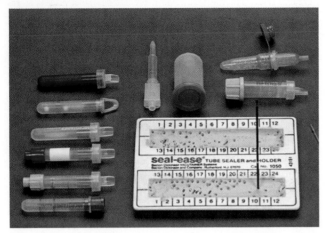

Fig. 1-9 Collection devices: microcontainer tubes, capillary tube in sealing clay, and Unopette system.

button is depressed. The skin is penetrated to a depth that is determined by the lancet blade size. The lancet holder is reusable, whereas the lancet is used only one time. These devices are intended mostly for single users, such as diabetic patients who perform their own skin punctures. Spring-loaded lancet devices in the medical office most often have a retractable blade, and some lock after use to prevent accidental reuse. Immediately after use, lancets are discarded in the sharps container.

Collection Containers

Capillary blood specimens can be collected in a variety of microcollection devices, including microcontainers, capillary tubes, on a glass slide, filter paper (as for phenylketonuria [PKU] testing) and in a Unopette (blood-diluting) system (Fig. 1-9).

- **Microcontainers** are small plastic tubes with a funnel-like top into which blood flows. These tubes use color-coded stoppers to identify the type of additive and laboratory use.
- **Capillary collection tubes** can be either plastic or glass-coated (although glass-coated tubes are not frequently used because of breakage) and are plain or contain **heparin** to prevent clotting.
- **Glass slides** can be used to collect a capillary blood sample for microscopic review.
- **Filter paper** can be used to blot an incised area to test for bleeding time or to collect a blood sample for PKU testing.

Patient Preparation

Medical assistants need to know how to prepare the patient for a capillary puncture, as follows:

1. The area to be punctured can be gently massaged to increase blood circulation.

2. Cleanse the site with an alcohol wipe and allow to air-dry, or wipe dry with a sterile gauze square.
3. When using the finger, puncture the skin at a slight angle and to the side of the fingerprint. This should be done on the middle or ring finger of the nondominant hand.
4. Do not squeeze the finger; squeezing might cause the red blood cells to *hemolyze* (break up). The blood must be free flowing.
5. Wipe away the first drop of blood with sterile gauze. This first drop of blood will contain tissue fluid and alcohol from the skin prep, which dilutes the specimen, causing the clotting process to begin and distorting test results.
6. Fill the required collection devices, and give the patient a sterile gauze square to hold against the puncture site to stop the bleeding. Apply an adhesive bandage if needed.

Procedure 1-10 outlines the proper technique for using a disposable automatic microlancet to collect a specimen in a capillary tube.

Venipuncture

Phlebotomy, another term for venipuncture, is accomplished by drawing blood directly from a vein. This process is considered an invasive procedure. In venipuncture, a sterile 18- to 22-gauge needle is inserted into a vein to remove a large specimen of blood for diagnostic testing. Venipuncture can be performed with a needle and syringe, winged infusion set ("butterfly"), or evacuated-tube system with a tube adapter (holder) and a multidraw (double-ended) needle.

Venipuncture Sites

Venipuncture is usually performed at the antecubital fossa (space) of either arm. Other acceptable sites are the cephalic or basilic veins or the forearm (Fig. 1-10). The site depends on the age of the patient and condition of the patient's veins. The median cephalic vein is most often used for a venipuncture. Areas to avoid are those that are scarred, bruised, freckled, edematous, or otherwise damaged (e.g., tattooed). A venipuncture should never be done in an arm that has impaired circulation (e.g., in patients with stroke) or poor lymphatic drainage (e.g., in patients with mastectomy).

Patient Preparation

Patient preparation is extremely important for venipuncture. Properly identifying the patient and explaining the procedure to minimize anxiety help prepare the patient for this procedure. The medical

Procedure 1-10 Use a Sterile Disposable Microlancet for Skin Puncture

TASK: Obtain a capillary blood specimen acceptable for testing using the index or middle finger.

EQUIPMENT AND SUPPLIES
- Nonsterile disposable gloves
- Alcohol wipe
- Sterile disposable microlancet with semi-automated lancet device, or semiautomatic, one-use lancet system (preferred)
- Sterile 2 × 2-inch gauze pads
- Sharps container
- Biohazardous waste container
- Bandage and adhesive

Supplies for Ordered Tests
Depending on the test ordered, the following supplies must be available (as appropriate):
- Unopette
- Microhematocrit capillary tubes
- Microcontainers
- Glass slides
- Glucometer or cholesterol device (as appropriate)
- Clay sealant tray

SKILLS/RATIONALE

STANDARD PRECAUTIONS ARE TO BE FOLLOWED.

1. **Procedural Step. Sanitize the hands.**
   Alcohol-based hand rub may be used instead of washing hands with soap and water, unless hands are visibly soiled.
   Rationale. Hand sanitization promotes infection control.

2. **Procedural Step. Assemble equipment and supplies and verify the order.**
   Depending on the test ordered and the age and size of the patient, select the lancet system that will achieve the correct depth of puncture.
   Rationale. It is important to have all supplies and equipment ready and available before starting any procedure to ensure efficiency. Lancet systems come in a variety of depths; selecting the correct depth ensures that a specimen will be correctly obtained with minimal discomfort and minimal damage to the tissue or underlying bone.

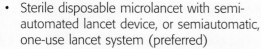

3. **Procedural Step. Greet and identify the patient, and escort the patient to the examination room.**

Rationale. Identifying the patient ensures the procedure is performed on the correct patient.

4. **Procedural Step. Explain the procedure to the patient.**
   If the test(s) ordered requires patient preparation such as fasting or medication restrictions, confirm that the patient has followed the preparation orders. If the preparation has not been followed, inform the physician and document "noncompliance" in the patient's medical record. Reschedule the test as office policy or the physician dictates.
   Rationale. Explaining the procedure to the patient promotes cooperation and provides a means of obtaining implied consent. Test results will be inaccurate if the patient has not followed the required preparation orders.

5. **Procedural Step. Open the sterile gauze packet and place the gauze pad on the inside of its wrapper.**

6. **Procedural Step. Open the sterile lancet system.**

7. **Procedural Step. Position the patient comfortably either sitting or lying down with the palmar surface of the hand facing up, and the arm supported.**
   The patient must be positioned comfortably with the arm secure and supported. If the patient informs you that he or she faints "at the sight of blood," position the patient in a reclining position.

8. **Procedural Step. Select the appropriate puncture site.**
   The preferred site is usually the lateral tip of the third or fourth finger of the nondominant hand. Another puncture site is the medial or lateral surface of the heel of an infant.

Continued

Procedure 1-10 Use a Sterile Disposable Microlancet for Skin Puncture—cont'd

Rationale. *The appropriate site selection will ensure adequate blood flow with minimal risk of injury to the patient.*

9. **Procedural Step. Warm the site to increase blood flow.**
   If the patient's finger is cold, it can be warmed by gently massaging the finger five or six times from the base to the tip, or by placing the hand in warm water for a few minutes.
   Rationale. *Blood flow will be greatly increased when the site is warm.*

10. **Procedural Step. Apply gloves.**

11. **Procedural Step. Cleanse the puncture site with an alcohol wipe, and allow it to air-dry. Do not touch or fan the area after cleansing. Tell the patient to not touch the cleansed area.**
   Rationale. *Allowing the site to air-dry prevents hemolysis of the specimen from the alcohol and lessens the stinging sensation that accompanies the puncture when alcohol is introduced into the tissues. If not allowed to dry completely, alcohol residue may interfere with the accuracy of test results.*

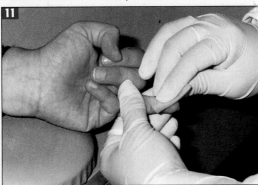

12. **Procedural Step. While the puncture site is drying, prepare the lancet by removing the cover or tab from the end.**
   Depending on the system used, the tab is either pulled straight out or twisted off.

13. **Procedural Step. Position the lancet and perform the puncture.**
   a. Hold the lancet between the first two fingers, and position it firmly against the puncture site.
   b. Place the thumb on the activation button at the top of the device housing, and firmly depress it to discharge the blade.

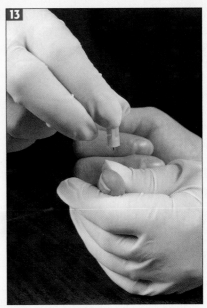

14. **Procedural Step. Dispose of the lancet.**
   When the blade is activated, it will puncture the skin and will retract automatically into the device housing. Immediately dispose of the lancet into the sharps container.
   Rationale. *Proper disposal of contaminated sharps is required by the OSHA standard to prevent exposure to blood-borne pathogens.*

15. **Procedural Step. Wipe away the first drop of blood with the dry gauze.**
   Rationale. *The first drop of blood is not collected because it usually contains more tissue fluid than blood, which will result in an inaccurate test result.*

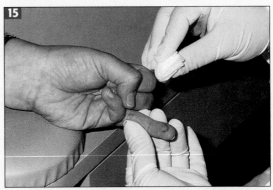

16. **Procedural Step. If necessary, massage the finger by applying gentle, continuous pressure from the knuckle to the puncture site to increase the blood flow.**

Procedure 1-10 Use a Sterile Disposable Microlancet for Skin Puncture—cont'd

Do not squeeze the finger; tissue fluid will dilute the specimen. Lowering the puncture site will allow gravity to assist with the blood flow.

NOTE: If the puncture is done correctly and at the right depth, the site will bleed properly. If not done properly, the procedure must be repeated at a new site with a new lancet. Performing the puncture correctly the first time is less traumatic to the patient.

17. **Procedural Step. Allow a second well-rounded drop of blood to form, and quickly collect the specimen in the correct manner for the test(s) ordered.**
    Rationale. Rapid collection is necessary to prevent coagulation.

18. **Procedural Step. After the sample has been collected, instruct the patient to apply pressure with a clean gauze square directly over the puncture site.**

19. **Procedural Step. Bandage the puncture site.**
    Check the puncture site to make sure it has stopped bleeding, and bandage it with a clean

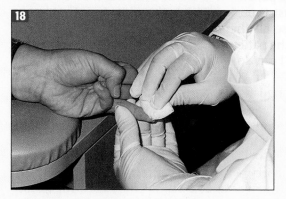

bandage to protect the wound. Discard any contaminated materials in the appropriate biohazardous waste container.

20. **Procedural Step. Remove gloves and sanitize the hands before transporting the specimen to the laboratory for processing.**
    Always sanitize the hands after every procedure or after using gloves.

Photos from Young AP, Kennedy DB: *Kinn's the medical assistant,* ed 9, Philadelphia, 2003, Saunders.

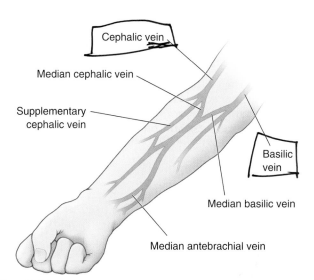

Cephalic vein

Median cephalic vein

Supplementary cephalic vein

Basilic vein

Median basilic vein

Median antebrachial vein

Fig. 1-10 Veins of the arm. (*From Stepp CA, Woods MA:* Laboratory procedures for medical office personnel, *Philadelphia, 1998, Saunders.*)

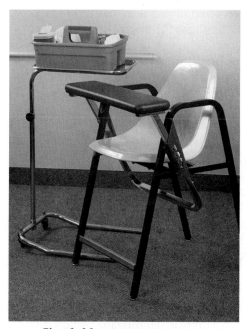

Fig. 1-11 Phlebotomy chair.

assistant must act in a professional manner and listen to the patient's concerns. If a patient tells you, "They usually draw my blood from here," listen to the patient. The patient is usually seated in a phlebotomy chair (Fig. 1-11). Ask the patient to lie down if previous episodes of fainting have occurred.

The medical assistant should have all supplies needed for the procedure readily available. This not only saves time but also projects an organized image. Having all supplies ready helps the patient feel relaxed and confident in the medical assistant's ability to

ipuncture. Being relaxed and confi-
nize the patient's discomfort. Never
I've never done this before," or "It's
r "I have trouble drawing blood,"
statements will cause anxiety for
nd the medical assistant. Do a self-
, and be confident.

Evacuated Tubes

With the **vacuum tube** system, once the vacuum tube needle has pierced the vein and the selected tube's colored stopper (cap), a vacuum pulls the blood into the tube. Vacuum tubes allow for the blood specimen to enter directly into a collection tube (the **evacuated tube**) to be used for testing purposes. Tubes come in different sizes (e.g., pediatric and adult) with different-colored stoppers, or tops. The color of the stopper identifies the type of test to be performed. The tubes are also marked with an expiration date and should be checked before use. Table 1-3 lists common stopper colors, additives, and laboratory uses.

Some tubes have an additive that, in most cases, acts as an anticoagulant. Hematology studies require tubes containing the anticoagulant ethylenediaminetetraacetic acid (EDTA). EDTA preserves the shape of the blood cells and prevents the platelets from clumping by removing calcium, thus preventing clotting. Chemistry and serology studies are drawn in a red or red-gray marbled stoppered tube, or gold Hemogard that has no additives.

Order of Draw

When several evacuated tubes are to be collected for multiple studies, there is a recommended **order of draw** for the tubes. The Clinical and Laboratory Standards Institute (CLSI), formerly the National Committee for Clinical Laboratory Standards (NCCLS), established the order of draw for quality control purposes. Following the order of draw minimizes the chance of additives from a previous tube getting into subsequent tubes when blood is drawn. The following color-topped tube order is recommended when the evacuated-tube (Vacutainer) system is used:

1. Yellow or blood culture tubes (sterile; special collection procedure required)
2. Light blue (sodium citrate)
3. Red (no additives)
4. Red-gray or Hemogard gold (silicone clot activator)
5. Light green (lithium heparin)
6. Green (sodium heparin)
7. Lavender (EDTA)
8. Gray (potassium oxalate)

To assist in remembering the order of draw, memorize the sentence in Fig. 1-12.

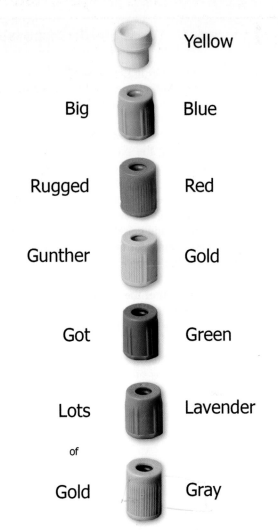

Big — Yellow
Big — Blue
Rugged — Red
Gunther — Gold
Got — Green
Lots — Lavender
of
Gold — Gray

Fig. 1-12 The order of drawing blood. Memorize "Big Rugged Gunther got Lots of Gold" to help remember the order, as shown. *(Modified from Sommer SR, Warekois RS: Phlebotomy: worktext and procedures manual, Philadelphia, 2002, Saunders.)*

Types of Equipment

Three types of equipment can be used in venipuncture: the evacuated-tube (Vacutainer) method, the syringe method, and the butterfly method.

VACUTAINER METHOD

The **evacuation blood collection system,** or **Vacutainer,** has a holder, a double-ended sterile needle of various lengths and gauges, and a tube with a color-coded stopper and a premeasured space with or without an additive. The Vacutainer system allows for several tubes of blood to be drawn from a single venipuncture. This minimizes the chance of labeling errors and hemolysis.

Needles are available as **multisample needles** (retractable rubber sleeve) (Fig. 1-13) or **single-sample needles.** When a multisample needle is used, the rubber sleeve retracts as the needle enters

TABLE 1-3 Common Stoppers, Additives, and Laboratory Uses

Vacutainer Colors*	Color	Hemogard Colors†	Additive and Function	Laboratory Use	Optimum Volume/ Minimum Volume
Adult Tubes					
Yellow		Yellow	SPS; prevents blood from clotting and stabilizes bacterial growth	Blood or body fluid cultures	5 mL/NA
Red		Red	None	Serum testing, chemistry tests, blood bank, serology	10 mL/NA
Red/gray (marbled)		Gold	None, but contains silica particles to enhance clot formation	Serum testing	10 mL/NA
Light blue		Light blue	Sodium citrate; removes calcium to prevent blood from clotting	Coagulation testing	4.5 mL/4.5 mL
Green		Green	Heparin (sodium, lithium, ammonium); inhibits thrombin formation to prevent clotting	Chemistry tests	10 mL/3.5 mL
Green/gray (marbled)		Light green	Lithium heparin and gel for plasma separation	Plasma determinations	2 mL/2 mL
Yellow/gray (marbled)		Orange	Thrombin	"Stat" serum demonstrations in chemistry studies	2 mL/2 mL
Lavender		Lavender	EDTA; removes calcium to prevent blood from clotting	Hematology testing	7 mL/2 mL
Gray		Gray	Potassium oxalate, sodium fluoride; removes calcium to prevent blood from clotting; fluoride inhibits glycolysis	Chemistry tests, especially glucose/alcohol levels	10 mL/10 mL
Royal blue		Royal blue	Sodium heparin (also sodium EDTA); inhibits thrombin formation to prevent clotting	Chemistry trace elements	7 mL
Pediatric Tubes‡					
Red		Red			2, 3, or 4 mL/NA
Lavender		Lavender			2 mL/0.6 mL; 3 mL/0.9 mL; 4 mL/1 mL
Green		Green			2 mL/2 mL
Light blue		Light blue			2.7 mL/2.7 mL

Modified from Young AP, Kennedy DB: *Kinn's the medical assistant,* ed 9, Philadelphia, 2003, Saunders.
*Stopper colors are based on Vacutainer tubes (Becton Dickinson).
†Hemogard closures provide a protective plastic cover over the rubber stopper as an additional safety feature.
‡Additives and function, and laboratory uses are the same as for adult tubes.
EDTA, Ethylenediaminetetraacetic acid; *NA,* not applicable; *SPS,* sodium polyanetholsulfonate.

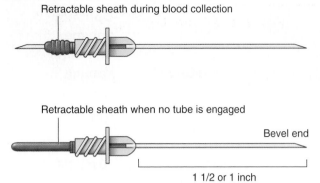

Retractable sheath during blood collection

Retractable sheath when no tube is engaged

Bevel end

1 1/2 or 1 inch

Fig. 1-13 A multisample needle. *(From Sommer SR, Warekois RS:* Phlebotomy: worktext and procedures manual, *Philadelphia, 2002, Saunders.)*

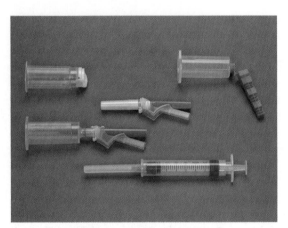

Fig. 1-14 Recapping safety devices.

How to assemble

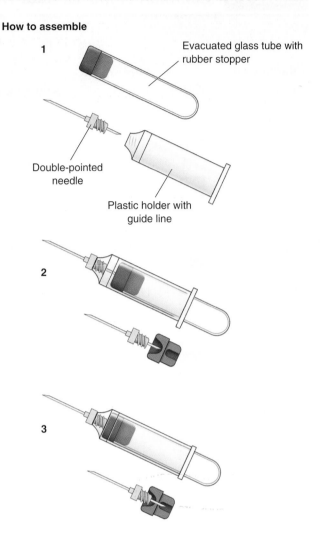

1

Evacuated glass tube with rubber stopper

Double-pointed needle

Plastic holder with guide line

2

3

Alternate method

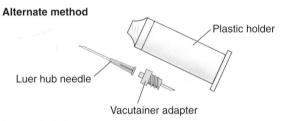

Plastic holder

Luer hub needle

Vacutainer adapter

Fig. 1-15 Venipuncture equipment using the evacuated-tube (Vacutainer) method. *(Courtesy Becton Dickinson.)*

the stopper, but then springs back to cover the needle when the tube is removed. Many manufacturers design needles with a recapping safety device to minimize the chance of an accidental needle stick (Fig. 1-14). The holder is available in either an adult or pediatric size. The single-sample needle does not have a rubber sleeve, therefore allowing blood to exit through the needle when the tube is removed.

The holder has a flange at one end for the medical assistant's fingers and a grooved opening on the other end for the needle. The barrel of the holder is marked with a stopper guideline (Fig. 1-15). It is only used one time and then disposed of in a biohazardous waste container, usually with the needle attached. The safety cap on the needle will be activated before disposal.

When the Vacutainer tube is pushed into the holder beyond the stopper guideline, the needle punctures the color-coded stopper, and the vacuum draws blood into the tube. Procedure 1-11 explains the process of venipuncture using the evacuated-tube method.

SYRINGE METHOD

The **syringe method** for venipuncture is used for patients with small or fragile veins (e.g., children, elderly persons). This method lessens the degree of pressure exerted on the vein to avoid the collapse of fragile veins. The medical assistant controls the vacuum created when the plunger of the syringe is pulled back slowly. When a blood sample is drawn with a needle and syringe, the blood sample must be transferred to the appropriate evacuated tube

Text continued on p. 47

Procedure 1-11 Perform Venipuncture Using the Evacuated-Tube Method (Collection of Multiple Tubes)

TASK: Obtain a venous blood specimen acceptable for testing using an evacuated-tube system.

EQUIPMENT AND SUPPLIES
- Nonsterile disposable gloves (latex-free)
- Personal protective equipment (PPE) as required
- Tourniquet (latex-free)
- Evacuated-tube holder
- Evacuated-tube multidraw needle (21 or 22 gauge, 1 or 1½ inch) with safety guards
- Evacuated blood tubes for requested tests with labels (correct nonadditive or additive required for ordered test)
- Alcohol wipe
- Sterile 2 × 2-inch gauze pads
- Bandage (latex-free), CoFlex, or nonallergenic tape
- Sharps container
- Biohazardous waste container
- Laboratory requisition form
- Patient's medical record

SKILLS/RATIONALE

STANDARD PRECAUTIONS ARE TO BE FOLLOWED.

1. **Procedural Step. Sanitize the hands.**
   An alcohol-based hand rub may be used instead of washing hands with soap and water, unless hands are visibly soiled.
   Rationale. Hand sanitization promotes infection control.

2. **Procedural Step. Assemble equipment and supplies and verify the order.**
   Select the required evacuated tubes according to the tests to be performed. Check the expiration date of the tubes. Arrange the tubes in order of draw. Tap powdered additive tubes lightly below the stopper to dislodge any additive caught on the tube stopper. Phlebotomy supplies are often kept in a portable sturdy tray that keeps everything together in one place and is easy to transport from one examination room to another. When a phlebotomy supply tray is used, make sure that the tray is stocked with all the needed supplies and a variety of color-topped evacuated tubes.
   Rationale. It is important to have all supplies and equipment ready and available before starting any procedure to ensure efficiency. Checking for the tube expiration date is important because outdated tubes may no longer contain a vacuum, and, as a result, they may not be able to draw blood into the tube. Outdated additives may cause inaccurate test results.

If an additive remains trapped in the stopper, inaccurate test results may occur.

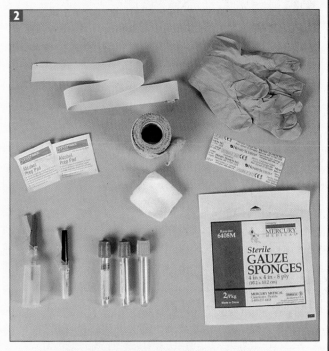

3. **Procedural Step. Greet the patient, introduce yourself, and confirm the patient's identity. Ask the patient to have a seat in the phlebotomy chair. If the patient states that he or she "faints" when blood is taken, place the patient in a supine position on the examination table.**

Continued

Procedure 1-11 Perform Venipuncture Using the Evacuated-Tube Method (Collection of Multiple Tubes)—cont'd

Rationale. Identifying the patient ensures the procedure is performed on the correct patient. Placing the patient in the supine position makes it less likely that the patient will faint.

4. **Procedural Step. Verify that any special diet instructions or restrictions have been followed (e.g., fasting) and explain the procedure to the patient.**

   If the test(s) ordered requires patient preparation such as fasting or medication restrictions, confirm that the patient has followed the preparation orders. When a patient is not properly prepared, the physician should be consulted for directions concerning how to proceed with the test.

   Rationale. Explaining the procedure to the patient promotes cooperation and provides a means of obtaining implied consent. Test results will be inaccurate if the patient has not followed the required preparation orders.

5. **Procedural Step. Prepare the evacuated-tube system.**

   Insert the rubber-tipped portion of the needle (posterior part of the needle) into the plastic holder. Screw the needle into the evacuated-tube holder, or insert it into a quick-release holder and tighten securely. Keep the cover on the needle.

   Rationale. The needle must be tightened securely or it may fall out of the holder or be pushed further than necessary into the patient's arm when the evacuated tube is pushed onto the needle.

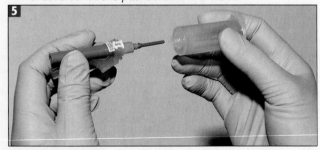

6. **Procedural Step. Prepare the gauze pad.**
   Open the sterile gauze packet and place the gauze pad on the inside of its wrapper, or obtain sterile gauze pads from a bulk package.

7. **Procedural Step. Position the remaining needed supplies.**
   Place the first tube loosely in the plastic holder with the label facing downward. Place the remaining supplies within comfortable reach of your nondominant hand. Do not remove the needle cap.

Rationale. Items used during the procedure should be positioned so that you do not have to reach over the patient, which may cause you to move the needle while it is still in the patient's arm. Puncturing the rubber stopper causes loss of tube's vacuum.

8. **Procedural Step. Position and examine the arm to be used in the venipuncture.**

   a. Ask the patient to extend both arms in a slightly downward position. Examine the antecubital area. If the patient has a preference, examine it first, but do not hesitate to select the other arm if it seems more acceptable. Select a suitable vein.

   b. The arm with the vein selected for the venipuncture should be in a downward position and not bent at the elbow. The arm should be supported on the armrest by a rolled towel or by having the patient place the fist of the other hand under the elbow.

   Rationale. Most adults have had previous venipunctures and know which veins are better for a successful draw. Asking a patient to state a preference gives the patient a sense of control over what is happening and increases patient comfort. Placing a rolled towel or having the patient place the fist under the elbow helps achieve proper positioning. Gravity helps to enlarge the veins.

9. **Procedural Step. Apply the tourniquet.**

   a. Apply the tourniquet 3 to 4 inches above the bend in the elbow and stretch it slightly. Cross the ends in the front of the arm so that each hand is holding the opposite end of the tourniquet. The tourniquet should be tight enough to allow arterial blood to flow while preventing venous return. It should be "tight, but not *too* tight."

   b. Grasp the tourniquet's middle, where the ends cross, between your thumb and forefinger. With the left hand, loop the "underneath" flap on the left over the top, and tuck it under the tightened crisscross, but do not push it all the way through. Then let go of the tourniquet. The friction on the rubber will hold the end in place. You should see a loop just above the antecubital space, and the end "flap" should be easy to grab. (You will pull this end to release the tourniquet when you have completed the venipuncture.)

   NOTE: The tourniquet should not be left on for longer than 1 minute to prevent venous

Procedure 1-11 Perform Venipuncture Using the Evacuated-Tube Method (Collection of Multiple Tubes)—cont'd

congestion, or excessive accumulation of blood in the vein (hemoconcentration). If you need to perform several assessments to locate the best vein, the tourniquet can be applied and reapplied as required.

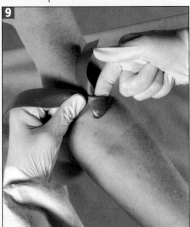

While holding the crossed area, tuck the top strap under the bottom strap so that the ends hang upward.

NOTE: Asking the patient to make a tight fist helps to locate deeper veins more easily. Do not leave the tourniquet on longer than 1 minute or have the patient pump (open and close) the fist because these techniques cause hemoconcentration (blood pooling) and lead to false test results. For example, the patient's potassium level could increase as much as 20%.

Rationale. The combined effect of the pressure of the tourniquet and the tightly clenched fist should cause the antecubital veins to stand out so that accurate selection of a puncture site can be made.

10. **Procedural Step. Apply gloves and personal protective equipment (PPE).**
   Rationale. Gloves and PPE are a precaution that provides a barrier against blood-borne pathogens.

11. **Procedural Step. Thoroughly palpate the selected vein.**
   Gently palpate the vein with the index finger to trace the direction of the vein and to estimate the size and depth of the vein. The vein feels like an elastic tube and gives under pressure while a tendon feels rigid, and a sclerosed or thrombosed vein feels cordlike.
   Rationale. The index finger is most sensitive for palpating a vein.

12. **Procedural Step. Release the tourniquet.**

13. **Procedural Step. Prepare the puncture site.**
   Cleanse the site with the alcohol wipe using a circular motion from the center and working outward. Allow the site to air-dry. Once the site has been cleaned, do not palpate it again.
   Rationale. The site must be cleansed in a circular motion from the puncture site outward to help remove contaminants from the site. The site must be allowed to dry to prevent alcohol from entering the blood specimen and contaminating it, causing inaccurate test results. Touching or fanning the area causes contamination, and the cleansing process must be repeated. In addition, if the alcohol is not allowed to dry completely, it may cause the patient to experience a stinging sensation. Also, the drying process helps to destroy microbes.

14. **Procedural Step. Reapply the tourniquet.**
   NOTE: According to the Clinical and Laboratory Standards Institute (CLSI), a tourniquet should not be reapplied for 2 minutes. If repalpation of the site chosen is necessary, cleanse the site again.

15. **Procedural Step. Position the holder.**
   a. Grasp the holder with all five fingers: the forefinger under the top of the holder; the middle, ring, and fifth fingers supporting the underside of the tube; and the thumb holding the top of the holder just below the flange.
   b. Remove the needle cover and inspect for barbs, and make sure the *bevel* of the needle is facing upward. Be sure the sheath on the safety device is flipped up and out of the way.
   c. Position the needle so that it follows the line of the vein. Twist the tube inside of the holder, without pushing onto the needle, so that the label is facing downward.
   Rationale. Positioning the needle with the bevel up allows for easier entry into the skin and the vein. With the label facing downward, you will be able to observe the blood as it fills the tube, which allows you to know when the tube is full.

16. **Procedural Step. Perform the venipuncture.**
   a. Warn that the patient will feel a little "stick."
   Rationale. Warning the patient before entering the vein prevents the element of surprise, which could cause the patient to pull away, causing the needle to be pulled out of the vein.

Continued

Procedure 1-11   Perform Venipuncture Using the Evacuated-Tube Method (Collection of Multiple Tubes)—cont'd

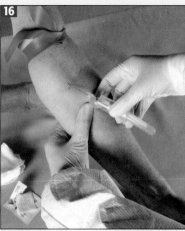

Anchor the vein with the nondominant hand and insert the needle with the dominant hand.

b. With the other hand, use your thumb to pull the skin taut below the intended puncture site to anchor the vein. Your thumb should be placed 1 to 2 inches below and to the side of the puncture site.

Rationale. Pulling the skin taut helps the needle glide in easily.

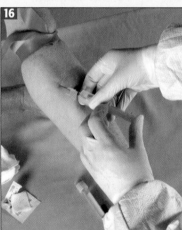

Push the Vacutainer tube into the needle holder with the thumb of the nondominant hand. Apply counterpressure on the flange of the Vacutainer holder with the fingers of the nondominant hand.

c. Following the direction of the vein, with one quick motion, smoothly pierce the skin and enter the vein at a small angle—about 15 degrees—and almost parallel to the skin.

Rationale. The angle of the needle is important because an angle of less than 15 degrees may cause the needle to enter above the vein, preventing puncture. An angle of more than 30 degrees may cause the needle to go through the vein, puncturing the posterior wall. This could result in a hematoma (blood in the tissues).

17. **Procedural Step. Secure the holder for blood collection.**
Support the holder on your middle finger by resting the middle finger against the patient's arm. Be careful to keep the holder steady in your dominant hand so that the needle does not move in the vein as you get ready to slide the tube "on." Then let go of the skin with the nondominant thumb, and anchor the forefinger and middle finger of the nondominant hand on the flange of the holder.
Rationale. Firmly grasping the holder prevents the needle from moving deeper into the vein when inserting an evacuated tube. Moving the needle is painful for the patient.

18. **Procedural Step. Push the bottom of the tube with the thumb of your nondominant hand carefully while holding the holder and needle steady, so that the needle inside the holder pierces the rubber stopper of the tube.**
If everything is done correctly, blood will begin to fill the tube.

19. **Procedural Step. Change tubes as required by test orders by repeating Steps 17 and 18.**
When the tube has stopped filling, grasp the bottom of the tube with the left hand. Push against the flange with the thumb and pull the tube from the holder. This lets the rubber sleeve slide back over the end of the needle and prevents blood from dripping into the holder. Invert the purple-top tube about 8 to 10 times (do not shake the tube; this applies to any tube with additives), then place it upright in a rack so that it will not roll.
Rationale. Anchor the tube and tube holder firmly before changing tubes to prevent the needle from being pulled out of the vein or being inserted deeper. Inverting tubes with additives activates the anticoagulant. Shaking the tube hemolyzes the blood and damages blood cells.

Procedure 1-11 Perform Venipuncture Using the Evacuated-Tube Method (Collection of Multiple Tubes)—cont'd

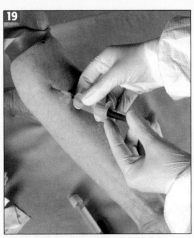

Pull out the tube with the fingers of the non-dominant hand while applying counterpressure against the flange with the thumb.

20 **Procedural Step. While the blood is filling the last tube, remove the tourniquet.**
With the dominant hand still holding the needle in place on the patient's arm, ask the patient to open the fist. Then release the tourniquet by pulling the loose left end upward with your other hand. This will allow blood to flow freely in the patient's arm again.

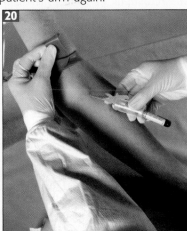

Remove the tourniquet as the last vacuum is filling.

21 **Procedural Step. Remove the needle and activate the safety needle device.**
After the last tube is removed and mixed, put it down, then pick up the sterile gauze with the nondominant hand and position the gauze over the needle. With one quick, smooth motion, remove the needle from the arm with the dominant hand and apply pressure with the gauze in the left hand immediately *after* you remove the needle. As you withdraw the

needle, flip the safety shield over the needle tip with your right thumb and direct the needle down and away from yourself and the patient.
NOTE: Do not place a gauze pad over the needle as it is being withdrawn because this can scratch the patient's arm or dig the needle into the arm, causing pain. Always withdraw the needle completely first, then apply the gauze pad to the site.
Rationale. Placing the gauze pad over the puncture site helps prevent tissue movement, absorbs small amounts of blood that ooze from the vein, and reduces patient discomfort. Careful withdrawal prevents further tissue damage. The needle sheath prevents needle sticks.

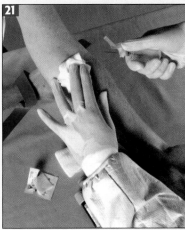

Place sterile gauze over the site. After the needle is removed, then apply pressure and activate then needle safety device.

22. **Procedural Step. Apply direct pressure on the venipuncture site to enhance the formation of a platelet plug. Secure the gauze dressing.**
Tell the patient to keep the arm straight to allow a good clot to begin forming over the puncture site.
Rationale. Keeping the arm straight prevents dislodging the plug that has formed and prevents the formation of a hematoma.

23. **Procedural Step. Instruct the patient to maintain pressure on the site for 1 to 2 minutes.**
NOTE: If any swelling or discoloration occurs, apply an ice pack to the site after bandaging it.
Rationale. Do not allow the patient to bend the arm at the elbow because this increases blood loss from the puncture site and causes bruising.

24. **Procedural Step. Activate the safety device and discard the entire Vacutainer system in the biohazard sharps container.**

Continued

Procedure 1-11   Perform Venipuncture Using the Evacuated-Tube Method (Collection of Multiple Tubes)—cont'd

25 **Procedural Step. Label the tubes.**
Include the patient's name, the date, time of draw, test to be performed, and your initials.
*Rationale. It is important to label the tubes **after** collecting the specimen but **before** leaving the patient. If an unlabeled tube is sent to the reference laboratory, it will be rejected.*

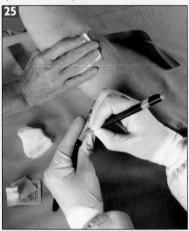

Label the tubes while the patient applies pressure to the puncture site.

26. **Procedural Step. After the tube(s) has been labeled, observe for any special handling procedures (e.g., frozen, chilled, warm) and place the tube(s) into the biohazard transport bag with the laboratory requisition.**

27 **Procedural Step. Check to make sure the patient's arm has stopped bleeding, and then place a latex-free bandage or CoFlex over the gauze to create a pressure dressing. Caution the patient not to lift anything for an hour.**
Rationale. A slight pressure bandage will help to prevent further bleeding. Lifting could cause further bleeding leading to a hematoma.
NOTE: Making certain that the bleeding has stopped is important for patients on anticoagulants. Continue with pressure until bleeding stops.

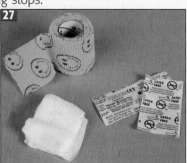

28. **Procedural Step. Remove and discard the alcohol wipe and gloves.**
Before removing gloves, grasp the alcohol wipe in the palm of one gloved hand so that the wipe is enveloped in the gloves as you take them off. Remove the disposable gloves and discard them in the biohazardous waste container because they may have come in contact with blood.

29. **Procedural Step. Sanitize the hands.**
Always sanitize the hands after every procedure or after using gloves.

30. **Procedural Step. Complete the laboratory requisition form to include the collection date and time and place the requisition in the biohazard transport bag with the specimen(s).**

31. **Procedural Step. Ask and observe how the patient feels.**
Observe breathing, color, and skin moisture, looking for signs that the patient may feel faint. If the patient states he or she feels fine and there are no signs of fainting, prepare to document the procedure in the patient's medical record.

32. **Procedural Step. Clean the work area using Standard Precautions.**

33. **Procedural Step. Document the procedure.**
Include the date and time, the test drawn, which arm and vein were used, and any unusual patient reaction.
NOTE: Some physician's offices keep a laboratory log for all outside testing that includes patient name, date, test required, outside laboratory receiving the specimen, results, and the medical assistant's initials.

Charting Example

Date	
8/10/xx	10:00 a.m. Venous blood specimen collected from Rt arm AC space for CBC; 1 EDTA tube collected for pickup by Medical Laboratory Corp.
	_____ V. Koszarek, CMA

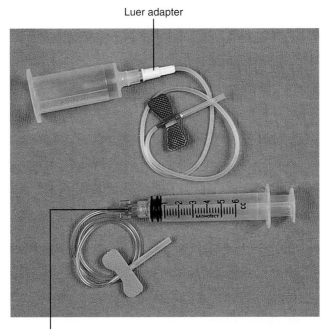

Luer adapter

Hub adapter

Fig. 1-16 Winged infusion set: Luer adapter with evacuated tube and hub adapter with syringe. *(From Bonewit-West K: Clinical procedures for medical assistants, ed 6, Philadelphia, 2004, Saunders.)*

(e.g., sterile, light blue, lavender, green, gray, red, red-gray). This is done by placing the syringe needle through the tube stopper. The vacuum exerted fills the tube automatically. Procedure 1-12 provides the steps for obtaining a blood specimen using the syringe method.

BUTTERFLY METHOD

The **butterfly method** uses a **winged infusion set** attached to plastic tubing. The plastic tubing attaches to either a syringe tip or a Vacutainer holder (Fig. 1-16). The butterfly method is used for infants, small children, or adults with small, difficult-to-find veins.

The "wings" make it easier to control and guide the needle. The medical assistant should make sure that he or she is actually holding the bottom, not just the top, of the wings for stability of draw. The forearm or hand is most often used in adults. A 23-gauge needle is typically used because this size will enter small veins easily and will not cause the vein to rupture. The most important step in a butterfly draw is to stabilize or anchor the vein before inserting the needle. The medical assistant then should "thread the vein" just under the skin in order to keep the needle inside the lumen of the vein while completing the draw. This is especially necessary when using the veins of the hand.

The butterfly method is more comfortable for the patient, but it takes longer to perform the actual

---

BOX 1-6 Reasons for Rejection of Specimen by Laboratory

- Incorrect or incomplete labeling of specimen
- Insufficient quantity or **quantity not sufficient (QNS)** of specimen *(short draw)* for the test ordered
- Collected in the wrong tube or container
- Blood sample hemolyzed
- Not refrigerated when required, or thawed and refrozen
- Patient not fasting when required

BOX 1-7 Failed Blood Draws

Do not be discouraged. On certain days or with certain patients, a failed draw will occur. The best strategy for missing a blood draw is that for riding a horse: "When you fall off, get back on and try again." Never take it as a defeat; rather, look at a failed draw as a challenge. As mentioned, make two attempts, then ask someone else to do it.

The more you practice, the better you will be. The most important task in being able to perform venipuncture is "finding the vein." If you can locate, stabilize, and enter the vein's lumen (opening), you will be successful at drawing blood.

---

blood draw. Procedure 1-13 explains how to obtain a venous blood specimen using the butterfly method.

Failed Draws

Regardless of the site or method chosen to perform the venipuncture, the patient must be prepared properly and the collection process done correctly. A partially filled tube, or *short draw,* is unacceptable because the ratio of additive to blood can produce inaccurate results. Box 1-6 lists other reasons that cause a laboratory to reject a collected specimen.

To become skilled and confident in venipuncture, the medical assistant must practice. Every venipuncture presents different challenges (e.g., an obese patient's veins will be deeper; an older patient's veins may collapse; large veins may roll more easily). No more than two venipuncture attempts should be done on a patient. If unsuccessful after two attempts, notify the physician or ask a co-worker to examine the patient's veins and perform the procedure. Various factors affect a successful draw, so not every attempt will be successful (Box 1-7). Fig. 1-17 illustrates various reasons for a failed draw.

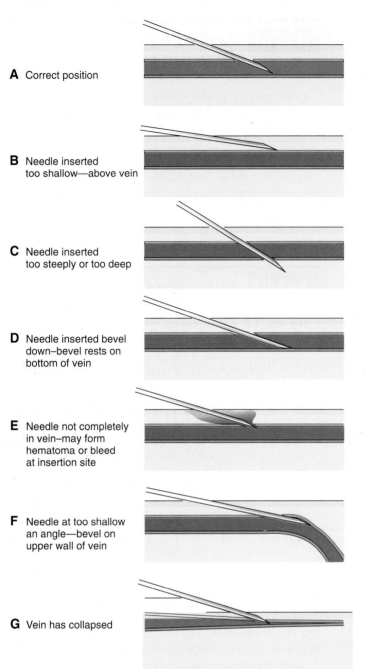

A Correct position

B Needle inserted
too shallow—above vein

C Needle inserted
too steeply or too deep

D Needle inserted bevel
down–bevel rests on
bottom of vein

E Needle not completely
in vein–may form
hematoma or bleed
at insertion site

F Needle at too shallow
an angle—bevel on
upper wall of vein

G Vein has collapsed

Fig. 1-17 Causes of failed draws. *(From Hunt SA: Saunders fundamentals of medical assisting, Philadelphia, 2002, Saunders.)*

Blood Culture Collection

When the body is in a diseased state, the blood may be invaded with microorganisms. When **bacteremia** (bacteria in the blood) is suspected, a blood sample is collected under sterile conditions. A venipuncture must be collected using a special aseptic technique to prevent possible contamination of the specimen from the skin.

For a **blood culture,** two blood samples are collected from different sites. Each site is cleaned with alcohol for 2 minutes, followed by cleaning with povidone-iodine. The blood sample is collected in either a yellow-stoppered tube or a special collection bottle with media designed to grow bacteria (Fig. 1-18). Sometimes physicians request that these samples be drawn at the outpatient or hospital laboratory to eliminate contamination factors.

Serum and Plasma Separation

If serum or plasma is required for a test, the blood specimen needs to be separated before transfer. The specimen is collected in a plain red, red/gray (marbled), or Hemogard gold Vacutainer tube containing serum separator, but no additives. After collection, the blood is allowed to sit for a minimum of 30 minutes to allow a clot (jelly-like mass) to

Procedure 1-12 **Perform Venipuncture Using the Syringe Method**

TASK: Obtain a blood specimen acceptable for testing using a syringe.

EQUIPMENT AND SUPPLIES
- Nonsterile disposable gloves
- Personal protective equipment (PPE)
- Tourniquet
- Test tube rack
- 10-cc (10-mL) syringe with 21- or 22-gauge needle with safety guards
- Evacuated blood tubes for requested tests with labels (correct evacuated tube required for designated test ordered)
- Alcohol wipe
- Sterile 2 × 2-inch gauze pads
- Bandage or nonallergenic tape
- Sharps container
- Biohazardous waste container
- Laboratory requisition form
- Patient's medical record

SKILLS/RATIONALE

STANDARD PRECAUTIONS ARE TO BE FOLLOWED.

1. **Procedural Step. Sanitize the hands.**
   An alcohol-based hand rub may be used instead of washing hands with soap and water, unless hands are visibly soiled.
   Rationale. Hand sanitization promotes infection control.

2. **Procedural Step. Assemble equipment and supplies and verify the order.**
   Be sure to select the proper evacuated tubes according to the tests to be performed. Check the expiration date of the tubes.
   Rationale. It is important to have all supplies and equipment ready and available before starting any procedure to ensure efficiency.

3. **Procedural Step. Greet and identify the patient, and escort the patient to the examination room.**
   Ask the patient to have a seat in the phlebotomy chair. If the patient states that he or she "faints" when having blood taken, place the patient in a supine position on the examination table.
   Rationale. Identifying the patient ensures the procedure is performed on the correct patient. Placing the patient in the supine position makes it less likely that the patient will faint.

4. **Procedural Step. Explain the procedure to the patient.**
   If the test(s) ordered requires patient preparation such as fasting or medication restrictions, confirm that the patient has followed the preparation orders. When a patient

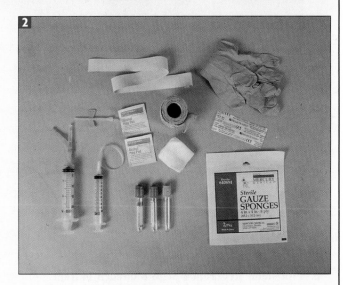

is not properly prepared, the physician should be consulted for directions concerning how to proceed.
Rationale. Explaining the procedure to the patient promotes cooperation and provides a means of obtaining implied consent. Test results will be inaccurate if the patient has not followed the required preparation orders.

5. **Procedural Step. Prepare the needle and syringe.**
   Make sure to keep the needle and the inside of the syringe sterile. Break the seal on the syringe by moving the plunger back and forth several times, being careful to keep the plunger within the syringe. Loosen the cap on the needle, and check to make sure that the hub is screwed tightly into the syringe.

Continued

Procedure 1-12   Perform Venipuncture Using the Syringe Method—cont'd

NOTE: Do not pull the cap straight off the needle, because this causes a "knee jerk" reaction and will cause you to stick yourself. Rock the cap gently back and forth at the hub of the needle, loosening it.

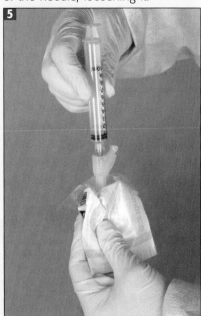

6. **Procedural Step. Place the evacuated tubes to be filled in a test tube rack on a work surface.**
   Make sure the tubes are placed in the correct order to be filled. If an evacuated tube contains a powdered additive, tap the tube just below the stopper to release any additive adhering to the stopper.
   Rationale. If an additive remains trapped in the stopper, inaccurate test results may occur.

7. **Procedural Step. Open the sterile gauze packet and place the gauze pad on the inside of its wrapper, or obtain sterile gauze from a bulk package.**

8. **Procedural Step. Follow Steps 8 through 14 from Procedure 1-11.**

9. **Procedural Step. Position the syringe.**
   Remove the cap from the needle. Hold the syringe by placing the thumb and index finger of the dominant hand near the needle hub while supporting the barrel of the syringe with the three remaining fingers. The needle should be positioned with the bevel facing up.
   Rationale. Positioning the needle with the bevel up allows for easier entry into the skin and the vein and allows the medical assistant to see when the needle enters the vein.

10. **Procedural Step. Perform the venipuncture.**
    a. Warn that the patient will feel a little "stick."

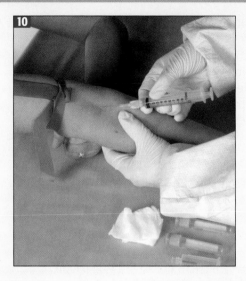

Rationale. Warning the patient before entering the vein prevents the element of surprise, which could cause the patient to pull away, causing the needle to be pulled out of the vein.

   b. With the other hand, pull the skin taut beneath the intended puncture site to anchor the vein. Your thumb should be placed 1 to 2 inches below and to the side of the puncture site.
   Rationale. Pulling the skin taut helps the needle glide in easily.

   c. Following the direction of the vein, with one quick motion, smoothly pierce the skin and enter the vein at a small angle—about 15 degrees—and almost parallel to the vein.
   Rationale. The angle of the needle is important because an angle of less than 15 degrees may cause the needle to enter above the vein, preventing puncture. An angle of more than 30 degrees may cause the needle to go through the vein, puncturing the posterior wall. This could result in a hematoma (blood in the tissues).

11. **Procedural Step. Grasp the syringe firmly between the thumb and the underlying fingers.**
    Blood may spontaneously enter the top of the syringe; this is called a "flash." If flash does not occur, gently pull back on the plunger of the syringe until blood begins to enter. Do not move the needle once the venipuncture has been made.
    NOTE: If no blood enters the syringe, slowly withdraw the needle, secure new supplies, and retry. The needle may not have threaded the vein or may have been resting on the vein wall.
    Rationale. Moving the needle is painful for the patient.

Procedure 1-12 Perform Venipuncture Using the Syringe Method—cont'd

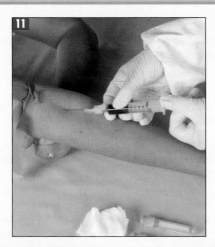

12. **Procedural Step. Anchor the syringe, and gently continue pulling back on the plunger until the required amount of blood is in the syringe.**
Be careful not to pull the needle out of the vein.
Rationale. Pulling back on the plunger causes a vacuum, which draws the blood into the syringe. The blood should be withdrawn slowly from the vein to prevent hemolysis and to prevent the vein from collapsing.

13. **Procedural Step. Release the tourniquet.**

14. **Procedural Step. Remove the needle.**
With one quick, smooth motion, remove the needle from the arm with the dominant hand and apply pressure with the gauze in the nondominant hand immediately *after* you remove the needle. As you withdraw the needle, flip the safety shield over the needle tip without locking with your dominant thumb and

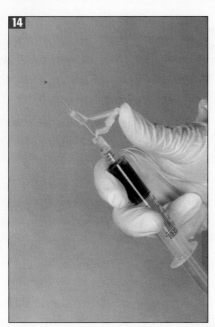

direct the needle down and away from yourself and the patient.
NOTE: Do not place a gauze pad over the needle as it is being withdrawn because this can scratch the patient's arm or dig the needle into the arm, causing pain. Always withdraw the needle completely first, then apply a gauze pad to the site.
Rationale. Placing the gauze pad over the puncture site helps prevent tissue movement, absorbs small amounts of blood that ooze from the vein, and reduces patient discomfort. Careful withdrawal prevents further tissue damage. The needle sheath prevents needle sticks.

15. **Procedural Step. Apply direct pressure on the venipuncture site, and instruct the patient to raise the arm straight above the head while continuing to apply pressure.**
Tell the patient to keep the arm straight while raised to allow a good clot to begin forming over the puncture site.
Rationale. Raising the arm straight above the head helps prevent a hematoma. Keeping the arm straight prevents dislodging the clot that has formed.

16. **Procedural Step. Instruct the patient to maintain pressure on the site for 1 to 2 minutes, with the arm raised straight up above the head.**
NOTE: If any swelling or discoloration occurs, apply an ice pack to the site after bandaging it.
Rationale. Maintaining pressure with the arm raised over the head will help speed up the clotting process and prevent a hematoma. Do not allow the patient to bend the arm at the elbow because this increases blood loss from the puncture site and causes bruising.

17. **Procedural Step. Transfer the blood to the evacuated tubes as soon as possible.**
a. Make sure the tubes are lined up in the correct order of fill in the tube rack. Transfer blood from the syringe into the tubes in the following order as needed (sterile, light blue, lavender, green, gray, red, and red/gray).
b. Insert the needle through the center of the rubber stopper and allow the vacuum to fill the tube. Do not apply pressure to the plunger of the syringe. Do not remove the tube cap.
c. If the blood is added to a tube containing an additive, it must be mixed immediately by gently inverting (rotating) the tube 8 to 10 times. Do not shake the tube.
Rationale. Blood must be transferred as soon as possible into evacuated tubes to avoid clotting of

Continued

Procedure 1-12 Perform Venipuncture Using the Syringe Method—cont'd

blood in the syringe. The suction action of the vacuum tube will automatically draw the blood into the tube. Pushing on the plunger causes hemolysis and increases the risk of aerosol spray when the needle is removed.

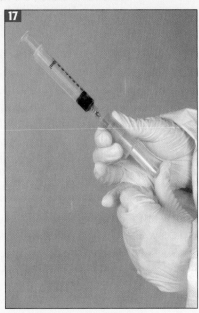

18. **Procedural Step. Discard the contaminated needle and syringe as one unit into the sharps container.** *Rationale. Proper disposal is required by the OSHA standard to prevent accidental needle stick injuries.*
19. **Procedural Step. Follow Steps 25 through 33 from Procedure 1-11.**

Charting Example

Date	
6/15/xx	12:00 p.m. Venous blood specimen collected from Ⓡ arm AC space. 1 EDTA tube for CBC to be picked up by Medical Laboratory Corp. ———————— S. Miller, CMA

Photos from Bonewit-West K: *Clinical procedures for medical assistants,* ed 6, Philadelphia, 2004, Saunders.

---

form. The tube is placed in the centrifuge and spun at the speed and time recommended by the manufacturer, usually 15 minutes.

The yellow liquid portion that is on top of the spun sample is serum. Serum is the liquid portion of blood minus the clotting factors. The serum should be **pipetted** (usually using a **pipette**) from the tube and placed in a properly labeled transfer tube for later testing. The serum specimen is either refrigerated or frozen to prevent chemical changes unless the specimen can be tested quickly. The use of a serum separator tube provides a silicone gel barrier that aids in separation and allows for pouring the serum into the transfer tube instead of pipetting it. Procedure 1-14 describes the process of separating serum from whole blood and transferring it to a transfer tube.

A lavender tube with EDTA is used to collect blood specimens for plasma or whole blood for blood counts. This type of specimen is not required to sit and can be centrifuged immediately after collection. The plasma is pipetted off in the same manner as serum and stored until collection (Fig. 1-19).

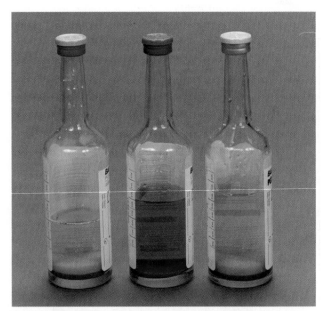

Fig. 1-18 Blood cultures may be collected in sterile yellow tubes or bottles that fit into the plastic holder.

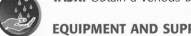

Procedure 1-13 Perform Venipuncture Using the Butterfly Method (Collection of Multiple Evacuated Tubes)

TASK: Obtain a venous blood specimen acceptable for testing using the butterfly method.

EQUIPMENT AND SUPPLIES

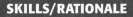

- Nonsterile disposable gloves
- Personal protective equipment (PPE)
- Tourniquet
- Test tube rack
- Winged-infusion set with Luer adapter and safety guard
- Multidraw needle (22 to 25 gauge) and tube holder, or 10-cc (10-mL) syringe
- Evacuated blood tubes for requested tests with labels (correct evacuated tube required for designated test ordered)
- Alcohol wipe
- Sterile 2 × 2-inch gauze pads
- Bandage or nonallergenic tape
- Sharps container
- Biohazardous waste container
- Laboratory requisition form
- Patient's medical record

SKILLS/RATIONALE

STANDARD PRECAUTIONS ARE TO BE FOLLOWED.

1. **Procedural Step. Sanitize the hands.**
   An alcohol-based hand rub may be used instead of washing hands with soap and water, unless hands are visibly soiled.
   Rationale. Hand sanitization promotes infection control.

2. **Procedural Step. Assemble equipment and supplies and verify the order.**
   Be sure to select the proper evacuated tubes according to the tests to be performed. Check the expiration date of the tubes.
   Rationale. It is important to have all supplies and equipment ready and available before starting any procedure to ensure efficiency.

3. **Procedural Step. Greet and identify the patient, and escort the patient to the examination room.**
   Ask the patient to have a seat in the phlebotomy chair. If the patient states that he or she "faints" when blood is taken, place the patient in a supine position on the examination table.
   Rationale. Identifying the patient ensures the procedure is performed on the correct patient. Placing the patient in the supine position makes it less likely that the patient will faint.

4. **Procedural Step. Explain the procedure to the patient.**

If the test(s) ordered requires patient preparation such as fasting or medication restrictions, confirm that the patient has followed the preparation orders. When a patient is not properly prepared, the physician should be consulted for directions concerning how to proceed.
Rationale. Explaining the procedure to the patient promotes cooperation and provides a means of obtaining implied consent. Test results will be inaccurate if the patient has not followed the required preparation orders.

5. **Procedural Step. Prepare the winged infusion set.**
   Remove the winged infusion set from its package. Extend the tubing to its full length and stretch it slightly to prevent it from coiling back up. Attach the winged infusion set to either a syringe or an evacuated-tube holder. If a holder is used, screw the adapter with the double-ended needle into the holder and tighten it securely. When using a syringe, tighten the Luer adapter onto the syringe.
   Rationale. Extending the tubing straightens it to permit a free flow of blood in the tubing. An unsecured needle or syringe can come loose or pop off during the draw.

6. **Procedural Step. Open the sterile gauze packet and place the gauze pad on the inside of its wrapper, or obtain sterile gauze pads from a bulk package.**

7. **Procedural Step. Position and examine the arm to be used in the venipuncture.**

Continued

Procedure 1-13 Perform Venipuncture Using the Butterfly Method (Collection of Multiple Evacuated Tubes)—cont'd

a. Ask the patient to extend both arms with the arms supported in a slightly downward position. Perform a preliminary assessment of both arms. If the patient has a preference, examine it first, but do not hesitate to select the other arm if it seems more acceptable. Often a winged infusion set is selected because the patient's veins are very small or fragile in the antecubital space. If this is the case, inspect the back of the patient's hands for a suitable vein.
Rationale. Most adults have had previous venipunctures and know which veins are better for a successful draw. Asking a patient to state a preference gives the patient a sense of control over what is happening and increases patient comfort.

b. The arm or hand with the vein selected for the venipuncture should be extended and placed in a straight line from the shoulder to the wrist with the antecubital veins facing anteriorly. The arm should be supported on the armrest by a rolled towel or by having the patient place the fist of the other hand under the elbow.

c. If the back of the hand is used, extend the arm with the back of the hand facing up. The hand should be placed on a flat surface. Have the patient grasp a hand roll with their hand and roll it toward you. This brings the veins closer to the surface. If using the forearm, position it over the towel in a similar fashion. The tourniquet is applied in the same manner but will be secured 3 to 4 inches above the venipuncture site (wrist or forearm).

8. **Procedural Step. Follow Steps 9 through 14 from Procedure 1-11.**

9. **Procedural Step. If drawing from the hand, ask the patient to make a fist or bend the fingers downward. Pull the skin taut with your thumb over the top of the patient's knuckles.**

10. **Procedural Step. Position the butterfly needle.** Grasp the "wings" and fold them together with the thumb and index finger of your dominant hand. Wrap the tubing from the medial aspect of your hand to the lateral aspect, allowing the tube holder or syringe to hang down loosely. Place evacuated tubes nearby if using the winged infusion set with a Luer adapter and tube holder.
Rationale. Holding the winged infusion set in this manner allows more freedom of movement to insert

the evacuated tube once the needle has been inserted into the vein.

11. **Procedural Step. Remove the protective shield from the needle of the infusion set, being sure the bevel is facing up.**
Rationale. Positioning the needle with the bevel up allows for easier entry into the skin and the vein.

12. **Procedural Step. Perform the venipuncture.**

a. Warn that the patient will feel a little "stick."
Rationale. Warning the patient before entering the vein prevents the element of surprise, which could cause the patient to pull away, causing the needle to be pulled out of the vein.

b. With the other hand, pull the skin taut beneath the intended puncture site to anchor the vein. Your thumb should be placed 1 to 2 inches below and to the side of the puncture site.
Rationale. Pulling the skin taut helps the needle glide in easily.

c. Following the direction of the vein, with one quick motion, smoothly pierce the skin and enter the vein at a small angle—about 15 degrees—and almost parallel to the vein.
Rationale. The angle of the needle is important because an angle of less than 15 degrees may cause the needle to enter above the vein, preventing puncture. An angle of more than 30 degrees may cause the needle to go through the vein by puncturing the posterior wall. This could result in a hematoma (blood in the tissues).

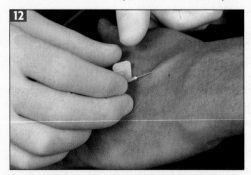

13. **Procedural Step. After penetrating the vein, decrease the angle of the needle to 5 degrees until a "flash" of blood appears in the tubing.** If no flash appears, thread the needle into the lumen of the vein a little further. If still no flash, release the tourniquet, slowly remove the needle, reassemble supplies, and try again.

Procedure 1-13 Perform Venipuncture Using the Butterfly Method (Collection of Multiple Evacuated Tubes)—cont'd

14. Procedural Step. Secure the needle for blood collection.

Seat the needle by slightly threading it up the lumen (central area) of the vein. This helps to prevent the needle from twisting out of the vein during the remainder of the procedure. Do not let go of the needle or allow it to move. Securely rest the needle flat against the skin.

Rationale. Seating the needle anchors the needle in the center of the vein. Moving the needle is painful for the patient.

15. Procedural Step. Insert the evacuated tube into the tube holder or gently pull back on the plunger of the syringe.

If using an evacuated tube system, keep the tube and holder in a downward position so that the tube fills from the bottom up and not near the rubber stopper. Push the bottom of the tube with the thumb of your nondominant hand carefully so that the needle inside the holder pierces the rubber stopper of the tube. If everything is done correctly, blood will begin to fill the tube.

Rationale. The tube must fill from the bottom up to prevent venous reflux.

16. Procedural Step. Change tubes as required by the test ordered.

When the tube has stopped filling, grasp the bottom of the tube with your nondominant hand. Push against the flange with the thumb, and pull the tube from the holder. This lets the rubber sleeve slide back over the end of the needle and prevents blood from dripping into the holder. Invert additive-containing tubes approximately 8 to 10 times, then place them upright in a rack so they will not roll. (Do not shake the tubes.)

17. Procedural Step. Release the tourniquet.

18. Procedural Step. Remove the needle.

With one quick, smooth motion, remove the needle from the arm with the dominant hand and apply pressure with the gauze in the left hand immediately *after* you remove the needle. As you withdraw the needle, flip the safety shield over the needle tip with your right thumb and direct the needle down and away from yourself and the patient.

NOTE: Do not place a gauze pad over the needle as it is being withdrawn because this can scratch the patient's arm or dig the needle into the arm, causing pain. Always withdraw the

needle completely first, then apply the gauze pad to the site.

Rationale. Placing the gauze pad over the puncture site helps prevent tissue movement, absorbs small amounts of blood that ooze from the vein, and reduces patient discomfort. Careful withdrawal prevents further tissue damage. The needle sheath prevents needle sticks.

19. Procedural Step. Apply direct pressure on the venipuncture site, and instruct the patient to raise the arm straight above the head.

Tell the patient to keep the arm straight while raised to allow a good clot to begin forming over the puncture site.

Rationale. Raising the arm straight above the head helps prevent a hematoma. Keeping the arm straight prevents dislodging the clot that has formed.

20. Procedural Step. Instruct the patient to maintain pressure on the site for 1 to 2 minutes, with the arm raised straight up above the head.

NOTE: If any swelling or discoloration occurs, apply an ice pack to the site after bandaging it.

Rationale. Maintaining pressure with the arm raised over the head will help speed up the clotting process and prevent a hematoma. Do not allow the patient to bend the arm at the elbow because this increases blood loss from the puncture site and causes bruising.

21. Procedural Step. If a syringe was used, transfer the blood to the evacuated tubes as soon as possible.

Refer to Step 17 in Procedure 1-12.

22. Procedural Step. Properly dispose of the winged infusion set.

Always drop the butterfly set and holder in a sharps container. When using a quick-release holder, disconnect the multisample needle from the infusion set. If the quick-disconnect holder is contaminated with blood, it should be discarded.

Rationale. Proper disposal of the needle is required by the OSHA standard to prevent accidental needle stick injuries.

23. Procedural Step. Follow Steps 25 through 33 from Procedure 1-11.

Charting Example

Date	
7/31/xx	10:30 a.m. Venous blood specimen collected for CBC from Ⓡ hand. Site without redness or edema. ——————— R. Green, CMA

Procedure 1-14 Separate Serum from a Blood Specimen

TASK: Transfer serum separated from blood by the process of centrifugation into a transfer tube.

EQUIPMENT AND SUPPLIES
- Nonsterile disposable gloves
- Personal protective equipment (PPE)
- Clotted blood specimen
- Laboratory requisition form
- Biohazardous waste container
- Sharps container
- Transfer tube
- Transfer pipette

SKILLS/RATIONALE

STANDARD PRECAUTIONS ARE TO BE FOLLOWED.

1. **Procedural Step. Sanitize the hands.**
   An alcohol-based hand rub may be used instead of washing hands with soap and water, unless hands are visibly soiled.
   Rationale. Hand sanitization promotes infection control.

2. **Procedural Step. Assemble equipment and supplies and verify the order.**
   Rationale. It is important to have all supplies and equipment ready and available before starting any procedure to ensure efficiency.

3. **Procedural Step. Apply gloves and other PPE.**

4. **Procedural Step. Verify orders against the laboratory requisition form and the specimen tube.**
   Rationale. All identification must match for accuracy.

5. **Procedural Step. Allow whole-blood specimens, collected in a red-top evacuated tube, to clot at room temperature for a minimum of 30 minutes, and no more than 45 minutes after collection.**
   Rationale. Specimens require a minimum of 20 minutes sitting upright in a tube rack to form a sufficient clot removing all clotting factors. After 45 minutes the specimen starts to lose its integrity.

6. **Procedural Step. Place two stoppered red-top tubes in the centrifuge to balance the centrifuge, and close and latch the centrifuge lid securely.**
   The centrifuge is balanced when tubes containing equal amounts of fluid are placed directly across from each other. If only one tube of blood is to be centrifuged, the second tube can be filled with an equal amount of water.
   Rationale. The tubes must remain stoppered during this process. If the centrifuge is not balanced, the

blood tube could break, creating a biohazardous situation.

7. **Procedural Step. Set the timer for 15 minutes.**

8. **Procedural Step. When the time has elapsed, allow the centrifuge to come to a complete stop before opening the lid and removing the tube.**
   Rationale. This prevents the potential of aerosol spray contamination.

9. **Procedural Step. Properly remove the stopper or apply a transfer device.**

10. **Procedural Step. Separate the serum from the top of the tube into a transfer tube using the transfer device or a disposable pipette.**
    If a red/gray (marbled) or Hemogard gold tube is used, the serum may be poured into a transfer tube.

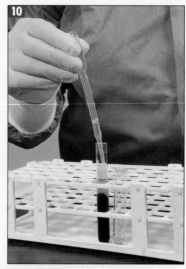

11. **Procedural Step. Label the tubes and attach the laboratory requisition form.**

Procedure 1-14 Separate Serum from a Blood Specimen—cont'd

12. **Procedural Step. Properly dispose of all waste material in the appropriate waste receptacle.**
    Any items contaminated with blood must be disposed of in a biohazardous waste container. Any items made of glass (tubes) must be disposed of in a sharps container. Items not contaminated with body fluids may be disposed of in regular waste containers.

13. **Procedural Step. Package the specimen for transport to the laboratory.**

14. **Procedural Step. Remove gloves and sanitize the hands.**
    Always sanitize the hands after every procedure or after using gloves.

Photo from Bonewit-West K: *Clinical procedures for medical assistants,* ed 6, Philadelphia, 2004, Saunders.

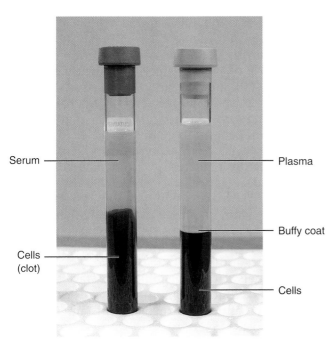

Serum

Plasma

Buffy coat

Cells
(clot)

Cells

Fig. 1-19 Blood separates into the layers shown here when there is no anticoagulant *(left tube)* and when an anticoagulant is present *(right tube). (From Bonewit-West K:* Clinical procedures for medical assistants, *ed 6, Philadelphia, 2004, Saunders.)*

PATIENT-CENTERED PROFESSIONALISM

- Why is it important for the medical assistant to know proper patient preparation and collection methods for a capillary puncture?
- Why must the order of draw be followed?

STOOL COLLECTION

The way **stool** specimens are transported depends on what testing is to be performed. For tests requiring an unpreserved stool specimen, the collection of feces (stool) should be done with a clean container that is not contaminated by urine, menstrual blood, or water. One method is to insert a paper plate in the toilet bowl and then transfer the stool to a smaller container. The type of container supplied by the laboratory will depend on the test being performed. No special patient preparation is usually required. Refer to Procedure 2-1 in the module C textbook for instructing the patient on collection of a stool sample.

Ova and Parasites

A special kit with two or three collection tubes is needed for ova and parasite collection. Each container has a different type of fixative. Each container is filled to the fill line on the label with stool from the initial collection container. Once filled, the container is closed, mixed, labeled with the patient's name, and kept at room temperature or refrigerated until testing occurs.

PATIENT-CENTERED PROFESSIONALISM

- Why would the medical assistant instruct the patient not to let the stool specimen become contaminated with urine, menstrual blood, or water?

SPUTUM COLLECTION

Sputum is the secretion from the lungs produced in the bronchi and throat. To collect a sputum specimen, the patient is first asked to rinse the mouth to remove food particles. Then the patient is instructed to take three deep breaths and cough deeply "from the lungs." The specimen is collected into a wide-mouthed container for culture and sensitivity testing. Upon awakening in the morning is an ideal time for collecting a specimen. Sputum testing is often done to rule out tuberculosis or determine the presence of blood (hemoptysis).

PATIENT-CENTERED PROFESSIONALISM

- Why is it important for the medical assistant to understand proper collection technique for a sputum collection?

CONCLUSION

Medical assistants are often involved in the collection, preparation for transport, and processing of the many types of specimens collected at the POL. The physician can analyze specimens collected from a patient to assess the patient's general health, as well as to diagnose and determine treatment plans.

The medical assistant must understand and follow federal, state, and office protocols for collecting and transporting specimens. These protocols help ensure that accurate results are obtained from testing. Accurate test results are crucial. Errors in specimen collection can cause delays in testing, diagnosis, and treatment, or even lawsuits in some situations. The knowledgeable, skilled medical assistant helps protect the patient and the medical office by performing all procedures accurately, efficiently, and in accordance with all guidelines and protocols.

SUMMARY

Reinforce your understanding of the material in this chapter by reviewing the curriculum objectives and key content points below.

1. Define, appropriately use, and spell all the Key Terms for this chapter.
   - Review the Key Terms if necessary.
2. Explain the purpose of the Clinical Laboratory Improvement Amendments of 1988 (CLIA 88).
   - CLIA 88 sets minimum performance standards for laboratories and defines three levels of complexity for performing laboratory testing.
3. List three factors that determine whether a medical office will perform and process a specimen.
   - The type of practice, the cost-effectiveness of the test, and the level of complexity of the test determine whether a medical office will perform and process a specimen or have the testing done elsewhere.

4. Briefly describe three CLIA-waived urine tests, six CLIA-waived blood tests, and seven CLIA-waived tests of other types.
   - Review Table 1-1.
5. Differentiate between quality assurance (QA) and quality control (QC) and briefly explain how each is accomplished in the medical office.
   - Quality assurance is designed to monitor and evaluate the quality of test results as processed by personnel.
   - Quality control is a process that provides the means to ensure that test results are accurate as processed by the equipment.
6. Demonstrate the correct procedure for using methods of quality control.
   - Review Procedure 1-1.
7. Explain the need for safety precautions in the medical office laboratory and how they protect both staff and patients.
   - Safety precautions help prevent cross-contamination from worker to patient and from patient to patient, and help protect employees from exposure to potentially biohazardous materials from patients' body fluids.
8. Identify the parts of a compound microscope, and explain its proper use and maintenance.
   - A microscope consists of a stand (arm and base), magnification system (objectives), stage, and light source.
   - Understanding magnification, stage use, light source function, and how to focus the microscope allows the medical assistant to use it properly.
   - Microscopes must be properly maintained to keep them in optimal working order by cleaning all nonglass surfaces using a soft cloth, using lens paper to clean all lenses, placing the microscope in a protective covering or cabinet for storage, holding the arm firmly during transport, and cleaning the oil-immersion lens with a special cleaner.
9. Demonstrate the procedure for successfully focusing a microscope from lower to higher power.
   - Review Procedure 1-2.
10. Explain the purpose and proper use of a centrifuge.
    - A centrifuge separates solid material from liquid through forced gravity.
    - The separation of materials allows all parts of a specimen to be studied.
    - Always counterbalance the centrifuge with tubes on opposite sides with the same specimen or a tube of equal size and shape and amount of fluid.

- Always follow the manufacturer's instructions for use and care of the centrifuge.
11. List six categories of laboratory tests and briefly explain the purpose of each.
    - Chemistry tests are performed on serum, plasma, urine, spinal fluid, and other body fluids to test levels of chemicals (e.g., glucose, cholesterol, electrolytes, proteins, drugs).
    - Hematology (and coagulation) studies assess formed elements of whole blood (white and red blood cells, platelets) in a blood sample.
    - Microbiology tests are performed on various body fluids to study bacteria, fungi, viruses, and parasites.
    - Serology tests are performed on serum to study the body's immune responses by detecting antibody and antigen reactions.
    - Blood bank tests involve studies for ABO blood groupings, Rh typing, and crossmatching of blood for surgical patients.
    - Urinalysis studies the physical, chemical, and microscopic structure of urine.
    - Medical assistants perform some, but not all, of these laboratory tests.
12. Explain the importance of effective patient preparation before laboratory tests are performed.
    - Effective patient preparation helps ensure the accuracy of test results.
    - Patients should be given time to ask questions, and medical assistants should make certain that patients understand all instructions.
13. Explain the importance of completing a laboratory request form accurately.
    - Incorrect paperwork can cause a laboratory test to be delayed or not run at all.
    - An inaccurate laboratory request form may result in the wrong test being completed.
14. Demonstrate the procedure for accurately completing a laboratory request form.
    - Review Procedure 1-3.
15. List three methods of specimen collection, and explain the need for collecting specimens accurately.
    - Three ways to collect specimens include collection and testing at the office, collecting at the office and testing at an outside lab, and collecting and testing at an outside lab.
    - Accurate collection of the specimen helps ensure the sample will produce accurate test results.
16. Demonstrate the procedure for accurately collecting a specimen for transport to an outside laboratory.
    - Review Procedure 1-4.

17. Explain the purpose of a laboratory report and why it must be accurate and transmitted to the physician in a timely manner.
    - The laboratory report assists the physician in diagnosis.
    - When the laboratory report is accurate and on time, the physician can make a more accurate, timely diagnosis.
18. Demonstrate the correct procedure for screening and following up on patient test results.
    - Review Procedure 1-5.
19. Demonstrate the correct procedure for collecting an uncontaminated throat specimen to test for group A beta-hemolytic streptococci.
    - Review Procedure 1-6.
20. Explain the purpose of a urinalysis and the need for avoiding sources of contamination and for processing urine specimens in the required time.
    - Urinalysis can detect kidney disease, infections in the urinary tract, and other disease states of the body.
    - Contamination of a specimen makes test results less accurate.
    - Processing of urine specimens must be done in a timely manner because bacteria will multiply rapidly unless the specimen is refrigerated (or a preservative is used).
21. List four instructions the medical assistant should give to a patient who is to collect a random urine specimen and bring it to the medical office.
    - Purpose of the collection.
    - Importance of not touching the inside of the container.
    - First morning specimen is best.
    - Urine specimen should be refrigerated until it can be transported.
22. Demonstrate the correct procedure for obtaining a urine specimen from an infant using a pediatric urine collector.
    - Review Procedure 1-7.
23. Demonstrate the correct procedure for providing patient instructions on collecting a midstream clean-catch urine specimen to ensure validity of test results.
    - Review Procedure 1-8.
24. Demonstrate the correct procedure for providing patient instructions on collecting a 24-hour urine specimen to ensure validity of test results.
    - Review Procedure 1-9.
25. Explain the special considerations for handling drug screenings and specimens that may be used as evidence in a court of law.
    - Chain of custody regulations specify how evidence should be collected and handled.

- Chain of evidence regulations specify how every detail of a forensic investigation should be handled from beginning to end.

26. List methods of collecting blood and give the three factors that determine which method will be used.
    - Venipuncture and capillary puncture are two methods of collecting blood.
    - The test to be performed and the age and condition of the patient determine which method will be used.

27. Explain the purpose of a lancet in capillary blood collection.
    - The sterile lancet makes a small puncture in the skin.
    - Lancets penetrate the skin at various depths depending on the patient and condition of the site.

28. Briefly describe five types of containers that can be used to collect capillary blood specimens.
    - Microcontainers, capillary tubes, glass slides, filter paper, and blood-diluting pipettes can be used to collect capillary blood specimens.

29. Demonstrate the correct procedure for obtaining a capillary blood specimen acceptable for testing using the index or middle finger.
    - Review Procedure 1-10.

30. List four acceptable sites for performing venipuncture and the two factors in selecting the site.
    - Venipuncture can be performed in the antecubital fossa of either arm, the cephalic veins, the basilic veins, or the forearm.
    - Site selection depends on the age of the patient and condition of the veins.

31. State two reasons for failed venipuncture draws.
    - Failed venipuncture draws can be caused by incorrectly positioning the needle or using the wrong angle.

32. List the order of draw for the evacuated-tube (Vacutainer) system recommended by the Clinical and Laboratory Standards Institute (CLSI).
    - Use the memory aid "Big Rugged Gunther Got Lots of Gold" to help you remember the order of draw (see Fig. 1-12).

33. Demonstrate the correct procedure for obtaining a venous blood specimen acceptable for testing using the evacuated-tube system.
    - Review Procedure 1-11.

34. Demonstrate the correct procedure for obtaining a venous blood specimen acceptable for testing using the syringe method.
    - Review Procedure 1-12.

35. Demonstrate the correct procedure for obtaining a venous blood specimen acceptable for testing using the butterfly method.
    - Review Procedure 1-13.

36. Demonstrate the correct procedure for successfully separating serum from a blood specimen and transferring the serum from the collection tube to a transfer tube.
    - Review Procedure 1-14.

37. Explain the considerations for collecting stool specimens.
    - A clean container (no urine, menstrual blood, or water) should be used to collect a stool sample.
    - No special patient preparation is necessary.
    - The type of container depends on the type of test being done.

38. Explain the considerations for collecting sputum specimens.
    - Sputum specimens are used for culture and sensitivity testing.
    - A good time for sputum collection is after awakening in the morning.

39. Analyze a realistic medical office situation and apply your understanding of the purpose and use of the physician office laboratory to determine the best course of action.
    - Medical assistants must understand and follow the procedures and policies associated with each laboratory procedure they perform.
    - Proper patient preparation is an important aspect of laboratory testing.

40. Describe the impact on patient care when medical assistants have a solid understanding of the processes and procedures used to collect specimens for testing in the medical office.
    - Accurate test results occur when the medical assistant properly collects or provides clear instructions to the patient for collection and follows proper processing procedures.
    - Patient care is enhanced when the medical assistant is knowledgeable about proper procedures for collecting and processing specimens.
    - Diagnosis and treatment of a patient begins sooner when test results are accurate.

FOR FURTHER EXPLORATION

Research the history of the microscope. The microscope is a valuable instrument in the physician office laboratory.

Keywords: Use the following keywords in your search: microscope, electron microscope.

LABORATORY TESTING IN THE PHYSICIAN OFFICE

21. Explain the purpose of the erythrocyte sedimentation rate (ESR) and list two common methods used in the POL to perform ESR.
22. Demonstrate the correct procedure for performing ESR using the Westergren method.
23. Explain the purpose of a differential blood cell count, and list five factors that affect the quality of a good blood smear.
24. Demonstrate the correct procedure for preparation of a blood smear slide.

Blood Chemistry
25. Explain how physicians use blood chemistry profiles.
26. Explain the purpose of cholesterol testing and list the desirable, borderline-high, and high cholesterol levels in test results.
27. Demonstrate the procedure for accurately collecting and processing a blood specimen for cholesterol testing.
28. Describe three tests performed to monitor a person's glucose level.
29. Demonstrate the procedure for accurately collecting and processing a blood specimen for glucose testing.

Serology and Immunology
30. Define serology and list seven types of serological or immunological testing.
31. List and describe four viewable reactions to additives that indicate positive results in serological testing.

Microbiology
32. Demonstrate the procedure for correctly obtaining a bacterial smear from a wound swab.
33. Explain the purpose of a Gram stain and briefly describe the staining process.
34. Explain why culture plates are inoculated, and briefly describe the process of streaking an agar plate.

Patient-Centered Professionalism
35. Analyze a realistic medical office situation and apply your understanding of laboratory testing in the physician office to determine the best course of action.
36. Describe the impact on patient care when medical assistants have a solid understanding of the purpose and procedures for laboratory tests performed in the medical office.

KEY TERMS

2-hour postprandial test Test measuring a patient's ability to metabolize food 2 hours after a meal.

acetone Chemical formed when fats are metabolized rather than glucose.

agar Seaweed extract used to make certain media solid for bacterial cultures.

agglutination Clustering or clumping together of cells as a result of an antigen-antibody reaction.

artifacts Structures not normally present in a urine specimen.

automated urine analyzer Equipment that uses light photometry to analyze a reagent test strip.

bacteria Microorganisms that may cause disease.

bacterial smear Placement of a bacterial specimen on a glass slide for microscopic review.

bacteriology Study of microorganisms.

bacteriuria Bacteria in the urine.

bilirubin Byproduct of hemoglobin breakdown; orange-yellow pigment of bile.

bilirubinuria Appearance of bilirubin in the urine.

C&S Culture and sensitivity; test to determine which antibiotic is most effective against cultured organisms.

casts Hardened protein material shaped like the lumen of a kidney tubule and washed out by urine.

cellular casts Hyaline casts that contain either white or red blood cells.

chemistry profile Blood test that details the chemical composition of the blood.

CLIA-waived tests Simple laboratory tests that can be performed in a licensed laboratory by nonlaboratory health care workers.

Clinical Laboratory Improvement Amendments of 1988 (CLIA 88) Legislation enacted to ensure the quality of laboratory results by setting performance standards.

complete blood count (CBC) Total count of each blood element.

confirmatory test Test that confirms the presence of a specific substance in a specimen.

crenated Shrunken; formation of notches on the edges of red blood cells.

crystals Translucent solids appearing in various shapes.

culture plate Covered container with nutritional substances that support growth of bacteria.

cystitis Inflammation of the urinary bladder.

diaphoresis Excessive sweating.

differential blood cell count Test that counts the types of white blood cells in a stained blood smear; "diff."

EDTA Ethylenediaminetetraacetic acid; anticoagulant used for preserving blood for hematology studies.

enzyme immunoassay (EIA) Pregnancy test that uses a color-change reaction.

erythrocyte sedimentation rate (ESR) Screening test that confirms an inflammatory process in the body by measuring how quickly red blood cells settle to the bottom of a calibrated tube; "sed rate."

fasting blood sugar (FBS) test Measurement of glucose present in the blood after fasting for 12 hours.

fatty casts Hyaline cast with fatty cells.

first morning specimen First voided urine specimen in the morning; most concentrated specimen, because it is in the bladder overnight.

galactosemia Galactose in the blood.

glucometer Device used to measure glucose in the blood.

glucose Sugar; end result of carbohydrate metabolism and the main producer of energy.

glucose reagent strip Chemical pad on a dipstick that tests for the presence of sugar.

glucose tolerance test (GTT) Test that determines the body's ability to metabolize glucose over a specific time period.

glycosuria Sugar in the urine.

glycosylated hemoglobin (GHb) test Hemoglobin A_{1c}; test that measures the amount of glucose attached to hemoglobin over a 3-month period.

Gram stain Staining method used to identify the shape and pattern of microorganisms.

granular casts Casts appearing microscopically as short, plump, and coarse.

HDL High-density lipoprotein; "good" cholesterol.

hematocrit (Hct) Measurement of the percentage of packed red blood cells in a volume of whole blood.

hematology Study of all blood elements.

hematuria Intact red blood cells in the urine.

hemoglobin (Hb) Red blood cell component that carries oxygen and gives blood its color.

hemoglobinuria Hemolyzed red blood cells in the urine.

hemolyzed Damaged, burst cells; hemolyzed red blood cells are colorless and cannot be seen under magnification.

high-power field (HPF) High magnification.

human chorionic gonadotropin (hCG) Hormone that is present only during pregnancy.

hyaline casts Common casts found in urine that are pale and transparent; appear in unchecked hypertension.

immunoassay Laboratory technique that measures the reaction of an antigen to a specific antibody.

immunological testing Tests used to measure antigen-antibody reactions.

immunology Study of how the immune system works to defend the body by antigen/antibody reaction.

ketone Chemical formed when fats are metabolized.

ketonuria Presence of ketones in the urine.

LDL Low-density lipoprotein; "bad" cholesterol.

leukocyte esterase Enzyme that is released from white blood cells.

low-power field (LPF) Low magnification.

lumen Opening in a vessel, intestines, or tube.

lysis Destruction, as of red blood cells.

media Nutritive substances used to grow bacteria and culture microorganisms; singular *medium.*

mucous threads Thin strands of mucus.

myoglobinuria Globin from damaged muscle cells in the urine.

nephron Basic functioning unit of the kidney.

nitrates Salts of nitric acid.

nitrites End products of nitrate metabolism from leukocyte metabolism.

parasites Organisms living on or within a host.

plaque Fat deposits on the inside wall of an artery.

platelet counts Total number of platelets in a blood sample.

point-of-care testing (POCT) Tests done in the physician office laboratory for immediate feedback.

precipitates Particles in a solution brought on by a chemical reaction.

proteinuria Protein in the urine.

qualitative Presence of a substance (e.g., hCG in a pregnant woman's urine or blood); positive or negative results.

quantitative Amount of a substance able to be measured; actual amounts.

random specimen Specimen taken anytime without special preparation.

reagent strip Dipstick containing several chemical pads that detect a specific substance in a body fluid.

reagent tablet Tablet that reacts to a specific substance, confirming its presence.

red cell indices Tests that determine the size, content, and hemoglobin concentration of red blood cells.

renal epithelial cells Epithelial cells released by the kidney indicating disease.

sediment Solid material that settles to the bottom of a urine specimen.

serological testing Testing of body fluids to analyze a reaction between an antigen and antibody.

serology Study of blood serum for antigen-antibody reactions.

serum cholesterol White, fatlike substance made in the liver.

specific gravity Measurement of the weight of dissolved substances in the urine compared with distilled water.

spermatozoa Reproductive cells of the male; sperm.

squamous epithelial cells Cells that appear as flat, irregular-shaped cells under magnification.

streak To inoculate or put a specimen onto a culture plate in an established pattern.

supernatant Top, liquid portion of a specimen that has been centrifuged to remove solid particles.

timed specimen Specimen collected in a specified time sequence.

total cholesterol Combined measurement of LDL and HDL cholesterol.

transitional epithelial cells Renal epithelial cells appearing in kidney disease.

turbid Not clear or transparent; particles floating within; cloudy.

urinalysis Analysis of urine specimen for physical, chemical, and microscopic properties.

urobilinogen Breakdown of bilirubin by intestinal bacteria.

urochrome Yellow pigment derived from urobilin that is left over when hemoglobin breaks down during red blood cell destruction.

viscosity Stickiness, or thickness, as of the blood; state of being viscous (sticky).

waxy casts Urinary casts that appear glassy and smooth with sawtooth edges under microscopic view.

Westergren method Method to measure ESR using a self-zeroing tube calibrated from 0 to 200.

Wintrobe method Method to measure ESR using a disposable tube calibrated from 0 to 100.

yeasts Oval-shaped fungi with small buds.

What Would You Do?

Read the following scenario and keep it in mind as you learn about laboratory testing in the physician office.

Dr. Carlson does not have a medical lab technician. Instead, she depends on the medical assistant to provide the test results of lab specimens that are ordered. Because of his training in a medical assisting program, Jerry is aware of the importance of quality control and quality assurance and that both should be done on a daily basis.

As part of the daily routine, Jerry, the medical assistant, is expected to perform physical and chemical testing of urine using reagent strips. Dr. Carlson also allows Jerry to examine specimens using a microscope to identify the urine sediment. Jerry completes hemoglobin testing using HemoCue and uses a centrifuge to spin hematocrits. As Jerry reads the hematocrit, he finds that the anticoagulated blood has separated into three layers, each of which has a specific characteristic.

Because CLIA-waived tests are often performed in a physician's office, Jerry and other medical assistants must be able to perform these tests on a daily basis. Would you be capable of performing these tasks?

The purpose of the **Clinical Laboratory Improvement Amendments of 1988 (CLIA 88)** was to establish minimum quality standards for laboratory testing. Any facility wanting to become certified to perform certain laboratory tests and procedures must submit an application with a fee. The laboratory must also follow all regulations on using quality control testing, hiring knowledgeable personnel, using quality assurance measures, and submitting to periodic inspections. The standards established by CLIA 88 help to ensure the reliability of testing results. This protects the patient by ensuring that employees are not performing tests without the proper educational training.

As discussed in Chapter 1, some laboratory tests are **CLIA-waived tests.** This "waived" status means these tests are simple and have minimal risk for error. CLIA provides a certificate to perform waived tests to a facility when it agrees to follow proper laboratory practices. CLIA-waived tests can be performed in physician offices, clinical laboratories, and long-term care facilities; at the bedside in an acute care setting; by insurance companies; and in other settings by nonlaboratory health care workers.

CLIA-waived tests are simple to perform, but care must be taken to follow quality control measures in order to minimize inaccurate test results.

This chapter discusses CLIA-waived urinalysis and blood testing as well as some non-CLIA-waived tests. Throat culture for group A beta-hemolytic streptococci is also a CLIA-waived test. Although some tests are not waived, the medical assistant should understand how they are done and their clinical significance (e.g., microscopic examination of urine sediment).

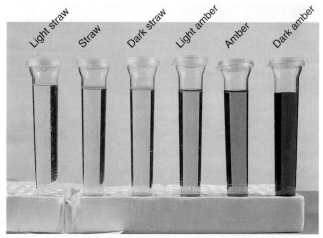

Fig. 2-1   Color of urine. *(From Bonewit-West K: Clinical procedures for medical assistants, ed 6, Philadelphia, 2004, Saunders.)*

URINALYSIS

Urinalysis is an examination of a urine specimen. It is one of the most common laboratory tests performed in the physician's office as part of a routine physical examination. Urinalysis involves the physical, chemical, and microscopic examination of the urine specimen. The medical assistant can perform the physical and chemical aspect of a urinalysis. However, a qualified member of the health care team must perform the microscopic portion because it is not a CLIA-waived procedure. (The microscopic aspect is only covered in this chapter to provide you with an overall understanding of the process.)

Physical Properties of Urine

A urinalysis can provide valuable diagnostic information concerning overall metabolic function of the kidneys and urinary tract. A visual inspection of the urine sample is made to assess its physical properties. This is the first step taken by the medical assistant when performing a urinalysis. Visual inspection includes observation of the color, appearance, and any distinctive odor from the specimen. A routine urinalysis does not require the medical assistant to record the amount or volume of the specimen, but the assistant needs to be aware if production amounts are within normal range (see Appendix A).

Color
Normal urine color can vary from pale yellow or light straw to amber (dark yellow) (Fig. 2-1). **Urochrome** is the yellow pigment (derived from urobilin) left over when hemoglobin breaks down during the destruction of red blood cells (RBCs). This is what gives urine its color.

Urine color is affected by food and fluid intake, medications, and waste products from a disease process. Usually a pale urine color indicates diluted urine, and a dark-yellow urine specimen indicates a concentrated specimen. In most cases, the more concentrated the specimen, the darker is the appearance.

Urine specimens may be collected at specific times of the day, which may affect the color, as follows:

- The **first morning specimen** is usually more concentrated because it has been in the bladder overnight.
- A **random specimen** (taken any time with no special preparation) may have less color because

TABLE 2-1	Urine Colors and Clinical Significance

Color	Clinical Significance
Pale yellow	High fluid consumption
	Diabetes mellitus
	Diabetes insipidus
	Diuretics
Straw	Normal
Amber	Concentrated specimen
	Dehydration
	Fever
	Excessive exercise
	Excessive fluid loss (diarrhea, vomiting)
Bright yellow	Excessive beta-carotene (carrots, high dose of vitamin A)
Orange-yellow	Drugs (e.g., phenazopyridine [Pyridium])
Yellow-brown	Bilirubin
	Liver disease
	Excessive destruction of red blood cells
	Iron preparations
Greenish-yellow	Bilirubin
	Drugs (e.g., senna, cascara)
Blue-green	*Pseudomonas* infection
	High ingestion of asparagus
	Vitamin B
Red	Blood (menstrual)
	High ingestion of beets
	Red blood cells (hemoglobin)
	Drugs

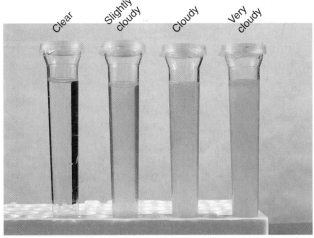

Fig. 2-2 Appearance of urine. *(From Bonewit-West K: Clinical procedures for medical assistants, ed 6, Philadelphia, 2004, Saunders.)*

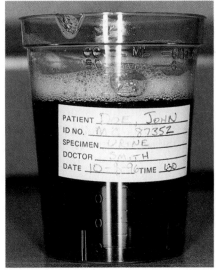

Fig. 2-3 Amber urine with foam may indicate increased protein and hematuria. *(From Young AP, Kennedy DB: Kinn's the medical assistant, ed 9, Philadelphia, 2003, Saunders.)*

foods and fluids taken throughout the day affect its concentration.

Chapter 1 provides more information on specific methods for urine collection. Table 2-1 lists the clinical significance of various colors of urine.

Appearance

The appearance of urine can be described in terms such as *clear* or *transparent, hazy* (slightly cloudy), *cloudy,* **turbid** (particles floating within), and *milky* (very cloudy). A fresh urine specimen should appear clear or transparent. A fresh specimen that appears cloudy or turbid could be contaminated with bacteria, pus, mucus, or yeast. Since refrigeration or standing at room temperature for long periods causes a specimen to become cloudy, its appearance should be observed and recorded as soon as possible (Fig. 2-2). Many factors can contribute to cloudi-

ness, including crystals, the change of the specimen's pH from acid to alkaline as it sits and cools, blood cells, bacteria, and other substances. Further examination of the specimen with a microscope will help determine the cause of the cloudiness.

Besides abnormal color, the presence of *foam* that does not rapidly disperse from a fresh specimen is clinically significant. White foam that stays on top of a freshly voided specimen may indicate an increase in proteins (proteinuria), a clinical symptom for complications of diabetes, and heart and renal disease. Greenish yellow foam on an amber specimen may indicate the presence of bilirubin in the urine specimen (bilirubinuria); this is one of the clinical signs of hepatitis and other liver disorders (Fig. 2-3).

TABLE 2-2	Abnormal Urine Odors
Smell	**Clinical Significance**
Fruity	Starvation
	Uncontrolled diabetes mellitus
Ammonia	Urinary tract infection (UTI)
	Long-standing specimen
Foul	Bacteria
"Musky"	Phenylketonuria (PKU) (metabolic disease)

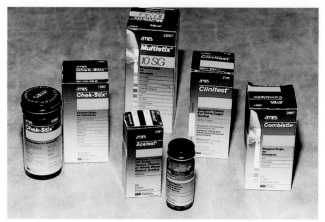

Fig. 2-4 Examples of reagent strips and reagent tablets. *(From Young AP, Kennedy DB:* Kinn's the medical assistant, *ed 9, Philadelphia, 2003, Saunders.)*

Odor

Normal urine is described as being "aromatic," or not having a distinctive smell. It develops an ammonia-like odor only on standing. To prevent urine from developing the ammonia-like odor, a specimen must be tested within 1 hour of collection. The ammonia smell is caused by bacteria breaking down urea in the specimen. Several factors can affect the odor of a fresh specimen, as follows (Table 2-2):

- Foods such as garlic and asparagus can produce a strong odor in urine.
- A strong unpleasant (foul) odor is brought on by bacteria from a urinary tract infection (UTI).
- A "sweet-smelling" (fruity) scent is characteristic of a patient with uncontrolled diabetes because of ketones (a byproduct of fat metabolism) in the urine.

Volume

The normal volume of urine produced by an adult in a 24-hour period is 750 to 2000 mL (0.75 to 2 L). Smaller amounts are normal for infants and children. The major factor affecting urine output is fluid intake.

Factors affecting low output of urine include the following:

- Inadequate fluid intake
- Fluids lost during episodes of diarrhea, vomiting, and profuse sweating **(diaphoresis)** causing dehydration

High urine output may be caused by the following:

- Excessive fluid intake
- Reduction in antidiuretic hormone (ADH) secreted
- Uncontrolled diabetes insipidus or renal disease

During the patient screening process, a medical assistant must listen carefully when the patient describes fluid intake and output. For example, if a patient off-handedly remarks that she seems to be thirstier lately and is constantly urinating, this information must be charted so that the physician can further investigate possible causes. The physician may then order a **timed specimen,** in which urine is collected for 24 hours and a small sample is removed and analyzed.

Chemical Properties of Urine

When the filtering ability of the kidneys is damaged, substances not normally found in the urine (e.g., protein, blood) are present. The chemical composition of a urine specimen is measured in the physician office laboratory (POL) to detect these substances. This can be done by using a **reagent strip** (dipsticks) or a **reagent tablet** (Fig. 2-4).

Differences between reagent strips and reagent tablets include the following:

- Reagent strips detect both the *presence* and approximate *amount* of these substances in the urine, whereas reagent tablet analysis detects only the *presence* of a particular substance (e.g., Acetest detects ketones) and not its quantity.
- Each chemical pad on the reagent strip tests for only one type of substance, whereas a reagent tablet can detect the presence of other related substances. For example, one chemical pad on the reagent strip detects only the presence of the sugar glucose in the urine, but a Clinitest (Ames) reagent tablet will detect the presence of other sugars (e.g., galactose, lactose, fructose). When galactose fails to convert to glucose, for example, a congenital disorder called

galactosemia is indicated. Reagent tablets can be used to confirm a particular substance in the urine (e.g., ketones, glucose).

Whether using a reagent strip or reagent tablet when performing laboratory tests, if the results do not fit with other test results or patient symptoms, the physician usually orders a retest. This can be done by (1) repeating the test on the same specimen or a new specimen, (2) performing a different test on the same specimen, or (3) running a test from a different type of specimen, such as blood.

Reagent Strips

The Multistix-10 SG (Bayer) reagent strip tests for glucose, bilirubin, ketones, specific gravity, blood, pH, protein, urobilinogen, nitrites, and leukocytes. The Chemstrip 9 (Boehringer Mannheim) tests for all the above except specific gravity. The type of reagent strip chosen by a medical practice depends on preference and the type of urine screening most often done in a particular medical office (e.g., an OB/GYN might use a reagent strip that tests for only glucose and protein).

QUALITY CONTROL

Accurate results require medical assistants to use an appropriate technique and follow the quality control program established by the facility. This includes (1) checking the expiration date on the bottle, (2) keeping the strips in their original container with the lid tight to prevent moisture and light from affecting the chemical pad, and (3) using a fresh specimen.

USING THE REAGENT STRIP

The reagent strip is dipped into the fresh urine specimen, wetting all pads. It is removed immediately, and any excess urine is removed by dragging (or tapping) the strip edge gently against the rim of the container as it is removed. The strip is then held horizontally to prevent the chemicals on each pad from mixing with the others. When the results are recorded, the color of each chemical pad at time intervals specified by the manufacturer is compared to a color scale located on the bottle. The medical assistant must be certain the specimen is fresh and must adhere to the times specified by the strip manufacturer because chemical reactions will continue to occur, resulting in elevated values.

Table 2-3 provides the normal values for each test, the clinical significance of each test, and possible reasons for false readings. Procedure 2-1 describes the proper technique for processing a urine specimen using a reagent technique. Box 2-1 reviews the necessary criteria for charting CLIA-waived tests.

> ### BOX 2-1 Documentation when Charting CLIA-Waived Tests
>
> 1. Date
> 2. Time
> 3. Name of test
> 4. Results
> 5. Patient reaction, if any
> 6. Proper signature and credential

Glucose. **Glucose** in the urine **(glycosuria)** may indicate that the patient has diabetes. It also can be present after a heavy meal, emotional stress, or high doses of vitamin C. The presence of glucose in the urine is recorded as a trace, +1, +2, +3, or +4. Absence of glucose in the urine is recorded as negative. The test is usually read 30 seconds after the strip has been dipped into the urine.

Bilirubin. The presence of **bilirubin** in the urine is **bilirubinuria.** Bilirubin, a byproduct of hemoglobin breakdown, is normally processed into bile by the liver and excreted by the intestines. Bilirubin appearing in the urine is a clear sign of liver or biliary tract dysfunction or disease.

The test values are recorded as negative, +1 (small amount), +2 (moderate amount), or +3 (large amount). The test is read 30 seconds after the strip is dipped into the urine.

Ketones. **Ketonuria** is the presence of **ketones** in the urine. When the body does not have an adequate intake of protein, carbohydrates, or other energy-producing elements, the body will burn fatty acids. Ketones are a waste product of fat metabolism. Ketones will be excreted when the patient is diabetic, dieting, suffering from anorexia, starving, experiencing excessive diarrhea, and vomiting.

The values are recorded as negative, trace, small, moderate, or large. The results are read 40 seconds after the strip has been dipped into the urine.

Specific Gravity. The kidneys function to regulate the amount of urine that is produced and to maintain the concentration of various substances that provide homeostasis. Urine **specific gravity** shows the amount of dissolved substances in the urine. This test indicates the kidney's ability to concentrate urine. The specific gravity of urine depends on a person's fluid intake, various disease states (e.g., dehydration, renal or liver disease, congestive heart failure, presence of protein or glucose in urine), and the ability of the kidneys to concentrate urine.

The specific gravity of urine is compared to that of distilled water (1). The normal range for specific

TABLE 2-3 Reagent Strip Tests

Test	Normal Values	Clinical Significance	Test Error	Causes of Error
Glucose	Negative	Diabetes mellitus Pancreatitis	False positive	High levels of vitamin C
		Gestational diabetes Hyperthyroidism	False negative	Increased SG Increased ketones
Bilirubin	Negative	Cirrhosis Hepatitis	False positive	Intestinal disease or disorder
		Bile duct obstruction	False negative	Exposure to light Vitamin C Increased nitrites
Ketones	Negative	Excessive vomiting	False positive, false negative	Medications
		Diabetic acidosis Starvation Screening of proper insulin levels		Red dyes Bacteria breakdown Incorrect timing
Specific gravity	1.01-1.025	Measures concentrating ability of kidneys	False positive False negative	Increased protein pH below 6.5
Blood	Negative	Glomerulonephritis Renal calculi	False positive False negative	Menses Increased SG with crenated RBCs
		Severe burns Trauma to kidney Strenuous exercise Muscle wasting Cystitis		Increased nitrites Increased vitamin C
pH	4.5-8	Metabolic disorders	False readings	Run allowed from one test pad onto another
		Acid-base respiratory diseases Renal calculi Crystals UTI treatment/drugs		
Protein	Negative	Renal disease (early)	False positive	Specimen contaminated with antiseptic solution Increased SG
		Muscle injury Severe infection or inflammation		
		Glomerular problems High-protein diet	False negative	Proteins other than albumin
Urobilinogen	2 mg/dL	Hemolytic diseases Hepatitis Cirrhosis	False positive	Metabolic disease Highly pigmented urine
		Liver cancer	False negative	Long-standing specimen Preservative (formalin)
Nitrites	Negative	Cystitis Pyelonephrosis	False positive	Long-standing specimen Preserved specimen done incorrectly
			False negative	Antibiotics Increased vitamin C Increased SG
Leukocytes	Negative	Cystitis Inflammation of urinary tract	False positive	Increased pigment in urine Preservative (formalin)
		Organ transplant rejection	False negative	Increased glucose, protein, and vitamin C Antibiotics

RBCs, Red blood cells; *SG,* serum glucose; *UTI,* urinary tract infection.

Procedure 2-1 Urinalysis Using Reagent Strips

TASK: Observe, record, and report the physical and chemical properties of a urine sample using Multistix 10 SG reagent strips.

EQUIPMENT AND SUPPLIES
- Nonsterile disposable gloves
- Personal protective equipment (PPE), as indicated
- Multistix 10 SG reagent strips
- Normal and abnormal quality control reagent strips
- Laboratory report form
- Quality control logsheet
- Urine specimen container
- Conical urine centrifuge tubes
- Digital timer or watch with second hand
- Paper towel
- 10% bleach solution
- Biohazardous waste container
- Patient's medical record
- Laboratory log

SKILLS/RATIONALE

STANDARD PRECAUTIONS ARE TO BE FOLLOWED.

1. **Procedural Step. Sanitize the hands.**
   An alcohol-based hand rub may be used instead of washing hands with soap and water, unless hands are visibly soiled.
   Rationale. Hand sanitization promotes infection control.

2. **Procedural Step. Assemble equipment and supplies and verify the order.**
   Check the expiration date of the reagent strips.
   Rationale. It is important to have all supplies and equipment ready and available before starting any procedure to ensure efficiency. Outdated reagent strips may lead to inaccurate test results.

3. **Procedural Step. Greet and identify the patient and escort the patient to the examination room or laboratory area.**
   Rationale. Identifying the patient ensures the procedure is performed on the correct patient.

4. **Procedural Step. Explain the procedure to the patient.**
   Rationale. Explaining the procedure to the patient promotes cooperation and provides a means of obtaining implied consent.

5. **Procedural Step. Ask the patient to collect a midstream clean-catch urine specimen.**
   Provide verbal and written instructions for the collection, as outlined in Procedure 1-8 (Chapter 1).

NOTE: Chemical analysis of urine is best performed on a well-mixed, uncentrifuged specimen at room temperature. The reagent pads are temperature sensitive. Cold urine may produce false-negative results.
Rationale. A freshly voided clean-catch specimen produces the most accurate results.

6. **Procedural Step. Apply gloves and other PPE as indicated.**

7. **Procedural Step. While waiting for the patient to collect the specimen, record the lot number and expiration date on the laboratory quality control logsheet.**
   The manufacturer displays this information on the outside of the bottle of reagent strips.
   Rationale. It is important to record the lot numbers and expiration dates of the reagent strips and controls. This gives the manufacturer and office a reference point in case the reagents or controls do not perform as expected.

8. **Procedural Step. Pour the controls from the manufacturer's container into the urine centrifuge tubes and record the lot number and expiration date on the tubes.**

9. **Procedural Step. Observe and record the physical properties of the control samples.**
   a. The color of urine is described as colorless, straw, yellow, or amber and is often assigned intensity from light to dark. The more concentrated the urine, the more the color intensifies.

Continued

Procedure 2-1 Urinalysis Using Reagent Strips—cont'd

b. Clarity is described as clear, slightly hazy, hazy, cloudy, or turbid (very cloudy) and is an indication of the amount of particulate matter in the sample. The cloudier the sample, the more particulate matter is present. The type of particulate matter is often identified on viewing urine sediment under the microscope.

c. Urine odor is not reported in most cases unless it is particularly foul. The smell of a specimen may indicate a disease process.

10. **Procedural Step. Open the jar of reagent strips and remove one strip. Recap the bottle immediately.**
Rationale. It is important to recap the bottle to prevent exposing the strips to environmental moisture, light, and heat, which can cause altered reagent reactivity.

11. **Procedural Step. Dip the strip in the abnormal control specimen, and draw it out along the edge of the tube top to remove excess urine.**
Briefly blot it on a paper towel by tapping the lengthwise edge to remove any of the sample that may be clinging to the strip.

12. **Procedural Step. Set the timer, or check the second hand on a watch to read the results after the recommended time has elapsed.**

13. **Procedural Step. After 30 seconds have elapsed, read the glucose and bilirubin results.**
Start by holding the reagent strip next to the color for the result of glucose and bilirubin. To

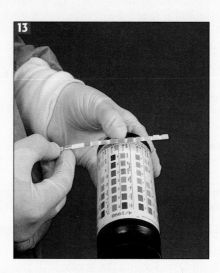

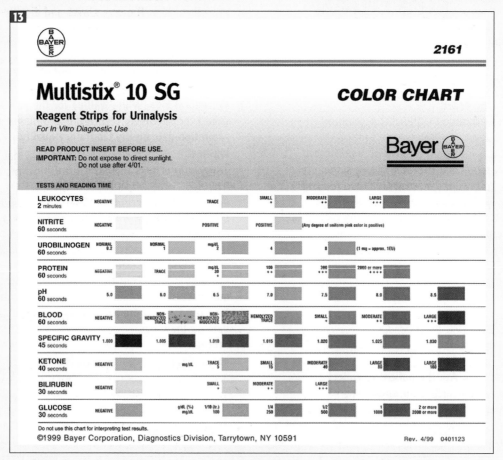

Multistix® 10 SG   **2161**

COLOR CHART

Reagent Strips for Urinalysis
For In Vitro Diagnostic Use

READ PRODUCT INSERT BEFORE USE.
IMPORTANT: Do not expose to direct sunlight.
Do not use after 4/01.

Bayer

TESTS AND READING TIME

TEST							
LEUKOCYTES 2 minutes	NEGATIVE		TRACE	SMALL +	MODERATE ++	LARGE +++	
NITRITE 60 seconds	NEGATIVE		POSITIVE	POSITIVE	(Any degree of uniform pink color is positive)		
UROBILINOGEN 60 seconds	NORMAL 0.2	NORMAL 1	mg/dL 2	4	8	(1 mg = approx. 1EU)	
PROTEIN 60 seconds	NEGATIVE	TRACE	mg/dL 30 +	100 ++	300 +++	2000 or more ++++	
pH 60 seconds	5.0	6.0	6.5	7.0	7.5	8.0	8.5
BLOOD 60 seconds	NEGATIVE	NON-HEMOLYZED TRACE	NON-HEMOLYZED MODERATE	HEMOLYZED TRACE	SMALL +	MODERATE ++	LARGE +++
SPECIFIC GRAVITY 45 seconds	1.000	1.005	1.010	1.015	1.020	1.025	1.030
KETONE 40 seconds	NEGATIVE	mg/dL	TRACE 5	SMALL 15	MODERATE 40	LARGE 80	LARGE 160
BILIRUBIN 30 seconds	NEGATIVE		SMALL +	MODERATE ++	LARGE +++		
GLUCOSE 30 seconds	NEGATIVE	g/dL (%) mg/dL	1/10 (tr.) 100	1/4 250	1/2 500	1 1000	2 or more 2000 or more

Do not use this chart for interpreting test results.
©1999 Bayer Corporation, Diagnostics Division, Tarrytown, NY 10591   Rev. 4/99 0401123

Procedure 2-1 Urinalysis Using Reagent Strips—cont'd

avoid contaminating the chart, the strip should not touch the chart.

14. **Procedural Step. After 40 seconds have elapsed, read the ketone results.**

15. **Procedural Step. After 45 seconds have elapsed, read the specific gravity results.**

    NOTE: Specific gravity is defined as the concentration of dissolved substances in a specimen compared with distilled water, which is free of dissolved substances. Specific gravity may be measured with a urinometer, refractometer, or reagent strip.

16. **Procedural Step. After 60 seconds have elapsed, read the blood, pH, protein, urobilinogen, and nitrite results.**

17. **Procedural Step. After 2 minutes have elapsed, read the leukocyte results.**

    Compare the reagent strip color with the chart color that most closely matches it.

18. **Procedural Step. After the reagent strip has been read and results interpreted on the logsheet, discard the reagent strip in the biohazardous waste container.**

    NOTE: Visual interpretation of color on the reagent strip is likely to vary among individuals, so some laboratories use automated instruments for consistency in the readings. The strip is placed in the analyzer and is moved into the path of a light beam. The amount of light reflected is analyzed by a microprocessor and converted into a digital reading that is printed out.

19. **Procedural Step. Repeat Steps 9 through 18 on the normal control specimen.**

20. **Procedural Step. After testing the controls, check them to make sure they are within the recommended ranges.**

    Rationale. The manufacturer tests each lot of controls to determine acceptable ranges of results for each test. These results are printed on the package insert, and your results should fall within the manufacturer's acceptable ranges. If they do, you know the reagent strips are acceptable for use with patient samples.

    If the controls do not fall within the acceptable ranges, the reagent strips cannot be used for patient samples until it is known why the controls are out of range and the problem has been fixed. Sometimes the reagent strips must be discarded.

21. **Procedural Step. Prepare to test the patient specimen.**

    Pour a portion of the clean-catch specimen into a urine centrifuge tube. Do not touch the cup to the tube. Save the remainder of the specimen, because the physician may decide to order a urine culture.

    Rationale. To maintain the integrity of the specimen, it is important to employ sterile technique by pouring from the collection container to the test tube without touching the container to the tube.

22. **Procedural Step. Perform Steps 9 through 18 on the patient sample and record the results on the laboratory report form.**

23. **Procedural Step. Clean and disinfect the work area with a 10% bleach solution.**

24. **Procedural Step. Remove gloves and dispose of in a biohazardous waste container.**

25. **Procedural Step. Sanitize the hands.**

    Always sanitize the hands after every procedure or after using gloves.

26. **Procedural Step. Report the result to the physician.**

    Depending on the results of the physical and chemical properties of the patient's urine specimen, the physician may request that you prepare a urine sediment for microscopic examination, as outlined in Procedure 2-2.

27. **Procedural Step. After the physician has reviewed the results, place the laboratory report form in the patient's medical record.**

---

gravity is 1.01 to 1.025. Specific gravity of urine is highest in the morning. The higher the specific gravity of the urine, the darker is the specimen's color. An exception occurs when a specimen is obtained from a diabetic patient. The specimen may have a high specific gravity because of glucose in the urine but may appear light yellow. The results are read after 45 seconds.

Blood. The chemical pad for blood on the reagent strip will react to three different forms of blood: intact RBCs, hemoglobin from RBCs, and myoglobin from muscle tissue.

- **Hematuria** is the presence of intact RBCs in the urine caused by an infection **(cystitis),** injury, or trauma to the urinary tract, such as a kidney stone.
- **Hemoglobinuria** is the presence of hemolyzed RBCs in the urine. This can be caused by a hemolytic transfusion reaction,

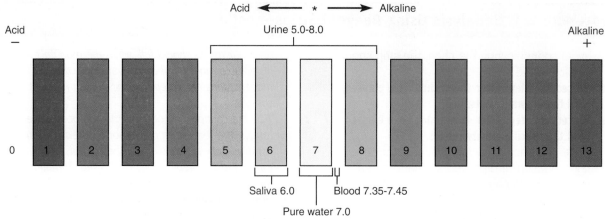

Fig. 2-5 The pH scale. *(Modified from Stepp CA, Woods MA:* Laboratory procedures for medical office personnel, *Philadelphia, 1998, Saunders.)*

drug reaction, severe burns, and other conditions.

- **Myoglobinuria** is the result of severe muscle injury caused by trauma (e.g., automobile accidents, sports injuries).

In a physician's office, most positive blood reactions result from intact RBCs. With women who are menstruating (or in the days before or after menses), blood may be present in the specimen. Ask the patient the date of her last menses to determine if this may be a factor. The results are recorded as negative, trace, +1 (small amount), +2 (moderate amount), or +3 (large amount). The color strip is read after 50 seconds.

pH. The kidneys regulate the amount of acids produced by the metabolism of blood and fluids, and the lungs regulate metabolism by the amount of carbon dioxide excreted. These two processes regulate the body's acid-base balance. The pH values of urine range from 5 (acid) to 8.5 (alkaline) (Fig. 2-5). An individual's urine is influenced by metabolic status, diet, medications, and any active disease process. For example, a diet high in proteins will produce acid urine, whereas a diet high in vegetables and dairy creates alkaline urine. Acid urine will become alkaline on standing because urea breaks down into ammonia. The chemical pad for pH is read after 60 seconds.

Protein. **Proteinuria** occurs when an increased amount of protein is excreted in the urine. It is an indicator of renal disease, complications of diabetes, congestive heart failure, or UTI. Proteinuria can also appear after heavy exercise, during pregnancy, and in newborns. The results are read after 60 seconds and recorded as negative, trace, +1, +2, +3, or +4.

Urobilinogen. Hemoglobin, when released from "worn out" RBCs, is converted to bilirubin in the liver. Intestinal bacteria break down bilirubin to form **urobilinogen.** Diseases of the liver (e.g., cirrhosis, hepatitis), bile duct obstruction, and antibiotic therapy increase the amount of urobilinogen in the urine. Because direct light breaks down bilirubin, the medical assistant must shield a specimen from light to avoid a false-negative reading. If the test does not detect a decrease in or absence of urobilinogen, the values are recorded as normal. An increase is recorded as positive. The strip is read 60 seconds after it has been dipped in urine.

Nitrites. Bacteria contain an enzyme that breaks down **nitrates** to **nitrites,** indicating **bacteriuria.** Common bacteria that infect the urinary tract are *Escherichia coli, Klebsiella, Proteus, Pseudomonas,* and *Staphylococcus.* The medical assistant should be aware that not all bacteria break down nitrates to nitrites, but that *E. coli* does and is the main cause of UTIs. Values are recorded as negative or positive. A color change of any degree is a positive sign for UTI. The reagent pad is read after 60 seconds.

Leukocytes. A reagent strip that tests positive for nitrites confirms the presence of **leukocyte esterase,** which is released from white blood cells (WBCs). Results are recorded as negative, trace, +1 (small), +2 (moderate), or +3 (large). A positive leukocyte reading without a positive nitrite reading may indicate a contaminated specimen. In this case, a fresh specimen should be obtained and the test redone. The results of the leukocyte reagent pad are not read for 2 minutes.

Automated Urine Analyzers

An **automated urine analyzer** uses the principle of light photometry to analyze a reagent test strip. The use of the analyzer eliminates the human error factor for color interpretation of a reagent strip. The Clinitek 50 Urine Chemistry Analyzer (Bayer), for

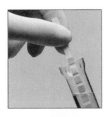
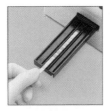
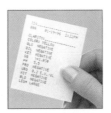

1. Dip reagent strip into sample and press the START button.

2. Blot side of reagent strip and place strip on test strip table.

3. Instrument analyzes, displays, and prints results at the rate of one test per minute.

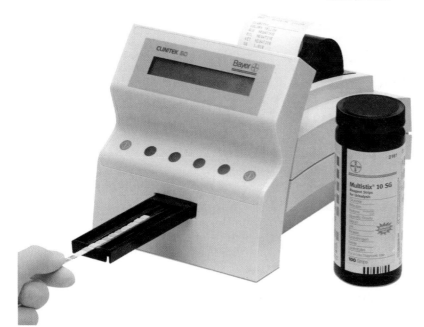

Fig. 2-6 Clinitek 50 urine chemistry analyzer is a semiautomated instrument designed to read the reagent strip. Results appear on the display panel and are printed on a paper printout. *(Courtesy Diagnostic Division, Bayer, Tarrytown, NY.)*

example, is a benchtop, semiautomatic instrument. As with any automated equipment, it is important to make certain that the quality control and quality assurance program of the facility is followed.

When the analyzer is turned "on," the feed table moves out to a ready position. A self-test cycle begins, and when the cycle is completed, a reagent strip can then be used. A reagent strip is immersed in urine, the edge of the strip is touched to a paper towel to remove excess urine, and then placed on the strip table, pad side up. It is automatically drawn into the instrument for analysis. Specimen results appear on a screen and are printed through a built-in printer (Fig. 2-6). The reagent strip should be removed and discarded, and the strip table should be gently wiped with a damp, lint-free tissue. Quality control measures must be followed closely (e.g., correct use of positive and negative control strips) to ensure accurate reporting of test results (see Table 2-3).

Reagent Tablets

Reagent tablets, as mentioned, test for only one specific substance. The advantage is that some reagent tablets can be used with specimens other than urine (e.g., Acetest for serum, plasma, whole blood, and urine). Accurate results require that the medical assistant follow the prepackaged instructions exactly for each type of reagent tablet used. Care must be taken to not handle the tablets. They must be poured into the cap, and then into the test tube or placed on the mat. The Clinitest is used most often for pediatric patients because sugars other than glucose can be detected. This test assists in the early detection of metabolic disorders in infants.

CONFIRMATORY TESTS

Reagent tablets are generally used for three **confirmatory tests:** Clinitest, used for glucose; Acetest, used for ketones; and Ictotest, used for bilirubin. As with reagent strips, reagent tablets must be kept in a dark bottle with the cap secure. Light or moisture can cause deterioration. The expiration date must be checked every time the tablets are used.

Glucose. The Clinitest 5-drop method can be used to confirm the presence of glucose and other types of sugars (e.g., fructose, lactose, galactose) in a urine specimen (Fig. 2-7). Results are compared to a color chart at 15 seconds and recorded as negative, ¼%, ½%, ¾%, 1%, 2%, or more. Certain types of medications, such as cephalexin (Keflex) and probenecid

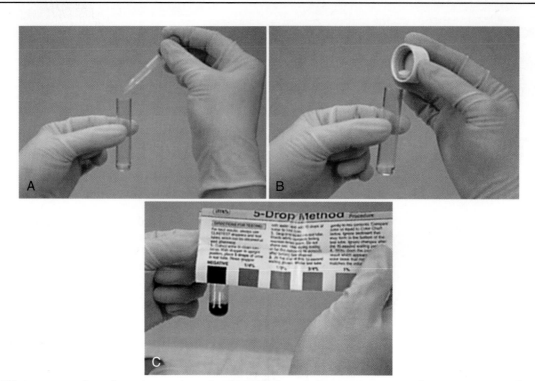

Fig. 2-7 Clinitest procedure for urine testing. **A,** Place 10 drops of water into test tube containing 5 drops of urine. **B,** Add one Clinitest tablet to test tube. **C,** Compare contents in test tube with color chart. *(From Zakus SM: Mosby's clinical skills for medical assistants, ed 4, St Louis, 2001, Mosby.)*

(Benemid), as well as high doses of vitamin C, may cause a false-positive reading.

Ketones. The Acetest reagent tablet confirms the presence of **acetone** (ketones) in urine, serum, plasma, or whole blood (Fig. 2-8). Results are determined after 30 seconds and recorded as negative, small, moderate, and large.

Bilirubin. The Ictotest confirms the presence of bilirubin in urine. Five drops of urine are placed on a small absorbent test mat. An Ictotest reagent tablet is placed in the center of the moistened mat. Two drops of distilled water are placed on the tablet. The results are negative if the mat shows no blue or purple color within 30 seconds. The results are positive for bilirubin if only these colors appear.

Microscopic Examination of Urine Sediment

Microscopic examination of urine sediment is not a CLIA-waived test. However, it is important for the medical assistant to understand the preparation of the specimen and the possible results. The purpose of microscopic examination of a urine sample is to identify cells and other formed elements present in urine. Casts, crystals, and other solids can be identified only by microscopic examination.

To perform this test, urinary **sediment** (solid material contained in the urine) is collected from a centrifuged urine specimen. The top liquid portion of the urine (the **supernatant**) is poured off, and the remaining sediment is examined under the microscope. A stain is often added to the sediment. This stain enables the health care professional to better visualize and identify structures.

The slide is first examined under **low-power field (LPF)** (10×) and low light for casts. The **high-power field (HPF)** (40×) is used to identify blood cells, crystals, bacteria, yeast, and parasites. Fig. 2-9 illustrates various formed elements that can be found in a microscopic examination of urine sediment. Procedure 2-2 explains the process of microscopic examination of urine.

Blood Cells

Red blood cells can be found in small numbers in normal urine (0-5 RBCs/HPF). More than this amount is a sign of urinary tract injury (e.g., kidney stones), renal disease (e.g., pyelonephritis), or a systemic disease (e.g., hemophilia). In dilute urine, a *hypotonic* solution, the cells may appear swollen and may hemolyze. In concentrated urine, a *hypertonic* solution, the cells are shrunken **(crenated).** An RBC that has **hemolyzed** is colorless and cannot be seen under the microscope. RBCs are counted in several fields (5-10), totaled, and divided by the number of fields examined.

White blood cells can be found in small numbers in normal urine (0-8 WBCs/HPF). Amounts greater than this are a clear indication of a contaminated specimen, UTI (e.g., cystitis, urethritis), kidney

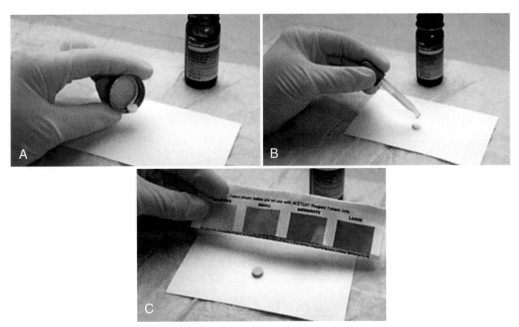

Fig. 2-8 Acetest reagent tablet detects the presence of acetone and acetoacetic acid in the urine. **A,** Place the tablet on clean paper. **B,** Place 1 drop of urine on the tablet. **C,** Compare the tablet with the color chart. *(From Zakus SM: Mosby's clinical skills for medical assistants, ed 4, St Louis, 2001, Mosby.)*

disease (e.g., pyelonephritis), or transplant rejection. WBCs are larger than RBCs and have a nucleus. WBCs are counted in several fields, totaled, and recorded as an average number per HPF.

Epithelial Cells

Epithelial cells line many structures in the body, including the urethra, bladder, and vagina. A few **squamous epithelial cells** found in a urine specimen are normal. Abnormally large numbers in women indicate vaginal contamination. These squamous cells appear as large, clear, flat, irregularly shaped cells, and they have a small nucleus.

Renal epithelial cells or **transitional epithelial cells** appearing in large numbers indicate a kidney problem. Renal epithelial cells are round to oval in shape and contain a large nucleus. When present in large numbers, tubular damage (e.g., tubular necrosis, glomerulonephritis) is suspected. Transitional epithelial cells appear pear shaped and line the urinary tract from the renal pelvis to the top of the urethra. Large amounts indicate diseases of the bladder or renal pelvis.

Casts and Crystals

Casts are microscopic protein materials that harden and take on the shape of the **lumen** of the tubule, where they are formed within the **nephron.** These materials are flushed out of the tubule and appear in the urine as casts. The presence of casts in the urine usually signifies a disease process. Names of casts represent their cell and substance composition (Table 2-4).

Finding casts in urinary sediment is significant. The light should be low because casts are transparent. They tend to settle toward the edges of the coverslip. The average number of casts per LPF should be reported after 5 to 10 fields have been counted. Although casts are counted using low light and LPF, HPF must be used to classify them.

Crystals are often found in urine sediment. The type and number depend on the pH of the urine. Acid crystals include amorphous urates, uric acid, and calcium oxalate crystals. Crystals found in alkaline urine include amorphous phosphate, triple phosphate, calcium phosphate, and ammonium urate crystals. Crystals considered abnormal are leucine, tyrosine, cystine, and cholesterol and are found in the urine of patients with metabolic disease or on sulfa drugs.

When crystals form, they do so as the urine cools. They are observed under HPF. Crystals are counted using 5 to 10 fields and then dividing by the number of fields used.

Other Structures

Other structures found in urine include bacteria, yeasts, and mucous threads.

- **Bacteria** are rod-shaped or spherical organisms that appear in a urine specimen only if it becomes contaminated during collection or if the patient has a UTI.
- **Yeasts** are oval shaped, vary in size, and have small buds. Yeast cells in the urine of a female patient are usually vaginal contaminants

CELLS IN URINE

Epithelial Cells   Three types of epithelial cells may appear in urine sediment: renal tubular, transitional and/or squamous. Other types of cells may appear in urine but are difficult to identify due to morphologic changes caused by urine. Tubular cells are approximately 1/3 larger than white blood cells. Transitional epithelial cells may arise from the renal pelvis, ureters, bladder or urethra. They tend to be pear-shaped. Squamous cells are large and flat with a prominent nucleus. They originate in the urethra.

RENAL TUBULAR

TRANSITIONAL

SQUAMOUS

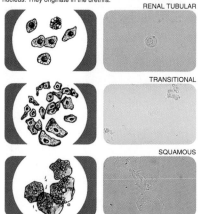

RBCs   Red blood cells may originate from any part of the renal system. The presence of large numbers of RBCs in the urine suggests infection, trauma, tumors, renal calculi, etc. However, the presence of 1 or 2 RBC/(HPF) in the urine sediment, or blood in the urine from menstrual contamination, should not be considered abnormal.

RBCs

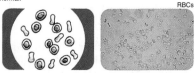

WBCs   White blood cells in the urine (pyuria) may originate from any part of the renal system. The presence of more than 5 WBCs per HPF may suggest infection, cystitis, or pyelonephritis.

RENAL TUBULAR & WBC (SEDI-STAIN*)

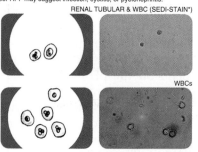

WBCs

CRYSTALS FOUND IN ACID, NEUTRAL AND ALKALINE URINE

Calcium Oxalate   Calcium oxalate crystals most frequently have an "envelope" shape and appear in acid, neutral or slightly alkaline urine. They appear in the urine after the ingestion of certain foods, i.e., cabbage, asparagus.

CALCIUM OXALATE (BRIGHTFIELD)

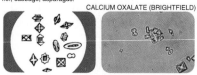

Hippuric Acid   Hippuric acid crystals are colorless or pale yellow. They occur as needles, six-sided prisms, or star-shaped clusters. They appear in urine after the ingestion of certain vegetables and fruits with benzoic acid content. They have little clinical significance.

HIPPURIC ACID (BRIGHTFIELD)

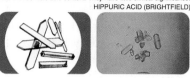

CASTS IN URINE

Hyaline Casts   Hyaline casts are formed from a protein gel in the renal tubule. Hyaline casts may contain cellular inclusions. Hyaline casts will dissolve very rapidly in alkaline urine. Normal urine sediment may contain 1 to 2 hyaline casts per low power field (LPF).

HYALINE

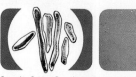

Granular Casts   Granular casts are casts with granules present throughout the cast matrix. They are quite refractile. If the granules are small, the cast is defined as a finely granular cast. If granules are large, it is termed a coarsely granular cast. Granular casts can appear in urine in normal or abnormal states.

GRANULAR

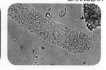

RBC Casts   RBC casts are pathologic and their presence is usually indicative of severe injury to the glomerulus. Rarely, transtubular bleeding may occur, forming RBC casts. RBC casts are found in acute glomerulonephritis, lupus, bacterial endocarditis and septicemias. "Blood" casts are granular and contain hemoglobin from degenerated RBCs.

RBC CASTS

WBC Casts   WBC casts occur when leukocytes are incorporated within the cast matrix. WBC casts will usually indicate an infection, most commonly pyelonephritis. They may also be seen in glomerular diseases. WBC casts may be the only clue to pyelonephritis.

WBC CASTS

CRYSTALS FOUND IN ALKALINE URINE

Ammonium Blurate or Ammonium Urates   Ammonium urates are yellow-brown in appearance and occur in urine as spheres or spheres with spicules ("thorny apples"). Both forms are frequently seen together. They appear in urine when there is ammonia formation in the urine present in the bladder. They are considered to have little clinical significance.

AMMONIUM URATES (BRIGHTFIELD)

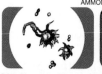

Triple Phosphate   Triple phosphate crystals are common in urine sediment. They have a "coffin-lid" shape, are colorless and appear in alkaline urine. The ingestion of fruit may cause triple phosphate to appear in urine.

TRIPLE PHOSPHATE (BRIGHTFIELD)

CRYSTALS FOUND IN ACID URINE

Uric Acid Crystals   Uric acid has birefringent characteristics; therefore, it polarizes light, giving multi-colors. Uric acid crystals are found in acid urine. Uric acid may assume various forms, e.g., rhombic, plates, rosettes, small crystals. The color may be red-brown, yellow or colorless. Although increased in 16% of patients with gout, and in patients with malignant lymphoma or leukemia, their presence does not usually indicate pathology or increased uric acid concentrations.

URIC ACID (BRIGHTFIELD)

URIC ACID (POLARIZED)

Leucine/Tyrosine Crystals   Leucine and tyrosine are amino acids which crystallize and often appear in the urine of patients with severe liver disease. Tyrosine usually appears as fine needles arranged as sheaves or rosettes and appear yellow. Leucine is usually yellow, oily-appearing spheres with radial and concentric striations.

TYROSINE (BRIGHTFIELD)

LEUCINE (BRIGHTFIELD)

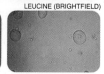

Cystine Crystals   Cystine crystals are thin, hexagonal-shaped (6-sided) structures. They appear in the urine as a result of a genetic defect. Cystine crystals and stones will appear in the urine in cystinuria and homocystinuria. Cystine crystals are frequently confused with uric acid crystals. Cystine crystals do not polarize light.

CYSTINE (BRIGHTFIELD)

CYSTINE (POLARIZED)

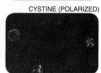

BACTERIA, FUNGI, PARASITES IN URINE

Bacteria   Bacteria in the urine (bacteriuria) can result from contaminants in collection vessels, from periurethral tissues, the urethra, or from fecal or vaginal contamination as well as from true urinary infection.

BACTERIA

Yeast   Yeast cells vary in size, are colorless, ovoid, and are often budding. They are often confused with RBCs. *Candida albicans* is often seen in diabetes, pregnancy, obesity and other debilitating conditions.

YEAST

Trichomonas Vaginalis   Trichomonas vaginalis is a flagellate protozoan which affects both males (urethritis) and females (vaginitis).

TRICHOMONAS VAGINALIS

Selected Photomicrographs credited to Bowman Gray School of Medicine, Wake Forest University, N.C. and Rachel Lehman, MS, MT (ASCP).

Fig. 2-9   Atlas of urine sediment. *(Courtesy Bayer, Elkhart, Ind.)*

Procedure 2-2 Prepare a Urine Specimen for Microscopic Examination

TASK: Prepare a urine sample for microscopic examination; mount a urine sediment sample on a microscope slide, and position the slide on the microscope stage.

EQUIPMENT AND SUPPLIES
- Nonsterile disposable gloves
- Personal protective equipment (PPE), as indicated
- Urine specimen container
- Conical urine centrifuge tubes with caps
- Disposable pipette
- Microscope slide and coverslip
- Centrifuge
- Paper towel
- Biohazardous waste container
- Laboratory logbook

SKILLS/RATIONALE

STANDARD PRECAUTIONS ARE TO BE FOLLOWED.

1. **Procedural Step. Perform Procedure 1-8 (Chapter 1) and then Procedure 2-1 in preparation for a microscopic urinalysis.**
2. **Procedural Step. Sanitize the hands.**
   An alcohol-based hand rub may be used instead of washing hands with soap and water, unless hands are visibly soiled.
   Rationale. Hand sanitization promotes infection control.
3. **Procedural Step. Put on gloves and other PPE as indicated.**
4. **Procedural Step. If the physician orders a microscopic examination of the patient's urine, prepare a urine sediment sample.**
   Pour 10 to 15 mL of the patient's specimen from the collection container into the urine centrifuge tube. When centrifuging specimens, the centrifuge must be balanced. Balance the

specimen as necessary by preparing a 10-mL tube of water to be placed opposite the urine tube. Visually compare the levels of urine and water in the tubes. If the same, the tubes will be balanced in the centrifuge. If not the same, adjust the levels by adding to or removing urine or water from one of the tubes.
Rationale. If the centrifuge is not balanced, the specimen will not be processed correctly.

5. **Procedural Step. Cap the tubes.**
   Rationale. It is important to cap the tubes to prevent contamination of the centrifuge by aerosol, or spray, from the urine.
6. **Procedural Step. Place the tubes in the centrifuge directly opposite each other for balance.**

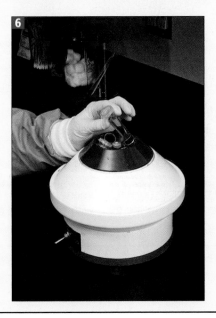

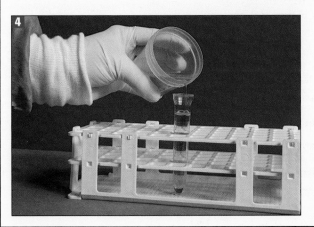

Continued

Procedure 2-2 Prepare a Urine Specimen for Microscopic Examination—cont'd

If the centrifuge is not balanced, it will make a loud noise and bounce around after it is turned on.

7. **Procedural Step. Close the lid, and set the timer on the centrifuge.**
The time and centrifuge speed vary according to laboratory policy and the specimen being spun. Typically, a urine sample is centrifuged for 5 minutes at a low speed. Some centrifuges start and stop automatically.
Rationale. The lid must be closed before starting the centrifuge to prevent aerosol or droplet contamination.

8. **Procedural Step. After the centrifuge stops, remove the cap from the specimen and discard it in the biohazardous waste container.**

9. **Procedural Step. Decant the supernatant (clear upper fluid).**
Suction it off with a plastic transfer pipette and discard it until there is about 1 mL of urine left in the bottom of the tube.

You may also pour off the supernatant from the top of the tube by inverting the tube over the sink. About 1 mL of sediment will remain in the bottom of the tube.

Be careful not to disturb the sediment while decanting.

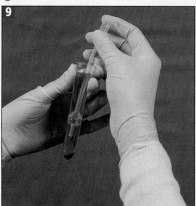

10. **Procedural Step. Mix the sediment with the remaining urine in the bottom of the tube.**
Suction it up and down with the transfer pipette.

You may also mix the sediment by gently tapping the side of the tube with your finger or on the countertop.

Rationale. Failure to mix the sediment properly will cause errors in the report because the elements in the sediment centrifuge at different rates.

11. **Procedural Step. Place a microscope slide on a paper towel, and dispense a small drop of the mixed urine sediment in the center of the slide.**
Rationale. The slide should be placed on a paper towel in case of spills.

12. **Procedural Step. Prepare the slide.**
Pick up a coverslip and hold it between the thumb and forefinger at two adjacent corners. Touch the opposite edge of the coverslip to the urine drop on the slide, and the drop will spread across the edge of the coverslip. Carefully lower the coverslip over the drop so that no air bubbles are under it.

13. **Procedural Step. Mount the slide on the microscope stage.**
Turn the coarse adjustment knob away from you to lower the stage, then place the slide between the spring-loaded clamps of the slide holder.
Rationale. The slide holder positions the slide over the opening in the stage, which allows the light to pass through the specimen and into the objective lens.

14. **Procedural Step. Remove gloves and dispose of in a biohazardous waste container.**

15. **Procedural Step. Sanitize the hands.**
Always sanitize the hands after every procedure or after using gloves.

16. **Procedural Step. Inform the physician that the slide is ready for viewing.**

17. **Procedural Step. Record the results in the laboratory logbook as reported by the physician.**

Charting Example—Laboratory Logbook

Date	
1/17/xx	Microscopic examination of clean-catch urine specimen as reported by Dr. Carlson.
	WBC: 0-16/HPF
	RBC: 0-2/HPF
	Hyaline casts: 0-4/HPF
	Crystals: – Uric acid, moderate
	Bacteria: Few
	Mucous: Occasional
	— W. Carter, RMA

Photos from Bonewit-West K: *Clinical procedures for medical assistants*, ed 6, Philadelphia, 2004, Saunders.

TABLE 2-4	**Types of Casts**	
Cast	**Appearance**	**Indication**
Hyaline casts	Colorless, cylinder-like structures with rounded ends	Occur in normal urine, after strenuous exercise, with unchecked hypertension, and with chronic renal disease
Granular casts	Hyaline casts that contain granules of disintegrated cells	Appear when patient has acute or chronic renal failure
Fatty casts	Cylinder-like structures that contain fat droplets	Appear in urine of diabetic patient or patient with nephrotic syndrome
Waxy casts	Appear glassy and smooth, and have sawtooth edges	Appear in urine during chronic renal disease and malignant hypertension
Cellular casts	Named according to what they contain (e.g., red blood cells, white blood cells, epithelial cells)	Appear in acute glomerulonephritis and other diseases

(Candida albicans) as found in diabetes mellitus, or may indicate UTI.

- **Mucous threads** from the urinary tract are normal in small amounts but indicate a urinary tract inflammation if found in large amounts. Microscopically they appear as long, waxy, threadlike structures with pointed ends. Mucous threads are best observed under LPF.
- **Spermatozoa** are normal in small numbers in male urine and should be reported as "present" only if found in large numbers. Sperm, if seen in a female patient, is not an indicator of disease when seen on microscopic examination. It only indicates that the patient has had intercourse.
- **Parasites** (e.g., *Trichomonas*) are considered a contaminant.

Artifacts

Artifacts are contaminants sometimes found in urine. Powder, hair, fibers, and similar substances are typical contaminants if a specimen is improperly collected. Care should be taken to encourage the patient to provide an uncontaminated specimen.

Pregnancy Tests

Two types of pregnancy tests are performed in the POL: enzyme immunoassay and agglutination. These are both CLIA-waived tests. All pregnancy tests are based on the **qualitative** presence or absence of a hormone called **human chorionic gonadotropin (hCG).** The hCG levels are detectable as early as 10 days after fertilization. Best results are obtained if the urine specimen is a first morning specimen and is obtained before the fourth month of pregnancy.

Enzyme immunoassay (EIA) pregnancy tests are available in commercially prepared kits. The color-change tests are very reliable and have a high sensitivity to color reaction. Procedure 2-3 outlines the process of performing a urine pregnancy color-reaction test.

The slide or test tube **agglutination** tests are *inhibition* immunoassay tests. When a urine specimen containing hCG is mixed with either latex beads (on a slide) or antiserum (in a tube), no agglutination (clumping action) takes place. The absence of agglutination indicates a positive reaction for pregnancy. Therefore when agglutination is visible, a negative reaction for pregnancy is recorded.

PATIENT-CENTERED PROFESSIONALISM

- What information is provided about a patient's state of health when a urinalysis is performed?
- Why must the medical assistant examine a urine specimen as soon as possible?

≋ BLOOD TESTS

The processing of blood samples in a POL usually falls into one of three categories: hematology, blood chemistry, and serology. Hematology is the study of blood cells, blood cell–forming tissues, and coagulation factors. Blood chemistry is the complete (quantitative) analysis of the chemical composition of the blood, including electrolytes, hormones, and glucose. Serology identifies the antigen and antibody reactions in the serum of blood. Microbiology is another category for processing blood samples. A medical assistant can perform simple hemoglobin

Procedure 2-3 Perform a Urine Pregnancy Test

TASK: Perform a urine pregnancy test using a commercially prepared CLIA-waived kit (QuickVue).

EQUIPMENT AND SUPPLIES
- Nonsterile disposable gloves
- Personal protective equipment (PPE), as indicated
- Urine specimen (preferably first-voided morning specimen)
- Urine pregnancy testing kit (QuickVue)
- Biohazardous waste container
- Laboratory logbook
- Patient's medical record

SKILLS/RATIONALE

STANDARD PRECAUTIONS ARE TO BE FOLLOWED.

1. **Procedural Step. Sanitize the hands.**
   An alcohol-based hand rub may be used instead of washing hands with soap and water, unless hands are visibly soiled.
   Rationale. Hand sanitization promotes infection control.

2. **Procedural Step. Assemble equipment and supplies and verify the order.**
   Check the expiration date on the urine pregnancy test. It should not be used if the expiration date has passed.
   Rationale. It is important to have all supplies and equipment ready and available before starting any procedure to ensure efficiency. An expired pregnancy test may produce inaccurate test results.

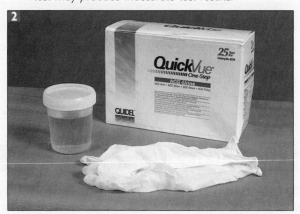

3. **Procedural Step. Perform the quality control test as recommended by the manufacturer and document in the laboratory logbook.**

4. **Procedural Step. Greet and identify the patient and escort the patient to the examination room.**
   (Escort the patient to the examination room only if the patient has not brought a urine specimen from home and a specimen is to be collected in the office.)
   Rationale. Identifying the patient ensures the procedure is performed on the correct patient.

5. **Procedural Step. If a urine specimen is to be collected in the office, explain the procedure to the patient.**
   Rationale. Explaining the procedure to the patient promotes cooperation and provides a means of obtaining implied consent.

6. **Procedural Step. Provide the patient with the collection container and instructions as needed.**
   The patient may have brought the first morning specimen from home for analysis, and this step may not be necessary.

7. **Procedural Step. Put on gloves and other PPE as indicated.**

8. **Procedural Step. Open the kit and remove one pregnancy test.**
   Remove the test cassette from the foil pouch and place it on a clean, dry, level surface.

9. **Procedural Step. Set up the test.**
   Using the disposable pipette included with the kit, add 3 drops of urine to the round sample well on the test cassette. Do not pick up or move the kit until you are ready to read the

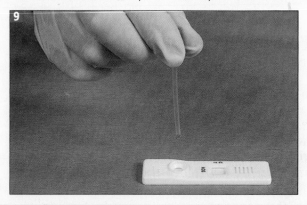

Procedure 2-3 Perform a Urine Pregnancy Test—cont'd

results. Dispose of the pipette in a biohazardous waste container.

Rationale. Moving the test cassette after the urine has been added may produce inaccurate test results.

10. **Procedural Step. Time the test for 3 minutes.**
11. **Procedural Step. Interpret the test results.**
    Observe for the following changes through the result window.
    Negative: The appearance of the blue procedural control line only next to the letter

"C" and no pink-to-purple test line next the to the letter "T."

Positive: The appearance of any pink-to-purple line next to the letter "T" along with a blue procedural control line next to the letter "C."

No Result: If no blue procedural control line appears, the test result is invalid, and the specimen must be retested.

12. **Procedural Step. Dispose of the test cassette in a biohazardous waste container.**
13. **Procedural Step. Remove gloves and dispose of in a biohazardous waste container.**
14. **Procedural Step. Sanitize the hands.**
    Always sanitize the hands after every procedure or after using gloves.
15. **Procedural Step. Document the results in the patient's medical record and the laboratory logbook.**
    Include date and time of the test, date of the patient's last menstrual period (LMP), name of the test, and results recorded (positive or negative).

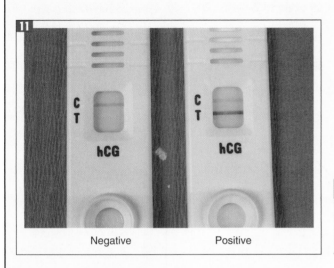

Negative   Positive

Charting Example

Date	
2/11/xx	10:30 a.m. LMP: 1/02/xx. QuickVue preg test: Positive. ——— T. Lane, CMA (AAMA)

---

analyses, microhematocrits, and manual (nonautomated) sedimentation rates.

Hematology

Hematology is the study of all blood components, including erythrocytes (RBCs), leukocytes (WBCs), and thrombocytes (platelets). RBCs carry oxygen throughout the body and transport carbon dioxide from the body's tissues to the lungs to be exhaled. WBCs defend the body against allergens, bacteria, and viruses. Platelets assist in blood clot formation.

Complete Blood Count

A **complete blood count (CBC)** is ordered to evaluate and monitor a patient's health and assist in the diagnosis of blood disorders (e.g., anemias, leukemias). The CBC is one of the most frequently performed laboratory tests on blood. It is not usually performed in the POL, but the medical assistant should be familiar with it and understand its importance. The CBC indicates the number of blood cells

present in a volume of blood. Blood is composed of formed elements that float in plasma. The RBCs are the largest number of blood cells in the body and are made in the red bone marrow. The WBCs are formed in bone marrow and in lymphoid tissue and are larger than RBCs, but fewer in number. Platelets are the least numerous type of cells in the blood.

Besides blood cell counts, CBC measures the size and shape of the cells, hemoglobin, hematocrit, and reticulocytes (immature RBCs) and provides a differential of WBC types. Table 2-5 lists CBC ranges.

Additional hematology tests often run by laboratories are **red cell indices** and **platelet counts.** Red cell indices determine the size, content, and hemoglobin concentration of RBCs, and they also include a mean cell volume (MCV, average size of RBCs), mean cell hemoglobin (MCH, average cell hemoglobin), and mean cell hemoglobin concentration (MCHC, average concentration of hemoglobin in a given volume of RBCs). RBC count, hemoglobin, and hematocrit are necessary to calculate the RBC indices. Red cell indices are useful in determining types of anemias.

TABLE 2-5 Complete Blood Count

Measurement	Range
Red Blood Cells	4.5-6 million/mm³
Hemoglobin (adult)	12-18 g/dL
Hematocrit (adult)	37%-52%
Reticulocytes	0%-1.5%
White Blood Cells	5000-10,000 mm³
Neutrophils	55%-70%
Eosinophils	1%-3%
Basophils	0.5%-1%
Lymphocytes	20%-35%
Monocytes	3%-8%
Platelets	150,000-300,000/mm³

TABLE 2-6 Hemoglobin and Hematocrit Values

Group	Range
Hemoglobin	
Men	13-18 g/dL
Women	12-16 g/dL
Child	10-14 g/dL
Infant	16-23 g/dL
Hematocrit	
Men	45%-52%
Women	37%-48%
Child to 6 years	34%-42%
Child to 1 year	32%-38%
Infant to 6 months	30%-40%
Infant to 1 month	35%-49%
Newborn	51%-61%

Cell analyzers are used to perform all the tests required of the CBC and require advanced training for operation.

Hemoglobin

Hemoglobin (Hb) is the component that gives RBCs their color. It carries oxygen to tissues and transports carbon dioxide to the lungs to be excreted. Hemoglobin measurement is used to detect blood loss and anemias. The test for hemoglobin can be performed on venous or capillary blood and can be measured as part of the CBC or as a separate test. Table 2-6 lists normal values.

Several automated devices are available to measure hemoglobin's oxygen-carrying capacity. The HemoCue hemoglobin analyzer is approved by CLIA 88 for use in the POL. The analyzer uses a photometer to measure blood hemoglobin, with the results displayed on a digital screen. The HemoCue uses a microcuvette that automatically draws the right amount of blood from a capillary puncture. A dry reagent on the microcuvette starts a chemical reaction to determine the hemoglobin. Procedure 2-4 provides instructions on obtaining a hemoglobin reading using a HemoCue.

Hematocrit

A **hematocrit (Hct)** reading can be performed on venous or capillary blood. The Hct is a measurement of the percentage of packed RBCs in a volume of whole blood. For example, an Hct of 45% indicates that every 100 mL (deciliter, dL) of blood contains 45 mL of packed RBCs (see Table 2-6).

To perform the Hct, an anticoagulated blood specimen is collected in a capillary tube, sealed at one end, and spun in a microhematocrit centrifuge (or a centrifuge with Hct-reading potential). The

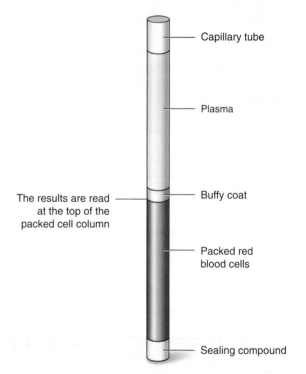

The results are read at the top of the packed cell column

— Capillary tube

— Plasma

— Buffy coat

— Packed red blood cells

— Sealing compound

Fig. 2-10 Hematocrit test results. The cellular elements are separated from the plasma by centrifuging an anticoagulated blood specimen, and the results are read at the top of the packed cell column. *(From Bonewit-West K: Clinical procedures for medical assistants, ed 6, Philadelphia, 2004, Saunders.)*

specimen separates into the following three layers (Fig. 2-10):

- Top layer = Plasma
- Middle layer = Buffy layer (coat) containing platelets and WBCs

Procedure 2-4 Determine a Hemoglobin Measurement Using a HemoCue

TASK: Accurately measure the hemoglobin of a blood specimen using a HemoCue.

EQUIPMENT AND SUPPLIES
- Nonsterile disposable gloves
- Personal protective equipment (PPE), as indicated
- Alcohol wipe
- Sterile disposable microlancet
- Sterile 2 × 2-inch gauze squares
- HemoCue
- Control cuvette

- Microcuvettes
- 10% bleach solution
- Sharps container
- Biohazardous waste container
- Patient's medical record
- Laboratory logbook
- Laboratory quality control logsheet

SKILLS/RATIONALE

STANDARD PRECAUTIONS ARE TO BE FOLLOWED.

1. **Procedural Step. Sanitize the hands.**
An alcohol-based hand rub may be used instead of washing hands with soap and water, unless hands are visibly soiled.
Rationale. Hand sanitization promotes infection control.

2. **Procedural Step. Assemble equipment and supplies and verify the order.**
Rationale. It is important to have all supplies and equipment ready and available before starting any procedure to ensure efficiency.

3. **Procedural Step. Perform the quality control test as recommended by the manufacturer and document in the laboratory quality control logsheet.**

4. **Procedural Step. Prepare the HemoCue analyzer.**
   a. Turn the power switch to the "on" position.
   b. Check that the meter reads zero.
   c. Place the control cuvette into the holder and push into the photometer.
   d. Validate the control values. If they are not within acceptable values, clean the test area and repeat the validation check.
   e. Fill a cuvette with a control solution.
   f. Place the cuvette into the holder and push into the photometer.
   g. Read the control result on the LED screen.
   h. Record the results.
   i. Dispose of the cuvette in a sharps container.

5. **Procedural Step. Greet and identify the patient and escort the patient to the examination room.**

Rationale. Identifying the patient ensures the procedure is performed on the correct patient.

6. **Procedural Step. Explain the procedure to the patient.**
Rationale. Explaining the procedure to the patient promotes cooperation and provides a means of obtaining implied consent.

7. **Procedural Step. Again sanitize the hands and apply gloves and PPE as indicated.**

8. **Procedural Step. Perform a capillary puncture (as outlined in Procedure 1-10), and dispose of the lancet in a sharps container.**
Rationale. Proper disposal of the lancet is required by OSHA standards to prevent exposure to blood-borne pathogens.

9. **Procedural Step. Wipe away the first drop of blood with a gauze pad.**
Rationale. The first drop of blood is not collected because it usually contains more tissue fluid than blood, which could cause an inaccurate test result.

10. **Procedural Step. Collect the specimen.**
Touch the cuvette to the second well-rounded drop of blood. Allow the cuvette to fill on its own by capillary action.
Rationale. Do not allow the patient's finger to touch the cuvette, only the drop of blood; the finger may break up or disintegrate cells and render the test inaccurate.

11. **Procedural Step. Wipe off any excess blood from the tip of the cuvette.**

12. **Procedural Step. Place the cuvette in its holder and push into the photometer.**

13. **Procedural Step. Read and record the hemoglobin value.**

Continued

Procedure 2-4 Determine a Hemoglobin Measurement Using a HemoCue—cont'd

14. **Procedural Step.** Discard the cuvette into the sharps container.
15. **Procedural Step.** Turn the equipment "off" as appropriate. Clean the equipment with a mild soap and water.
16. **Procedural Step.** Disinfect the work area with 10% bleach solution.
17. **Procedural Step.** Remove gloves and sanitize the hands.

    Always sanitize the hands after every procedure or after using gloves.

18. **Procedural Step.** Document the results in the patient's medical record and the laboratory logbook.

    Include date and time of the test, name of the test, and results.

Charting Example

Date	
7/13/xx	9:00 a.m. Hb 16 g/dL per HemoCue. ———— ———————————————— J. Duarte, CMA

- Bottom layer = Packed RBCs that have settled to the bottom because they are heavier than the other cells

The specimen is measured using a microhematocrit reader.

A patient's Hct should be approximately three times the value of the patient's hemoglobin (Hb). For example, if a patient's Hb is 12 g/dL, multiply by 3 to obtain the patient's Hct ($12 \times 3 = 36\%$, ±3). If you know the patient's Hct, you divide by 3 to obtain the Hb. A low reading may indicate anemia, and a high reading could be the result of polycythemia. Results other than the 1:3 ratio would require a retest. Procedure 2-5 explains the steps in performing a hematocrit.

Erythrocyte Sedimentation Rate

The **erythrocyte sedimentation rate (ESR),** or "sed rate," is a nonspecific screening test that confirms an inflammation is present somewhere in the body (e.g., respiratory infections, arthritis, pregnancy). ESR is a measurement of how fast RBCs settle to the bottom of a tube. The average rate is 1 mm every 5 minutes.

In a healthy person, ESR is slow and RBCs do not fall far. If inflammation is present, the test will show RBCs falling very quickly. The medical assistant will collect a venous blood specimen in a lavender tube (**EDTA,** the anticoagulant ethylenediaminetetraacetic acid). Two common ESR methods used in the POL are the Westergren tube method and the Wintrobe tube method.

The **Westergren method** uses a disposable self-zeroing tube calibrated from 0 to 200. A blood sample from a blood tube containing EDTA is transferred to the tube, mixed with sodium citrate solution, and set upright in a sedimentation rack for 1 hour (Fig. 2-11). Procedure 2-6 describes this

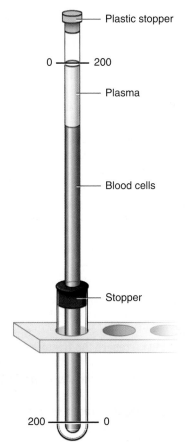

Fig. 2-11 Westergren erythrocyte sedimentation rate (ESR) system. This closed system protects against exposure to body fluids. In exactly 1 hour, the distance the red blood cells have dropped is determined. The tubes used in the Westergren system are much longer than those used in the Wintrobe method. *(Modified from Stepp CA, Woods MA: Laboratory procedures for medical office personnel, Philadelphia, 1998, Saunders.)*

Procedure 2-5 Perform a Microhematocrit Test

TASK: Accurately collect a capillary blood sample to spin and measure, and read a microhematocrit.

EQUIPMENT AND SUPPLIES
- Nonsterile disposable gloves
- Personal protective equipment (PPE), as indicated
- Microhematocrit capillary tubes (heparinized)
- Sealing compound
- Alcohol wipe
- Sterile disposable microlancet
- Sterile 2 × 2-inch gauze squares
- 10% bleach solution
- Microhematocrit centrifuge
- Hematocrit reader
- Sharps container
- Biohazardous waste container
- Patient's medical record
- Laboratory logbook

SKILLS/RATIONALE

STANDARD PRECAUTIONS ARE TO BE FOLLOWED.

1. **Procedural Step. Sanitize the hands.**
   An alcohol-based hand rub may be used instead of washing hands with soap and water, unless hands are visibly soiled.
   Rationale. Hand sanitization promotes infection control.

2. **Procedural Step. Assemble equipment and supplies and verify the order.**
   Rationale. It is important to have all supplies and equipment ready and available before starting any procedure to ensure efficiency.

3. **Procedural Step. Greet and identify the patient and escort the patient to the examination room or laboratory area.**
   Rationale. Identifying the patient ensures the procedure is performed on the correct patient.

4. **Procedural Step. Explain the procedure to the patient.**
   Rationale. Explaining the procedure to the patient promotes cooperation and provides a means of obtaining implied consent.

5. **Procedural Step. Apply gloves and PPE as indicated.**

Collecting the Specimen

6. **Procedural Step. Perform a capillary puncture (as outlined in Procedure 1-10), and dispose of the lancet in a sharps container.**
   Rationale. Proper disposal of the lancet is required by OSHA standards to prevent exposure to blood-borne pathogens.

7. **Procedural Step. Wipe away the first drop of blood with a gauze pad.**
   Rationale. The first drop of blood is not collected because it usually contains more tissue fluid than blood, which could cause an inaccurate test result.

8. **Procedural Step. Collect the specimen.**
   Allow another drop of blood to accumulate, and touch the end of the capillary tube to it. Keep the tip of the capillary tube in the blood, and do not allow it to press against the skin of the patient's finger. The blood will be drawn into the tube through capillary action. Continue filling the tube until it is about three-quarters full. Fill the second capillary tube in the same way.

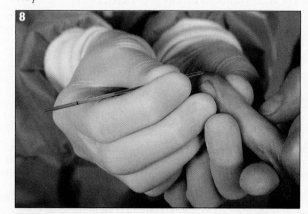

   Rationale. Removing the capillary tube from the drop of blood may result in air bubbles within the tube, causing inaccurate test results. Allowing the capillary tube to press against the skin will close off the

Continued

Procedure 2-5 Perform a Microhematocrit Test—cont'd

opening of the capillary tube and will not allow blood to enter the tube.

9. **Procedural Step. After the sample has been collected, instruct the patient to squeeze a clean gauze square for direct pressure to the puncture site.**

10. **Procedural Step. Seal the dry end of the capillary tubes with clay (e.g., Critoseal, Hemato-Seal).**
    To avoid splashing blood from the end used to collect the sample while sealing the tube, tilt the capillary tube slightly to allow air to enter the end of the tube used to fill it. When the dry end is sealed, air will be displaced instead of blood.
    Rationale. The capillary tubes must be properly sealed to prevent leakage of the blood specimen during centrifugation.

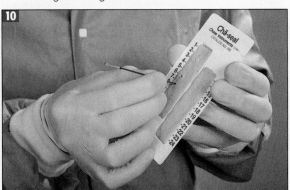

11. **Procedural Step. Leave the capillary tubes embedded in the sealing clay to prevent damaging them.**
    The clay board can be transported to the laboratory for the specimen to be processed.

12. **Procedural Step. Check the puncture site.**
    Make sure it has stopped bleeding, and bandage it with a clean strip bandage to protect the wound. Discard any contaminated materials in the appropriate biohazardous waste container.

13. **Procedural Step. Remove gloves, and sanitize the hands.**
    Always sanitize the hands after every procedure or after using gloves.

Testing the Specimen

14. **Procedural Step. Place the specimens in the centrifuge.**
    Apply gloves and remove the patient samples from the clay. Place the capillary tubes opposite each other in the centrifuge for balance. Make

sure the sealed end is placed against the outer rim, and record the location of the patient samples in the centrifuge in the logbook.
NOTE: Commercial controls of known values, or *quality controls,* are not usually processed with patient samples for spun hematocrit measurements because no chemicals are needed to perform the test. For *quality assurance,* patient samples are run in duplicate, and the results of the two readings must agree within 2%.
Rationale. When more than one patient's samples are being spun, recording the locations of the tubes is the only way to tell them apart after they are placed in the centrifuge.

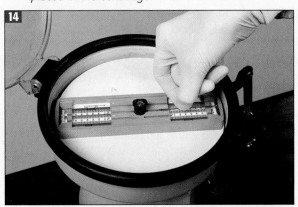

15. **Procedural Step. Secure the locking top by placing it over the threaded bolt on the centrifuge head and turning the fastener until tight.**

16. **Procedural Step. Close and latch the lid of the centrifuge, and spin for 5 minutes at 2500 rpm or the high setting.**
    Most microhematocrit centrifuges are preset to the appropriate speed, so all that needs to be done is to set the timer for 5 minutes.
    Rationale. Spinning separates the blood into cells and plasma.

17. **Procedural Step. Wait until the centrifuge comes to a complete stop before unlatching the lid, and remove the locking top.**
    Rationale. The centrifuge must be stopped completely to prevent injury when removing the tubes.

18. **Procedural Step. Position one of the tubes in the hematocrit reader.**
    Remove one of the tubes from its slot, taking care to note the number of the slot. Place the tube in the hematocrit reader with the junction of the clay and red blood cells against the zero line.

Procedure 2-5 Perform a Microhematocrit Test—cont'd

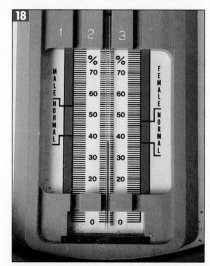

19. Procedural Step. Adjust the reader to read the results.
Rotate the outer disk to the 100% line. Then rotate the inner disk until the reading line is even with the bottom of the meniscus of the plasma. This defines 100% of the sample and includes red blood cells, white blood cells, and plasma.

20. Procedural Step. Determine what percentage of the sample is made up of red blood cells.
Rotate the inner and outer disks together by grasping just the outer disk. Turn the disks until the reading line is at the junction of the red blood cell layer and white blood cell layer.

21. Procedural Step. Record the number on the outer disk as the percentage of red blood cells in the sample, or the hematocrit.

22. Procedural Step. Discard the capillary tube in a sharps container.

23. Procedural Step. Repeat the reading for the second capillary tube.

24. Procedural Step. Average the two results, and record the average value as the patient result.
The two readings should not vary by more than 2%. If they do, repeat the collection and run the test again.

25. Procedural Step. Disinfect the work area with 10% bleach solution.

26. Procedural Step. Remove gloves and sanitize the hands.
Always sanitize the hands after every procedure or after using gloves.

27. Procedural Step. Document the results in the patient's medical record and the laboratory logbook.
Include date and time of the test, name of the test, and results.

Charting Example

Date	
6/12/xx	1:00 p.m. Hct: 42%. —————— R. Bair, RMA

Photos from Bonewit-West K: *Clinical procedures for medical assistants,* ed 6, Philadelphia, 2004, Saunders.

---

process in detail using the Sed-Pac system (Futura Medical Corp.).

The **Wintrobe method** requires that an EDTA blood sample be transferred to a disposable tube. The Wintrobe tube is smaller than the Westergren tube, and it is calibrated from 0 to 100. The tube is placed in a sedimentation rack for 1 hour. The distance that the RBCs have fallen is recorded (Fig. 2-12).

Table 2-7 compares the reference values of the Wintrobe and Westergren methods.

Blood Slide Differential

Another routine hematology procedure is the microscopic examination of blood. This involves the preparation, staining, and examination of a dried blood specimen on a glass slide. In most cases, only licensed laboratory technicians can perform these tests because they are not CLIA waived. However,

TABLE 2-7	Erythrocyte Sedimentation Rate (ESR) Values	
	Westergren Method	**Wintrobe Method**
Men		
<50 years	0-15 mm/hr	0-7 mm/hr
>50 years	0-20 mm/hr	5-7 mm/hr
Women		
<50 years	0-20 mm/hr	0-15 mm/hr
>50 years	0-30 mm/hr	25-30 mm/hr

Procedure 2-6 Determine Erythrocyte Sedimentation Rate (ESR, Non-Automated) Using the Westergren Method

TASK: Properly fill a Westergren tube and observe and report ESR results accurately.

EQUIPMENT AND SUPPLIES

- Nonsterile disposable gloves
- Personal protective equipment (PPE), as indicated
- Supplies to perform venipuncture
- EDTA-anticoagulated blood specimen (lavender-top tube)
- Sed-Pac ESR system (reservoir, diluent, Dispette tube) with rack
- Transfer pipette
- Timer
- 10% bleach solution
- Biohazardous waste container
- Patient's medical record
- Laboratory logbook

SKILLS/RATIONALE

STANDARD PRECAUTIONS ARE TO BE FOLLOWED.

1. **Procedural Step. Sanitize the hands.**
   An alcohol-based hand rub may be used instead of washing hands with soap and water, unless hands are visibly soiled.
   Rationale. Hand sanitization promotes infection control.

2. **Procedural Step. Assemble equipment and supplies and verify the order.**
   Rationale. It is important to have all supplies and equipment ready and available before starting any procedure to ensure efficiency.

3. **Procedural Step. Greet and identify the patient and escort the patient to the examination room or laboratory area.**
   Rationale. Identifying the patient ensures the procedure is performed on the correct patient.

4. **Procedural Step. Explain the procedure to the patient.**
   Rationale. Explaining the procedure to the patient promotes cooperation and provides a means of obtaining implied consent.

5. **Procedural Step. Apply gloves and PPE as appropriate.**

6. **Procedural Step. Perform a venipuncture.**
   Collect one EDTA tube (lavender top) of blood. Follow Procedure 1-12.

7. **Procedural Step. Transport the specimen to the physician office laboratory.**

8. **Procedural Step. Transfer the specimen.**
   Remove the stopper on the prefilled ESR vial, and fill the reservoir to the indicated line with blood using a transfer pipette. Mix well.

9. **Procedural Step. Insert the Dispette tube into the reservoir, and push down until the tube touches the bottom of the reservoir.**
   The Dispette tube will auto-zero the blood, and any excess will flow into the closed reservoir compartment.

10. **Procedural Step. Place the ESR tube in a rack, making certain it remains vertical.**
    Rationale. Results will be inaccurate if the ESR tube is not kept vertical.

11. **Procedural Step. Set the timer for 1 hour.**

12. **Procedural Step. Read the results.**
    Observe the level of the meniscus of the blood in the tube after 1 hour. The scale is measured in millimeters; each line equals 1 mm.

13. **Procedural Step. Properly dispose of the ESR tube in a biohazardous waste container.**

14. **Procedural Step. Disinfect the work area using 10% bleach solution.**

15. **Procedural Step. Remove gloves and sanitize the hands.**
    Always sanitize the hands after every procedure or after using gloves.

16. **Procedural Step. Document the results in the patient's medical record and the laboratory logbook.**
    Include date and time of the test, name of the test, and results.

Charting Example

Date	
3/10/xx	2:15 p.m. ESR 9 mm/hr (Westergren).
	J. Apollo, CMA (AAMA)

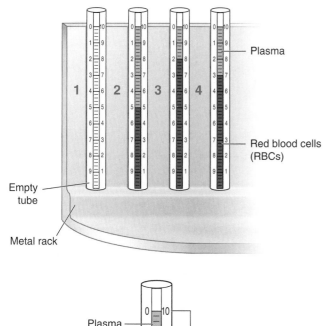

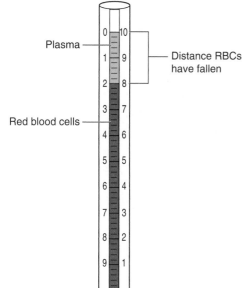

Fig. 2-12 Wintrobe ESR system. As with the Westergren method, the distance the red blood cells have dropped is determined in exactly 1 hour. *(Modified from Stepp CA, Woods MA: Laboratory procedures for medical office personnel, Philadelphia, 1998, Saunders.)*

the medical assistant can prepare the blood smear in preparation for the procedure.

A **differential blood cell count,** or "diff," is an important diagnostic test. An increase or decrease in one or several types of cells may occur in various disease conditions. The test differentiates WBCs (counts them by type) as a percentage per 100 cells. It also observes the shape of the RBCs and estimates the number of platelets.

When first learning this procedure, the medical assistant must remember that slide preparation takes time, patience, and practice. If the blood smear is too thick, the cells cannot be seen clearly, and it may not stain correctly. If it is too thin, the cells

will be spread out, and the time needed to count increases. The medical assistant must be able to "feather" the blood smear to one cell layer thick.

The specimen can be from a capillary puncture, a freshly drawn specimen using a syringe, or an EDTA blood specimen. Basically, a drop of blood is pushed across a slide with another slide, as follows:

1. A medium-sized drop of blood is placed near the frosted edge of the slide, with the spreader slide at a 30-degree angle just in front of the drop of blood.
2. The spreader slide is pulled back until the edge comes in contact with the drop of blood.
3. The blood should spread evenly across the width of the spreader slide.
4. The spreader slide is then pushed toward the opposite end of the slide and disposed of in a sharps container.
5. The slide should be placed on a flat surface immediately and allowed to air-dry. This prevents blood cell shrinkage.

The following factors can affect the quality of a good blood smear:

1. *Size* of the drop of blood. A small drop may produce a short, thick smear. A large drop can produce a longer, thinner specimen. A large drop can also produce too much blood so that the smear has cells stacked on top of each other.
2. *Angle* of the spreader slide. An angle less than 30 degrees produces a long, thin slide. An angle greater than 30 degrees produces a shorter, thicker blood smear.
3. *Pressure* used. Pressure must be even during the process. The greater the pressure, the thinner is the smear. Uneven pressure creates ridges or gaps in the blood smear.
4. *Speed* of the spreading movement. Too much or too little speed can increase or decrease the thickness of the blood smear. The spreading movement must be smooth and continuous to achieve the desired thickness.
5. *Viscosity* (blood stickiness, or thickness). **Viscosity** can affect how evenly the smear can be done. If the blood is too thick or sticky, only masses of RBCs will be visible, and WBCs will not be seen.

Making a blood smear correctly depends on adjusting the technique according to the problem. Procedure 2-7 describes proper preparation of a blood smear.

TASK: Prepare a blood smear for a differential count.

EQUIPMENT AND SUPPLIES
- Nonsterile disposable gloves
- Personal protective equipment (PPE), as indicated
- Supplies to perform capillary puncture or venipuncture
- Glass slides (frosted end)
- Pipette or Diff-Safe
- Slide holder
- Pencil
- 10% bleach solution
- Sharps container

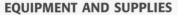

SKILLS/RATIONALE

STANDARD PRECAUTIONS ARE TO BE FOLLOWED.

1. **Procedural Step. Sanitize the hands.**
   An alcohol-based hand rub may be used instead of washing hands with soap and water, unless hands are visibly soiled.
   Rationale. Hand sanitization promotes infection control.

2. **Procedural Step. Assemble equipment and supplies and verify the order.**
   Slides must be clean and free from chips or cracks.
   Rationale. It is important to have all supplies and equipment ready and available before starting any procedure to ensure efficiency.

3. **Procedural Step. Greet and identify the patient and escort the patient to the examination room or laboratory area.**
   Rationale. Identifying the patient ensures the procedure is performed on the correct patient.

4. **Procedural Step. Explain the procedure to the patient.**
   Rationale. Explaining the procedure to the patient promotes cooperation and provides a means of obtaining implied consent.

5. **Procedural Step. Apply gloves and PPE, as indicated.**

6. **Procedural Step. Label two slides on the frosted end, using a pencil, with the patient's name and the date.**
   Rationale. Two slides will be smeared. Labeling the slides identifies the patient's specimen.

7. **Procedural Step. Perform a venipuncture.**
   Collect one EDTA tube (lavender top) of blood. Follow Procedure 1-12, or perform a capillary puncture following Procedure 1-10.

8. **Procedural Step. Place a well-rounded medium-sized drop (1-2 mm) of fresh whole blood on each slide as follows:**

From a *venipuncture.* The blood specimen can be transferred to the slide in one of three ways:

a. Blood is obtained from the fresh whole blood left in the needle after performing a venipuncture. This is done by depositing a drop of blood left in the multidraw needle onto each glass slide, immediately after withdrawing the needle from the patient's arm, approximately ¼ inch from the frosted edge of the slide. This method is difficult and requires much practice and experience as well as proficiency in making accurate slides every time.

b. The lavender-top tube is carefully removed, and a drop of blood is transferred to each glass slide using a disposable pipette. This is the least favored method because it poses the greatest risk of aerosol and droplet contamination.

c. Blood is collected into an EDTA tube, and the specimen is transported to the POL, where a Diff-Safe is inserted into the top of the blood tube. The Diff-Safe with the attached tube is pushed down on top of each glass slide, releasing the drop of blood. This is the most accurate and safest method because it provides a measured drop of blood accurately and consistently, and the risk is minimal.

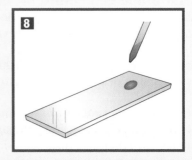

From a *skin puncture.* Perform a capillary puncture and wipe away the first drop of blood. Place a drop of blood from the patient's finger onto each slide approximately ¼ inch from the frosted edge of the slide. Do not allow the patient's finger to touch the slide.

If only a differential and perhaps one other point-of-care test are ordered, a capillary puncture will provide a sufficient amount of blood. Again, this requires a great amount of skill and proficiency in smearing the slide. If a slide cannot be made from the first drops of blood, it may require a second puncture. With time and experience, however, this is an efficient method of collection and requires only a minimal amount of blood.

NOTE: The patient's finger must not touch the slide; it may cause hemolysis of the specimen and inaccurate test results. It may also cause the specimen to spread prematurely, and moisture and oils from the patient's skin can interfere with test results.

9 Procedural Step. Spread the drop of blood back.
Once the drop of blood is placed on the glass slide, take a second glass slide or "spreader" slide in your dominant hand. Place it directly in front of the drop of blood at a 45-degree angle. Slowly back the spreader slide into the drop of blood. Allow the drop of blood to spread evenly across the width of the slide.
Rationale. This ensures an even smear.

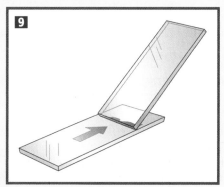

10 Procedural Step. Spread the drop of blood forward.
Lower the angle of the spreader slide to 30 degrees, and quickly push the slide forward along the length of the stationary glass slide.

This movement is much like striking a match.
Rationale. If the angle is greater than 30 degrees, the smear will be too thick and will be difficult to read because the cells will be overlapping. If the

angle is less than 30 degrees, the smear will be too thin, and the cells will be too spread out.

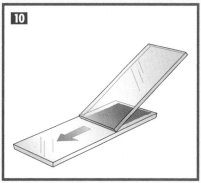

11 Procedural Step. Evaluate the slide.
The smear should be approximately one half the slide's length. The blood smear will be heavier at the blood drop end of the slide, gradually thinning out to a feathered edge.

When held up to the light, a rainbow should be visible in the feathered end. The feathered end of the slide is only one cell thick and is the area where the physician will "read" the differential.

The smear should be free from holes, lines, clumps, or jagged edges. The feathered end should be free from streaks and spikes of blood extending from the feathered edge.

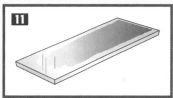

12. **Procedural Step. Repeat Steps 9 to 11 for the second glass slide.**
13. **Procedural Step. Allow both slides to air-dry standing at an angle, with the frosted end of the slide or the blood end down.**
    Rationale. If the blood end of the slide is up, the blood may run down the slide and destroy the smear.
14. **Procedural Step. Dispose of the spreader slide in a sharps container, and dispose of all other contaminated or regular waste appropriately.**
15. **Procedural Step. Once the slides are completely dry (a minimum of 20 minutes), both slides can be placed in slide holders and transported to the laboratory.**
16. **Procedural Step. Disinfect the work area using 10% bleach solution.**
17. **Procedural Step. Remove gloves and sanitize the hands.**
    Always sanitize the hands after every procedure or after using gloves.

Blood Chemistry

Blood chemistry is the **quantitative** (measurable, pertaining to amount) analysis of chemicals in the blood. Most blood chemistry tests are performed on serum. The test ordered will depend on the physician's diagnosis or the patient's present symptoms. The medical assistant must be conscious of the type of specimen required for each test ordered. Table 2-8 provides a reference range for various blood chemistry tests.

Specimens are frequently sent to an outside laboratory for processing so that qualified personnel and analyzers can perform the tests (Fig. 2-13). A **chemistry profile** provides the physician with information about the patient's general state of health and includes lipid and carbohydrate metabolism and liver, thyroid, kidney, and cardiac function. Other profiles can be ordered to address a particular body system (e.g., liver, renal, cardiac, lipid).

Point-of-care testing (POCT) involves tests done in the physician's office for immediate feedback and can be performed by medical assistants. Such tests include cholesterol and glucose measurements. These tests require only a small sample of blood, so a capillary puncture is adequate. Blood glucose tests are performed for the diagnosis and control of diabetes mellitus. Cholesterol testing in the POL is used to monitor the patient's general health status and the effectiveness of cholesterol-lowering medications. "Protimes" (coagulation and bleeding times or PT and PTT) are also done on site to assist the physician with warfarin (Coumadin) adjustments. CLIA 88 requires that two levels of controls be performed daily: normal control and high level. This validates the accuracy of the equipment and reagents.

Cholesterol Testing

The body makes **serum cholesterol,** a white, fatlike substance, in the liver. Cholesterol is also metabolized from foods (e.g., organ meats, dairy products). It is contained within cell membranes. The body needs cholesterol for normal functioning and uses it to produce hormones and bile. Higher-than-normal levels of cholesterol in the blood cause narrowing of the blood vessels, leading to heart disease and stroke. The following three levels of cholesterol are measured:

- **Total cholesterol** is a combined measurement of the amount of LDL cholesterol and HDL cholesterol in the blood.
- **LDL** (low-density lipoprotein), the "bad" cholesterol, picks up cholesterol from ingested fats and the liver and takes it to the blood

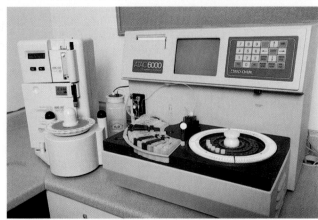

Fig. 2-13   Blood chemistry analyzer. *(ATAC Lab System by BioMed.)*

vessels and muscles. When it builds up on the walls of blood vessels, LDL cholesterol causes heart disease.
- **HDL** (high-density lipoprotein), the "good" cholesterol, removes excess cholesterol from the body cells and takes it to the liver to be excreted.

Cholesterol test results are as follows:
Desirable cholesterol level:	<200 mg/dL
Borderline-high cholesterol level:	200-240 mg/dL
High cholesterol level:	>240 mg/dL

The primary use of cholesterol testing is to screen for high levels of blood cholesterol related to heart disease. The total amount of cholesterol, the amount of LDL and HDL cholesterol in the blood, and the ratios of each provide a good indicator of risk for artery disease. Cholesterol testing is often used to monitor liver and thyroid function. Procedure 2-8 explains the process of performing cholesterol testing.

Glucose Testing

The end result of carbohydrate metabolism is glucose, or sugar. Glucose is the main source of energy for the body. The body functions best if the blood glucose level remains constant. When not used for energy, glucose is stored in muscles and the liver as glycogen. When an overload of glucose is present, it can be stored as fat in the adipose tissue.

The hormone *insulin* allows glucose to enter the cells and be converted to energy. A person's blood glucose rises after an ingestion of glucose but should return to normal range after 2 hours.

FASTING BLOOD SUGAR TEST

The **fasting blood sugar (FBS) test** measures the glucose level in a blood sample. The patient is

TABLE 2-8	Normal Blood Chemistry Values
Test	**Reference Range for Adults**
Alanine aminotransferase (ALT)	6-37 U/L
Albumin	3.5-5.5 g/dL
Alkaline phosphatase (ALP)	0.8-2 BLB unit
Amylase	95-290 U/L
Anion gap (R factor) (AG)	10-18 mEq/L
Aspartate transaminase (AST)	5-30 U/L
Bilirubin, total	0.2-1.2 mg/dL
Bilirubin, conjugated	0.1-0.3 mg/dL
Blood urea nitrogen (BUN)	5-20 mg/dL
Calcium (Ca)	8.4-10.2 mg/dL
Carbon dioxide (CO_2)	22-29 mEq/L
Chloride (Cl)	98-106 mEq/L
Cholesterol, total (CH, Chol)	Desirable: <200 mg/dL Borderline: 200-240 mg/dL High: >240 mg/dL
Cholesterol, low-density lipoprotein (LDL)	Desirable: <170 mg/dL Borderline: 170-199 mg/dL High: >200 mg/dL
Cholesterol, high-density lipoprotein (HDL)	Men: 29-60 mg/dL Women: 38-75 mg/dL
Creatine kinase (CK)	Men: 15-160 U/L Women: 15-130 U/L
Creatinine	Men: 0.6-1.2 mg/dL Women: 0.5-1.1 mg/dL
Glucose, fasting (fasting blood sugar, FBS)	70-110 mg/dL
Glucose, 2-hour postprandial (PPBS)	<140 mg/dL
Glucose tolerance test (GTT)	FBS: 70-110 mg/dL 30 min: 110-170 mg/dL 1 hr: 120-170 mg/dL 2 hr: 70-120 mg/dL 3 hr: <120 mg/dL
Iron (Fe)	40-160 mcg/dL
Iron-binding capacity, total (TIBC)	250-400 mcg/dL
Lactate dehydrogenase (LD, LDH)	100-200 U/L
Lipase	0-1 U/mL
Magnesium (Mg, Mag)	1.3-2.1 mEq/L
Phosphorus (P)	2.7-4.5 mg/dL
Potassium (K)	3.5-5.1 mEq/L
Protein, total (TP)	6.2-8.2 g/dL
Sodium (Na)	136-146 mEq/L
Triglycerides (TG, Trig)	10-190 mg/dL
Uric acid	Men: 3.5-7.2 mg/dL Women: 2.6-6 mg/dL

required to refrain from eating and drinking (except water) for at least 12 hours before testing. A blood sample is drawn, tested, and compared to the normal range of 70 to 110 mg/dL of glucose in the blood.

TWO-HOUR POSTPRANDIAL TEST
The **2-hour postprandial test** is used to screen for diabetes mellitus and to monitor the effects of a patient's insulin regimen. A patient is required to fast, then either eat a special meal or drink a glucose

Procedure 2-8 Perform Cholesterol Testing

TASK: Collect and process a blood specimen accurately for cholesterol testing using the Cholestech LDX analyzer.

EQUIPMENT AND SUPPLIES
- Nonsterile disposable gloves
- Personal protective equipment (PPE), as indicated
- Capillary puncture supplies
- Cholesterol testing device (Cholestech LDX)
- Cholesterol testing kit (capillary tube with plunger, test cassette)
- 10% bleach solution
- Sharps container
- Biohazardous waste container
- Quality control logsheet
- Patient's medical record
- Laboratory logbook

SKILLS/RATIONALE

STANDARD PRECAUTIONS ARE TO BE FOLLOWED.

1. **Procedural Step. Sanitize the hands.**
   An alcohol-based hand rub may be used instead of washing hands with soap and water, unless hands are visibly soiled.
   Rationale. Hand sanitization promotes infection control.

2. **Procedural Step. Assemble equipment and supplies and verify the order.**
   Check the expiration dates of the test kits.
   Rationale. It is important to have all supplies and equipment ready and available before starting any procedure to ensure efficiency. Expired test kits may produce inaccurate test results.

3. **Procedural Step. Prepare the test kit and analyzer.**
   Remove the test kit from the refrigerator and warm to room temperature. Prepare the analyzer according to the manufacturer's instructions.

4. **Procedural Step. Perform a quality control test as recommended by the manufacturer, and document in the laboratory quality control logsheet.**

5. **Procedural Step. Greet and identify the patient, and escort the patient to the examination room or laboratory area.**
   Rationale. Identifying the patient ensures the procedure is performed on the correct patient.

6. **Procedural Step. Explain the procedure to the patient.**
   Rationale. Explaining the procedure to the patient promotes cooperation and provides a means of obtaining implied consent.

7. **Procedural Step. Apply gloves and PPE as indicated.**

8. **Procedural Step. Perform a capillary puncture (follow Procedure 1-10).**

9. **Procedural Step. Wipe away the first drop of blood.**

10. **Procedural Step. Collect the blood specimen in a capillary tube.**
    NOTE: The capillary specimen must be inserted into the cassette within 4 minutes of collection.

11. **Procedural Step. Prepare the specimen.**
    Place the end of the capillary tube in the sample well of the cassette, and dispense the blood by pushing down on the plunger.

12. **Procedural Step. Insert the cassette into the Cholestech LDX analyzer and activate the timer.**

13. **Procedural Step. When the timer stops, read the results.**

14. **Procedural Step. Discard the cassette, capillary tube, and plunger into a sharps container.**

15. **Procedural Step. Turn off the analyzer and wipe it with a damp cloth.**

16. **Procedural Step. Disinfect the work area using 10% bleach solution.**

17. **Procedural Step. Remove gloves and sanitize the hands.**
    Always sanitize the hands after every procedure or after using gloves.

18. **Procedural Step. Document the results in the patient's medical record and the laboratory logbook.**
    Include date and time of the test, name of the test, and results.

Charting Example

Date	
4/30/xx	11:15 a.m. Cholesterol level 210 mg/dL using Cholestech LDX.
	— L. Carter, CMA (AAMA)

solution containing 100 g of glucose. Two hours after ingestion, a blood sample is drawn and compared to the normal range.

GLUCOSE TOLERANCE TEST

The **glucose tolerance test (GTT)** is more sensitive to the patient's ability to metabolize glucose. The patient fasts, blood and urine specimens are collected, and the patient ingests a special glucose drink. After this, blood and urine specimens are collected at 30 minutes, 1 hour, 2 hours, and 3 hours. Urine specimens are collected to measure the amount of glucose and ketones filtered out by the kidneys. The blood test determines if the glucose level has returned to within a normal range. The patient should be encouraged to drink water so the necessary specimens can be provided.

GLUCOMETER

Measuring the amount of glucose in the blood is frequently performed in the medical office with a **glucometer** (Fig. 2-14). On-site testing requires no special patient preparation and provides immediate feedback to the physician on the patient's status. This allows the physician to monitor the effectiveness of diabetic medications and diets.

GLUCOSE REAGENT STRIP

Several manufacturers offer machines for home and clinical use that have a **glucose reagent strip** to test for glucose levels in blood. The medical assistant must follow the manufacturer's instructions for the specific device used in the medical office. Typically, a small drop of whole blood, usually obtained by capillary puncture, is applied to a reagent test strip. A glucometer uses a photometer to read the color change in the reagent paper. The result is automatically calculated and displayed in the window of the meter (see Fig. 2-14).

Box 2-2 lists reasons why a blood glucose reading could be inaccurate. Procedure 2-9 explains how to collect and process a blood specimen accurately for glucose testing.

GLYCOSYLATED HEMOGLOBIN TEST

The **glycosylated hemoglobin (GHb) test** monitors diabetes treatment and control by measuring the amount of hemoglobin A_{1c} in the blood. When glucose is not used for energy and remains in the bloodstream, it attaches to the hemoglobin. Because the life span of an RBC is 120 days, GHb can be measured and an average glucose level obtained for the past 3 months.

Serology and Immunology

Serology is the laboratory study of blood serum for signs of antibodies produced by the antigen-

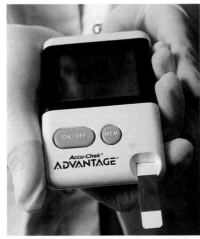

Fig. 2-14 Glucometer. *(From Bonewit-West K:* Clinical procedures for medical assistants, *ed 6, Philadelphia, 2004, Saunders.)*

BOX 2-2   Reasons for Errors in Glucose Readings

Errors in Procedure
- Not enough blood on test strip
- Not wiping away the first drop of blood on the patient
- Touching the finger to the test strip (allows substances from finger to be included in the reading)
- Using expired test strips
- Touching the pad on the test strip while taking the strip from the bottle
- If the test has a code, not checking that the code matches the strips

Other Reasons for Errors
- Hematocrit readings that fall below or that exceed the normal range can cause an inaccurate low glucose reading
- High levels of cholesterol and triglycerides may influence the blood glucose result

---

antibody reaction. The body's immune system provides a defense against infection by producing antibodies against a disease-producing organism. When the body senses a foreign object or organism (antigen), it may produce antibodies to neutralize the offending organism. The body also produces antibodies against bacterial toxins, allergens, and blood allergens. **Immunology** is the study of how the immune system works to defend the body.

The testing of body fluids is referred to as **serological testing, immunological testing,** and **immunoassays.** Serological testing done in the POL involves the use of prepackaged test kits that analyze a reaction between an antigen and an anti-

Procedure 2-9 Perform Glucose Testing

TASK: Accurately collect and process a blood specimen for glucose testing using Accucheck.

EQUIPMENT AND SUPPLIES
- Nonsterile disposable gloves
- Personal protective equipment (PPE), as indicated
- Capillary puncture supplies
- Glucose testing device (Accucheck)
- Test strip
- Control solution
- 10% bleach solution
- Sharps container
- Biohazardous waste container
- Patient's medical record
- Laboratory quality control logsheet
- Laboratory logbook

SKILLS/RATIONALE

STANDARD PRECAUTIONS ARE TO BE FOLLOWED.

1. **Procedural Step. Sanitize the hands.**
   An alcohol-based hand rub may be used instead of washing hands with soap and water, unless hands are visibly soiled.
   Rationale. Hand sanitization promotes infection control.

2. **Procedural Step. Assemble equipment and supplies and verify the order.**
   Check the expiration dates of the test kits, and check the Glucometer to make sure it is functioning properly.
   Rationale. It is important to have all supplies and equipment ready and available before starting any procedure to ensure efficiency. Expired test kits may produce inaccurate test results. The glucometer should be on a maintenance schedule for cleaning and battery replacement.

3. **Procedural Step. Prepare the analyzer according to the manufacturer's instructions.**
   Calibrate the glucometer by matching the glucometer code numbers to the code numbers on the vial of test strips. Adjust if necessary according to the manufacturer's instructions.

4. **Procedural Step. Perform a quality control test as recommended by the manufacturer, and document in the laboratory quality control logsheet.**
   The manufacturer displays the lot numbers and expiration dates on the outside of the bottle of test strips. Insert a control strip into the Accucheck glucometer. Apply a drop of control solution. Verify the accuracy of the control strip. Discard the control strip.

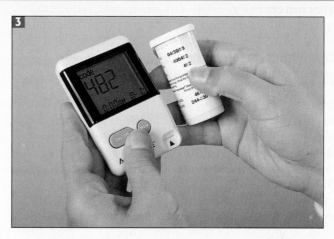

Rationale. It is important to record the lot numbers and expiration dates of the test strips and controls. This provides a reference point in case the reagents or controls do not perform as expected. Recording the acceptable ranges of the controls lets you know immediately if the result obtained is acceptable.

5. **Procedural Step. Greet and identify the patient and escort the patient to the examination room or laboratory area.**
   Rationale. Identifying the patient ensures the procedure is performed on the correct patient.

6. **Procedural Step. Explain the procedure to the patient.**
   Rationale. Explaining the procedure to the patient promotes cooperation and provides a means of obtaining implied consent.

7. **Procedural Step. Apply gloves and PPE as indicated.**

8. **Procedural Step. Insert a test strip into the test strip slot.**

Procedure 2-9 Perform Glucose Testing—cont'd

After the monitor displays the code key number, it signals when to insert a test strip. Some models use a flashing icon of a test strip, others sound a beep, and still others use both a beep and a visual symbol. Within 30 seconds of the signal, insert a test strip in the slot.

Some models have metal colored bars at one end of the test strip. The test strip is inserted into the slot bars first, yellow pad facing up. When the flashing drop appears, the sample can be applied to the strip.

9. **Procedural Step. Ask when the patient last had something to eat or drink (besides water).**
   Rationale. *The interval between the last consumption of food or beverage and the blood test for glucose may become a factor in the health care provider's evaluation of the result. If the last time the patient had anything to eat or drink was 12 hours or longer, the patient is considered to be fasting. The patient who has consumed food or a beverage within the last 12 hours is considered to be nonfasting.*

10. **Procedural Step. Perform a capillary puncture (refer to Procedure 1-10).**
    Wipe away the first drop of blood.

11. **Procedural Step. Apply a rounded drop of blood from the capillary puncture to the test strip.**

Make certain the test area is completely covered.

12. **Procedural Step. When the glucometer timer stops, read the results.**

13. **Procedural Step. Discard the test strip into the biohazardous container.**

14. **Procedural Step. Turn off the glucometer and wipe it with a damp cloth.**

15. **Procedural Step. Disinfect the work area using 10% bleach solution.**

16. **Procedural Step. Remove gloves and sanitize the hands.**
    Always sanitize the hands after every procedure or after using gloves.

17. **Procedural Step. Document the results in the patient's medical record and the laboratory logbook.**
    Include date and time of the test, name of the test, and results.

Charting Example

Date	
11/22/xx	9:45 a.m. NON-FBS: 110 mg/dL. ————————
	———————— B. Carter, CMA (AAMA)

BOX 2-3 Serological Tests

Hepatitis test. Detects viral hepatitis and determines what type of hepatitis.

Syphilis test. Screening test for the syphilis antibodies (VDRL or RPR). Any active reaction results in a positive test result being recorded. Further tests are done to confirm a diagnosis of syphilis (e.g., FTA absorption test).

Mononucleosis test. Detects the presence of infectious mononucleosis using serum, plasma, and sometimes whole blood (see Fig. 2-16).

Rheumatoid test. Detects rheumatoid factor (RF) in patients with rheumatoid arthritis.

Antistreptolysin O test. Detects ASO antibodies in the serum of a patient with a streptococcal infection or a disease occurring as a secondary infection (e.g., rheumatic fever, bacterial endocarditis).

C-reactive protein (CRP) test. Detects an abnormal protein (CRP) in the blood during inflammation and tissue destruction. This screening test assists with the diagnosis of bacterial infections, malignancy, heart disease, and arthritis. Some research indicates that the buildup of **plaque** (fatty deposits) on the arterial walls is a result of an inflammatory response.

ABO and Rh blood typing. Determines a patient's blood type and the presence or absence of the Rh factor.

---

body. Those performed in the medical office are for diseases seen most frequently by the physician (Box 2-3). Results are recorded as a reaction (positive) or lack of reaction (negative) to an additive. To be considered positive, the reaction must be viewable and measurable. Viewable reactions include the following:

• *Agglutination.* As discussed earlier in this chapter, agglutination means "clumping." Think of the

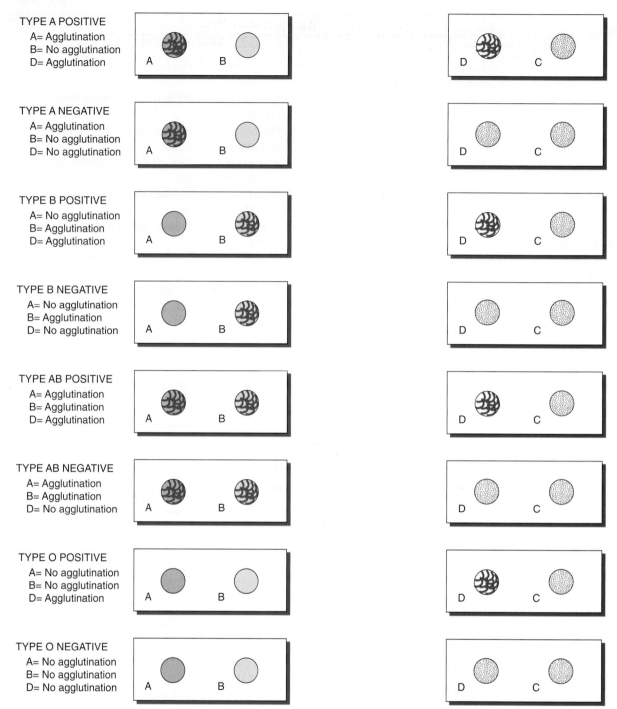

TYPE A POSITIVE
A= Agglutination
B= No agglutination
D= Agglutination

TYPE A NEGATIVE
A= Agglutination
B= No agglutination
D= No agglutination

TYPE B POSITIVE
A= No agglutination
B= Agglutination
D= Agglutination

TYPE B NEGATIVE
A= No agglutination
B= Agglutination
D= No agglutination

TYPE AB POSITIVE
A= Agglutination
B= Agglutination
D= Agglutination

TYPE AB NEGATIVE
A= Agglutination
B= Agglutination
D= No agglutination

TYPE O POSITIVE
A= No agglutination
B= No agglutination
D= Agglutination

TYPE O NEGATIVE
A= No agglutination
B= No agglutination
D= No agglutination

Fig. 2-15 Blood can be tested for blood type by combining a drop of blood with anti-*A,* anti-*B,* and anti-*D* (contains antibodies to Rh factor) solutions. If antigens are present in the blood, agglutination will result. *C* is the control (negative). *(From Hunt SA:* Saunders fundamentals of medical assisting, *Philadelphia, 2002, Saunders.)*

agglutination process as how a magnet attracts items. The antigen is the magnet, and it attracts antibodies to it. Fig. 2-15 illustrates the agglutination process in blood typing.

- *Color change.* The color change technique is based on the use of an enzyme to test specifically for antigen-antibody sensitivity. Fig. 2-16 provides an example of a product insert

used to perform the mononucleosis test on whole blood using the color-change technique.

- *Precipitation* is a visible reaction between the antigen and antibody that produces a solid residue **(precipitates).**
- **Lysis** is the destruction of RBCs caused by an antibody-antigen response.

QuickVue® + Mononucleosis Test

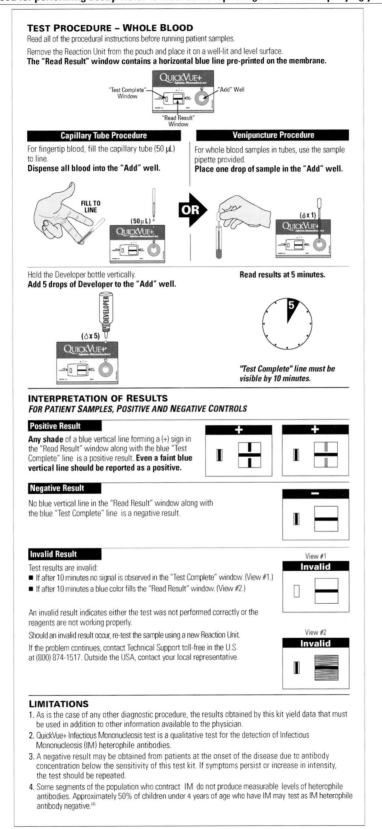

TEST PROCEDURE – WHOLE BLOOD

Read all of the procedural instructions before running patient samples.

Remove the Reaction Unit from the pouch and place it on a well-lit and level surface.
The "Read Result" window contains a horizontal blue line pre-printed on the membrane.

Capillary Tube Procedure	Venipuncture Procedure
For fingertip blood, fill the capillary tube (50 µL) to line. **Dispense all blood into the "Add" well.**	For whole blood samples in tubes, use the sample pipette provided. **Place one drop of sample in the "Add" well.**

OR

Hold the Developer bottle vertically.
Add 5 drops of Developer to the "Add" well.

Read results at 5 minutes.

"Test Complete" line must be visible by 10 minutes.

INTERPRETATION OF RESULTS
FOR PATIENT SAMPLES, POSITIVE AND NEGATIVE CONTROLS

Positive Result

Any shade of a blue vertical line forming a (+) sign in the "Read Result" window along with the blue "Test Complete" line is a positive result. **Even a faint blue vertical line should be reported as a positive.**

Negative Result

No blue vertical line in the "Read Result" window along with the blue "Test Complete" line is a negative result.

Invalid Result

Test results are invalid:
■ If after 10 minutes no signal is observed in the "Test Complete" window. (View #1.)
■ If after 10 minutes a blue color fills the "Read Result" window. (View #2.)

An invalid result indicates either the test was not performed correctly or the reagents are not working properly.

Should an invalid result occur, re-test the sample using a new Reaction Unit.

If the problem continues, contact Technical Support toll-free in the U.S. at (800) 874-1517. Outside the USA, contact your local representative.

LIMITATIONS

1. As is the case of any other diagnostic procedure, the results obtained by this kit yield data that must be used in addition to other information available to the physician.
2. QuickVue+ Infectious Mononucleosis test is a qualitative test for the detection of Infectious Mononucleosis (IM) heterophile antibodies.
3. A negative result may be obtained from patients at the onset of the disease due to antibody concentration below the sensitivity of this test kit. If symptoms persist or increase in intensity, the test should be repeated.
4. Some segments of the population who contract IM do not produce measurable levels of heterophile antibodies. Approximately 50% of children under 4 years of age who have IM may test as IM heterophile antibody negative.[4]

Fig. 2-16 Procedure for performing the QuickVue + Mononucleosis Test. *(Courtesy Quidel, San Diego.)*

Microbiology

Bacteriology is the study of microorganisms, especially pathogenic (disease-producing) organisms. When a physician suspects a particular disease or infection, or wants to identify a microorganism causing an infection, the physician may request that a specimen be collected of a particular substance for microbiological review. The medical assistant or other health care professional may collect body fluids (e.g., urine, blood) or other specimens from the throat, wound, or lungs (sputum). The medical assistant may send these to an outside reference laboratory for processing, or they may be processed in-house by a licensed laboratory technician. The preparation of bacterial smears and Gram staining may be done in the POL. Cultures may also be prepared.

Bacterial Smears

A direct bacterial smear may be taken from the patient using a sterile swab in the POL or may be cultured on an agar plate in an outside laboratory and transferred as a colony (cluster) to a glass slide. The specimen is then dried and stained to assist viewing under the microscope. Procedure 2-10 explains how to prepare a **bacterial smear** from a swab.

Gram Staining

The purpose of the **Gram stain** is to separate bacteria into two groups: gram positive and gram negative. The coloring of the cells of the bacteria allows for easier identification. Gram-positive microorganisms stain purple, and gram-negative microorganisms stain pink-red (Fig. 2-17). Table 2-9 lists and illustrates staining properties of various bacteria. Fig. 2-18 provides instructions for Gram staining.

If the specimen is sent to the laboratory for identification, it is often collected with a sterile swab. After collection, the swab is placed in a tube containing transport medium. This substance keeps the specimen moist until it can be processed (Fig. 2-19).

Cultures

Inoculating a **culture plate** is done (when ordered) to identify which bacteria are causing the infection or which antibiotic to use for treatment. The successful growth of bacteria depends on the correct nutrients and environmental conditions. Most often, the cultures taken in the POL are for group A *Streptococcus* (throat), *E. coli* (urine), and *Staphylococcus* (wound).

Substances that support the growth of microorganisms are called **media.** Media selected could be a broth (liquid), a semisolid, or a solid **(agar)** type.

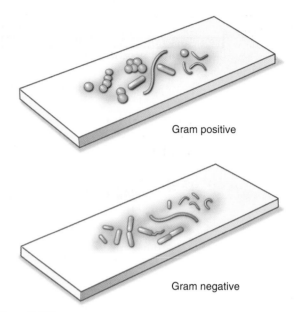

Fig. 2-17 Gram-positive and gram-negative bacteria. *(From Stepp CA, Woods MA:* Laboratory procedures for medical office personnel, *Philadelphia, 1998, Saunders.)*

The agar could be either in a tube or on a Petri dish (culture plate). Some media are specific for particular organisms, whereas others support the growth of all bacteria. Throat cultures are usually cultured on a blood agar medium because this allows the *Streptococcus* bacteria to use the RBCs for growth. Urine cultures are either done on eosin–methylene blue agar or MacConkey agar specific for *E. coli.* Table 2-10 lists common culture media used to identify infectious bacteria.

To inoculate, or **streak,** the culture medium (in an agar plate, swab, or other collection device), the specimen is passed over the medium in a zigzag pattern (Fig. 2-20). After the inoculation is complete, the Petri dish is turned upside down (to discourage condensation) and placed in an incubator for 24 hours at 99° F (37° C). Sometimes, antibiotic disks are placed on the inoculated plate before incubation. With this test, the physician orders a **C&S** (culture and sensitivity) to determine the antibiotic to which the organism is most sensitive (Fig. 2-21).

PATIENT-CENTERED PROFESSIONALISM

- How would the medical assistant explain the function of hematology testing to a patient?
- How would the medical assistant explain liver and cardiac profiles to a patient?
- What are the advantages of point-of-care testing for the patient?

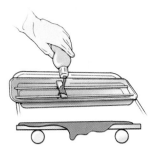

A Pour crystal violet stain onto one end of the slide until the slide is covered.

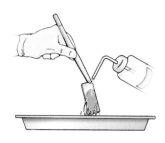

B Lift one end of the slide and rinse gently with distilled or deionized water.

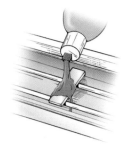

C Flood the slide with iodine solution.

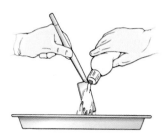

D Hold the slide at an angle and decolorize with an acetone/alcohol mixture.

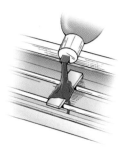

E Flood the slide with safranin.

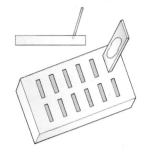

F Drain the slide and air-dry it in a slide dryer.

Fig. 2-18 Gram stain technique. *(From Stepp CA, Woods MA:* Laboratory procedures for medical office personnel, *Philadelphia, 1998, Saunders.)*

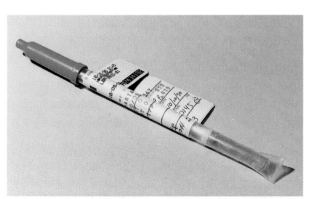

Fig. 2-19 Labeled collection tube to be sent to the laboratory. *(From Stepp CA, Woods MA:* Laboratory procedures for medical office personnel, *Philadelphia, 1998, Saunders.)*

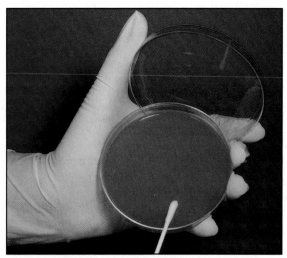

Fig. 2-20 Method for streaking with culture swab. *(From Chester GA:* Modern medical assisting, *Philadelphia, 1998, Saunders.)*

Procedure 2-10 Obtain a Bacterial Smear from a Wound Specimen

TASK: Collect a sample of wound exudates, using sterile collection supplies, without contaminating the specimen. Prepare the specimen for transport to the laboratory.

EQUIPMENT AND SUPPLIES
- Nonsterile disposable gloves
- Personal protective equipment (PPE), as indicated
- Laboratory requisition form
- Plastic-backed paper towel
- Biohazard transport bag
- Sterile gauze (4 × 4 inch)
- Bottle of antiseptic solution
- Surgical tape
- Bandage roll
- Marking pen
- Agar-gel transport system (sterile tube with sterile swab and semisolid solution in the bottom)
- 10% bleach solution
- Biohazardous waste container
- Patient's medical record

SKILLS/RATIONALE

STANDARD PRECAUTIONS ARE TO BE FOLLOWED.

1. **Procedural Step. Sanitize the hands.**
   An alcohol-based hand rub may be used instead of washing hands with soap and water, unless hands are visibly soiled.
   Rationale. Hand sanitization promotes infection control.

2. **Procedural Step. Assemble equipment and sterile supplies and verify the order.**
   Check expiration date on the swab.
   Rationale. It is important to have all supplies and equipment ready and available before starting any procedure to ensure efficiency. Transport medium may dry up and lose its effectiveness past the expiration date.

3. **Procedural Step. Prepare a laboratory requisition form for submitting the specimen to the microbiology department.**

4. **Procedural Step. Greet and identify the patient and escort the patient to the examination room.**
   Rationale. Identifying the patient ensures the procedure is performed on the correct patient.

5. **Procedural Step. Explain the procedure to the patient.**
   Rationale. Explaining the procedure to the patient promotes cooperation and provides a means of obtaining implied consent.

6. **Procedural Step. Apply gloves and PPE as indicated.**

7. **Procedural Step. Position the patient for easiest access to the area from which the specimen will be collected.**

8. **Procedural Step. Remove the patient's old dressing and dispose of it in a biohazardous waste container.**

9. **Procedural Step. Change gloves.**
   Rationale. Clean gloves are necessary when obtaining a specimen to prevent cross-contamination after the dressing is removed.

10. **Procedural Step. Inspect the wound for odor, color, amount of drainage, and depth.**
    Make a mental note of these characteristics for documentation later.

11. **Procedural Step. Obtain the specimen.**
    Carefully remove the sterile swab from the agar-gel tube so that it does not touch the sides of the tube as it is withdrawn. Being careful not to touch surrounding skin or anything other than the inside of the wound, insert the sterile swab into the wound where the drainage is most abundant.

12. **Procedural Step. Move the swab around from side to side.**
    Rationale. This ensures an adequate sample collection that will produce pathogens representative of any that may be causing the infection.

13. **Procedural Step. Carefully return the swab to the tube.**
    Make certain it does not touch the sides or the opening of the tube. Firmly slide the swab into

Procedure 2-10 Obtain a Bacterial Smear from a Wound Specimen—cont'd

the agar-gel so that the entire swab is suspended in the transport medium. If the transport medium is encapsulated, crush the ampule to moisten the swab to keep it in optimal condition during transport.

14. **Procedural Step. Label the specimen.**
Indicate the patient's name, identification number, date and time of collection, tests requested, site of collection, and physician's name. If you are using a computer system that generates a label, apply the label to the specimen instead.

15. **Procedural Step. Place the agar-gel transport tube in a biohazard transport bag and seal the bag.**

16. **Procedural Step. Apply a clean bandage to the wound site.**

17. **Procedural Step. Dispose of all waste material appropriately, and disinfect the work area using 10% bleach solution.**

18. **Procedural Step. Remove gloves and sanitize the hands.**
Always sanitize the hands after every procedure or after using gloves.

19. **Procedural Step. Complete the laboratory requisition form and transport the specimen as soon as possible to the laboratory.**

20. **Procedural Step. Document the procedure.**
Include date and time of the procedure and condition of the wound.

Charting Example

Date	
1/20/xx	11:45 a.m. Lesion Ⓛ ankle. Copious amounts of purulent discharge. Specimen obtained and sent to lab for culture. ———————————————— K. Contrea, CMA (AAMA)

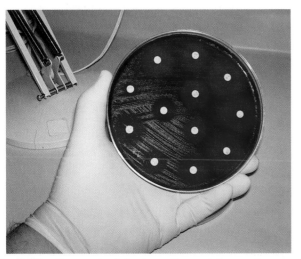

Fig. 2-21 Zones of inhibition of bacterial growth around sensitivity disks. The greenish lines are bacterial colonies. *(From Stepp CA, Woods MA:* Laboratory procedures for medical office personnel, *Philadelphia, 1998, Saunders.)*

〰 CONCLUSION

The purpose of any laboratory testing is to aid the physician in diagnosis, treatment, or maintenance of the patient's current health status. All laboratory-testing procedures must follow established guidelines in order for the results to be considered valid. Medical assistants need to be aware of the types of CLIA-waived tests and procedures because these can be performed in physician offices. Even though these tests have a minimal risk for error, they must be performed carefully to produce results that will be helpful to the physician.

SUMMARY

Reinforce your understanding of the material in this chapter by reviewing the curriculum objectives and key content points below.

1. Define, appropriately use, and spell all the Key Terms for this chapter.
   • Review the Key Terms if necessary.
2. Explain what causes urine's color and what causes urine to have an abnormal color.
   • Urochrome is the yellow pigment derived from urobilin in urine; it is left over when hemoglobin breaks down.
   • Fluid intake, medications, and waste products from a disease process can cause urine to have an abnormal color.
3. Describe the normal appearance of urine, and explain what causes urine to have an abnormal appearance.
   • Normal urine should appear clear or transparent.
   • Crystals, change of pH, blood cells, bacteria, and other substances can cause urine to have an abnormal appearance.

TABLE 2-9	Identification of Bacteria Using Staining Techniques

Shape	Arrangement	Reaction	Appearance	Genus/Species
Sphere (Diplococci)	Pairs and singles	Gram positive		Enterococcus species
		Gram negative		Neisseria gonorrhoeae
Sphere (Streptococci)	Chains	Gram positive		Streptococcus pyogenes
Sphere (Staphylococci)	Clusters	Gram positive		Staphylococcus aureus
Rod (Bacilli)	Singles and chains	Gram positive		Bacillus anthracis Clostridium tetani
		Gram negative		Escherichia coli
		Acid fast		Haemophilus influenzae Pseudomonas aeruginosa Mycobacterium tuberculosis, M. leprae
Spiral (Spirilla)		Gram negative		Treponema pallidum

From Hunt SA: *Saunders fundamentals of medical assisting,* Philadelphia, 2002, Saunders.

4. Explain why various odors occur in urine.
   • An ammonia smell is the result of bacteria breaking down urea in a specimen.
   • Foods can also produce odor in urine.
   • Odor can also be caused by bacteria, uncontrolled diabetes, and infection.
5. List two causes of low urinary output and three causes of high urinary output.
   • Low urinary output can be caused by low fluid intake or excessive fluid loss through diarrhea, vomiting, or sweating.
   • High urinary output can be caused by high fluid intake, reduced secretion of ADH, and uncontrolled diabetes.

6. State two testing differences between a reagent strip and a reagent tablet.
   • Reagent strips detect the presence and amount of substances; reagent tablets detect only the presence of substances, not the amount.
   • Reagent tablets test for only one substance; reagent strips detect the presence of one or several substances.
7. Demonstrate the correct procedure for processing a urine specimen using a reagent technique.
   • Review Procedure 2-1.
8. List 10 tests performed during a routine urinalysis.

TABLE 2-10   Primary Plating Media Typically Used in Culture Growths to Identify Infectious Bacteria

Medium	Form Used	Expected Isolates	Comments
Anaerobic CDC blood agar *(Brucella)* (BRUC, BRU)	Plate	All types of aerobic and anaerobic and gm(+) and gm(−) bacteria	Supports growth of all strict anaerobic and facultatively anaerobic bacteria
Anaerobic colistin–nalidixic acid agar (ANA-CAN, CNA)	Plate and biplate	Growth of most gm(+) and gm(−) anaerobes; inhibits facultatively anaerobic gm(−) bacteria	
Anaerobic kanamycin–bile-esculin agar (KBE)	Plate and biplate	*Bacteroides fragilis* group	Provides presumptive identification of *B. fragilis* group
Anaerobic kanamycin-vancomycin laked blood agar (KVLB, LKV)	Plate	*Bacteroides* species; pigmented anaerobic gm(−) rods, or *F. mortiferum*	Yeasts and kanamycin-resistant gm(−) bacilli may grow on this medium
Chocolate/modified Thayer-Martin agar (CHOC/MTM)	Biplate	CHOC: *Haemophilus influenzae, Neisseria gonorrhoeae, N. meningitides* MTM: *N. gonorrhoeae, N. meningitidis*	CHOC: see Chocolate agar MTM: vancomycin inhibits gm(+) and colistin gm(−) bacteria; nystatin inhibits yeast
Blood agar (BAP)	Plate	Both gm(+) and gm(−) organisms	
Chocolate agar (CHOC)	Plate	*H. influenzae, N. meningitidis*	Low agar content provides increased moisture
Hektoen enteric agar (HE)	Plate	*Salmonella* and *Shigella* species	Has lactose, sucrose, and salicin, and most Enterobacteriaceae ferment one of these Detects H$_2$S
Löwenstein-Jensen agar (LJ)	Slant	Isolation of acid-fast bacilli	
MacConkey agar (MAC)	Plate	Gm(−) enteric bacilli	Bile salts inhibit gm(+) organisms
Streptococcus selective agar (SXT)	Plate	Isolation of beta-hemolytic streptococci	Most gm(−) organisms are inhibited

Source: Stepp CA, Woods MA: *Laboratory procedures for medical office personnel,* Philadelphia, 1998, Saunders. *gm*(+), gram-positive; *gm*(−), gram-negative; H$_2$S, hydrogen sulfide.

- Glucose, bilirubin, ketones, specific gravity, blood, pH, protein, urobilinogen, nitrites, and leukocytes are tested for during a routine urinalysis.
9. Explain how an automated urine analyzer processes reagent test strips.
   - The automated urine analyzer eliminates the human error factor by using light photometry to analyze a reagent test strip.
10. List three brands of reagent tablets and their use in confirmatory tests.

- Clinitest reagent tablets confirm the presence of glucose.
- Acetest tablets confirm ketones.
- Ictotest tablets confirm bilirubin.
11. Explain why microscopic examination of urine sediment may be done.
    - Casts, crystals, and other solids can be identified only by microscopic examination.
12. Demonstrate the correct procedure for microscopic examination of urine.
    - Review Procedure 2-2.

13. List seven types of structures typically found in urine.
    - Red blood cells, white blood cells, epithelial cells, casts, crystals, artifacts, and other substances (e.g., bacteria, yeast, mucous threads, spermatozoa, parasites) can be found in urine.
14. Demonstrate the correct procedure for performing a urine pregnancy color-reaction test.
    - Review Procedure 2-3.
15. Differentiate among hematology, serology, blood chemistry, and microbiology.
    - Hematology is the study of blood cell–forming tissues and coagulation factors.
    - Serology is the study of antigen and antibody reactions in blood serum.
    - Blood chemistry is the complete quantitative analysis of the chemical composition of the blood.
    - Microbiology is the study of all microorganisms in the blood (bacteriology focuses on bacteria).
16. State the purpose of a complete blood count (CBC) and list six types of information it provides.
    - A CBC indicates the number of blood cells present in a volume of blood.
    - The CBC measures blood cell counts, hemoglobin, hematocrit, and reticulocytes; generates a differential of white blood cell types; and measures the size and shape of the cells.
17. State the purpose of measuring hemoglobin and list one automated device approved by CLIA for this use in the physician office laboratory (POL).
    - Hemoglobin measurement is used to detect blood loss and anemias.
    - HemoCue is an automated device approved by CLIA for use in the POL for analyzing hemoglobin.
18. Demonstrate the correct procedure for obtaining a hemoglobin reading.
    - Review Procedure 2-4.
19. Explain the purpose of a hematocrit and what a low reading and a high reading may indicate.
    - Hematocrit (Hct) is a measurement of the percentage of packed blood cells in a volume of whole blood.
    - A low Hct reading may indicate anemia; a high Hct reading could be the result of polycythemia.
20. Demonstrate the correct procedure for obtaining an accurate hematocrit value.
    - Review Procedure 2-5.

21. Explain the purpose of the erythrocyte sedimentation rate (ESR) and list two common methods used in the POL to perform ESR.
    - ESR confirms an inflammation is present somewhere in the body; it measures how quickly red blood cells settle in a tube.
    - The Westergren and Wintrobe tube methods are commonly used in the POL.
22. Demonstrate the correct procedure for performing ESR using the Westergren method.
    - Review Procedure 2-6.
23. Explain the purpose of a differential blood cell count, and list five factors that affect the quality of a good blood smear.
    - The differential blood cell count ("diff") is a test that differentiates white blood cells, observes the shape of red blood cells, and estimates the number of platelets.
    - Size of the drop of blood, angle of the pusher slide, pressure, speed, and viscosity affect the quality of the smear.
24. Demonstrate the correct procedure for preparation of a blood smear slide.
    - Review Procedure 2-7.
25. Explain how physicians use blood chemistry profiles.
    - Blood chemistry profiles give the physician information about the patient's general state of health.
    - Blood profiles can be ordered to address particular body systems.
26. Explain the purpose of cholesterol testing and list the desirable, borderline-high, and high cholesterol levels in test results.
    - Cholesterol is screened because high levels of blood cholesterol are related to heart disease.
    - Cholesterol is also used to monitor liver and thyroid function.
    - Desirable cholesterol level: less than 200 mg/dL; borderline-high level: 200 to 240 mg/dL; high level: greater than 240 mg/dL.
27. Demonstrate the procedure for accurately collecting and processing a blood specimen for cholesterol testing.
    - Review Procedure 2-8.
28. Describe three tests performed to monitor a person's glucose level.
    - Fasting blood sugar (FBS) test measures glucose level in a blood sample. The patient refrains from eating and drinking (except water) for at least 12 hours before testing. A blood sample is drawn, tested, and compared to normal range of 70 to 110 mg/dL of glucose.
    - Two-hour postprandial test is used to screen for diabetes mellitus and to monitor the

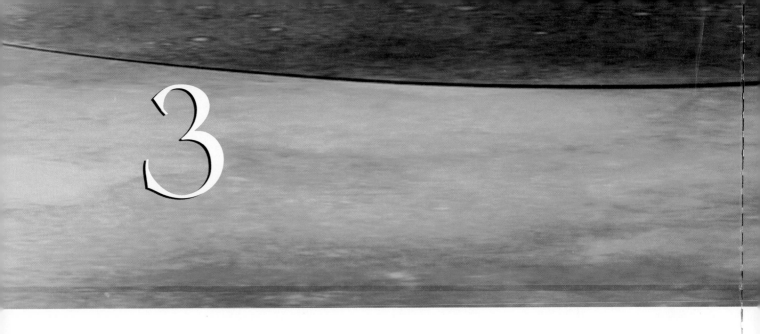

3

"What is man, when you come to think about him, but a minutely set, ingenious machine for turning with infinite artfulness, the red wine of Shiraz into urine?"
—Isak Dinesen

OBJECTIVES

1. Recognize and use terms related to the anatomy and physiology of the urinary system.
2. Recognize and use terms related to the pathology of the urinary system.
3. Recognize and use terms related to the diagnostic procedures for the urinary system.
4. Recognize and use terms related to the therapeutic interventions for the urinary system.

MEDICAL TERMINOLOGY OF THE URINARY SYSTEM

CHAPTER AT A GLANCE

ANATOMY AND PHYSIOLOGY

bladder	nephron	urethra
hilum	renal pelvis	urinary meatus
kidneys	trigone	urination
micturition	ureters	voiding

KEY WORD PARTS

PREFIXES	SUFFIXES	COMBINING FORMS
an-	-cele	azot/o
dys-	-dipsia	cyst/o
poly-	-graphy	gluc/o, glyc/o
	-pexy	kal/i
	-ptosis	lith/o
	-scope	natr/o
	-scopy	nephr/o
	-tripsy	pyel/o
	-uria	ren/o
		ureter/o
		urethr/o
		urin/o, ur/o
		vesic/o

KEY TERMS

catheter	dysuria	polydipsia	urination
cystocele	hemodialysis	polyuria	vesicoureteral reflux
cystoscope	incontinence	pyelonephritis	voiding
diabetes insipidus	lithotripsy	retention	voiding cystourethrography
diabetes mellitus	micturition	urgency	
diuresis	nephrolithotomy	urinalysis	

BE CAREFUL!

-uria is a suffix that means a condition of the urine; *urea* is a chemical waste product.

FUNCTIONS OF THE URINARY SYSTEM

The major function of the urinary system is to continually maintain a healthy balance of the amount and content of **extracellular fluids** within the body. Biologists use the term *homeostasis* to describe this important process. The process of metabolism changes food and liquid (with its requisite fats, carbohydrates, and proteins) into building blocks, energy sources, and waste products. To operate efficiently, the body needs to monitor and rebalance the amounts of these substances constantly in the bloodstream. The breakdown of proteins and amino acids in the liver leaves chemical wastes, such as urea, creatinine, and uric acid, in the bloodstream. These wastes are toxic nitrogenous substances that must be excreted in the urine. The act of releasing urine is called **urination, voiding,** or **micturition** (mick ter RIH shun).

Succinctly phrased by Homer William Smith in 1939, "It is no exaggeration to say that the composition of the blood is determined not by what the mouth ingests but by what the kidneys keep; they are the master chemists of our internal environment, which, so to speak, they synthesize in reverse."

COMBINING FORMS FOR THE URINARY SYSTEM	
MEANING	**COMBINING FORM**
cell	cellul/o, cyt/o
scanty, few	olig/o
same	home/o
urine, urinary system	ur/o, urin/o

PREFIXES AND SUFFIXES FOR THE URINARY SYSTEM	
PREFIX/SUFFIX	**MEANING**
extra-	outside
-stasis	controlling, stabilizing
-uria	condition of the urine

◇ Exercise 3-1: FUNCTIONS OF THE URINARY SYSTEM

Circle the correct term.

1. Through the process of *(homeostasis, deglutition)* the body monitors the *(intracellular, extracellular)* fluid and removes the waste products of *(carbohydrates, proteins)* from the body called *(uria, urea)*, creatinine, and uric acid. The process of *(forming, excreting)* urine is termed *urination.*

ANATOMY AND PHYSIOLOGY

The urinary system is composed of two kidneys, two ureters, a urinary bladder, and a urethra (Figs. 3-1 and 3-2). The work of the urinary system is done by a specialized tissue in the **kidneys** called **parenchymal** (pair EN kuh mul) **tissue.** The **ureters** (YOOR eh turs) are thin, muscular tubes that move urine in peristaltic waves from the kidneys to the bladder. The urinary **bladder** is the sac that stores the urine until it is excreted, and the **urethra** (yoo REE thrah) is the tube that conducts the urine out of the body. The opening of the urethra is called the **urinary meatus** (YOOR in nair ee mee ATE us). The triangular area in the bladder between the ureters' entrance and the urethral outlet is called the **trigone** (TRY gohn). The ureters, bladder, and urethra are all **stromal** (STROH mul) **tissue,** which is a supportive tissue.

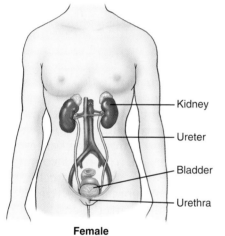

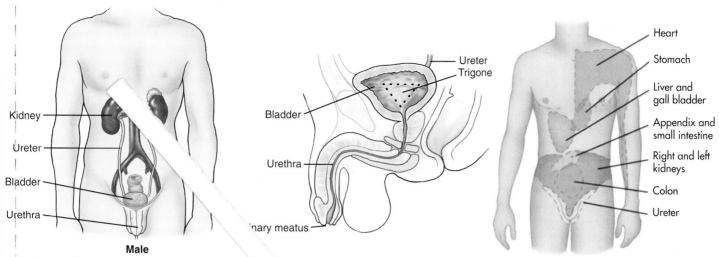

Fig. 3-1 Male urinary system. Areas of pain radiation. *(From Patton KT, Thibodeau GA: Anatomy & Physiology, ed 7, St. Louis, 2010, Mosby.)*

Fig. 3-2 Female urinary system.

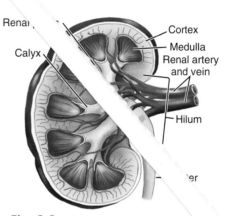

Fig. 3-3 Cross section of a kidney.

⊗ **BE CAREFUL!**

Calic/o and *cali/o* are the combining forms for calyx, but *calc/o* is the combining form for calcium.

⊗ **BE CAREFUL!**

It is easy to confuse the combining forms *perone/o*, which means fibula; *perine/o*, which means the space between external genitalia and the anus; and *periton*, which means the abdominal lining.

The Kidney

Because the kidneys are primarily responsible for the functioning of the urinary system, it is helpful to look at them in more detail. Each of the two kidneys is located high in the abdominal cavity, tucked under the ribs in the back and behind the lining of the abdominal cavity (retroperitoneal). The normal human kidney is about the size of a fist. If a kidney were sliced open, the outer portion, the **cortex** (KORE tecks) (*pl.* cortices), and the inner portion, called the **medulla** (muh DOO lah) (*pl.* medullae), would be visible (Fig. 3-3). The **renal pelvis** and **calyces** (KAL ih seez) (*sing.* calyx) are an extension of the ureter inside of the kidney. The term **renal** means *pertaining to the kidneys.*

The **hilum** (HYE lum) (*pl.* hila) is the location on the kidney where the ureter and renal vein leave the kidney and the renal artery enters. The cortex contains tissue with millions of microscopic units called **nephrons** (NEFF rons) (Fig. 3-4). Here in the tiny nephrons, blood passes through a continuous system of urinary filtration, reabsorption, and secretion that measures, monitors, and adjusts the levels of substances in the extracellular fluid.

The Nephron

The nephrons filter all of the blood in the body approximately every 5 minutes. The **renal afferent arteries** transport unfiltered blood to the kidneys. Once

DID YOU KNOW?

The term *gross* in *gross anatomy* refers to those structures that can be seen with the naked eye as opposed to a microscope.

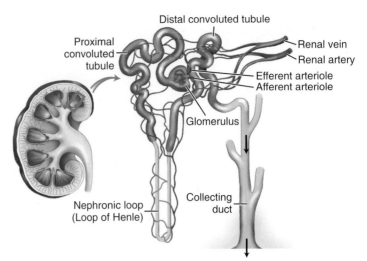

Fig. 3-4 The nephron.

in the kidneys, the blood travels through small arteries called **arterioles** (ar TEER ree ohls) and finally into tiny balls of renal capillaries, called **glomeruli** (gloh MER yoo lye) (*sing.* glomerulus). These glomeruli cluster at the entrance to each nephron. It is here that the process of filtering the blood to form urine begins.

The nephron consists of four parts: (1) the **renal corpuscle** (KORE pus sul), which is composed of the glomerulus and its surrounding Bowman's capsule; (2) a **proximal convoluted tubule;** (3) the **nephronic loop,** also known as the loop of Henle; and (4) the **distal convoluted tubule.** As blood flows through the capillaries, water, electrolytes, glucose, and nitrogenous wastes are passed through the glomerular membrane and collected. The most common electrolytes are sodium (Na), chloride (Cl), and potassium (K). Blood cells and proteins are too large to pass through the glomerular membrane. Selective filtration and reabsorption continues along the renal tubules, with the end result of urine concentration and subsequent dilution occurring in the renal medulla. From there, the urine flows to the calyces and exits the kidney, flowing through the ureter into the bladder, where it is stored until it can be expelled from the body through the urethra.

COMBINING FORMS FOR ANATOMY AND PHYSIOLOGY

MEANING	COMBINING FORM	MEANING	COMBINING FORM
calyx	calic/o, cali/o	peritoneum	peritone/o
chloride	chlor/o	potassium	potassi/o, kal/i
cortex	cortic/o	renal pelvis	pyel/o
glomerulus	glomerul/o	sodium	natr/o
hilum	hil/o	trigone	trigon/o
kidney	nephr/o, ren/o	ureter	ureter/o
meatus	meat/o	urethra	urethr/o
medulla	medull/o	urinary bladder	cyst/o, vesic/o

◈ Exercise 3-2: THE URINARY SYSTEM

Match the combining form with its term.

_____ 1. opening of the urethra

_____ 2. tubes connecting kidneys and bladder

_____ 3. tube conducting urine out of the bladder

_____ 4. same as ren/o

_____ 5. sac that stores urine

_____ 6. area between ureters coming in and urethra going out in the sac that stores urine

_____ 7. urine, urinary system

_____ 8. renal pelvis

_____ 9. outer portion of the kidney

_____ 10. inner portion of the kidney

_____ 11. artery

_____ 12. renal calyx

_____ 13. location where ureter and renal vein leave kidney and renal artery enters

A. nephr/o
B. ur/o, urin/o
C. meat/o
D. urethr/o
E. cyst/o, vesic/o
F. ureter/o
G. trigon/o
H. medull/o
I. calic/o, cali/o
J. cortic/o
K. hil/o
L. pyel/o
M. arteri/o

Circle the correct term.

14. The basic working unit of the kidney is the *(hilum, nephron)*.
15. The nephron is located in the *(cortex, medulla)* of the kidney.
16. The name of the ball of capillaries within the nephron is the *(calyces, glomerulus)*.
17. The capsule that surrounds these capillaries is called *(Bowman, Henle)* capsule.
18. Blood is carried to the nephron through the *(afferent, efferent)* arteriole.
19. *(Water and electrolytes, Blood and proteins)* are normally too large to pass through the glomerular membrane into its surrounding capsule.
20. Place the following terms in order, showing the normal direction of the flow of urine from structures within the kidney to when it leaves the body.

ureter, renal pelvis, urinary meatus, renal cortex, urethra, urinary bladder, renal medulla

_____→_____→_____→_____→_____→_____→

_____→_____

〜 PATHOLOGY

Terms Related to Urinary Conditions Ending in -uria

TERM	WORD ORIGIN	DEFINITION
Albuminuria al byoo mih NOOR ee ah	*albumin/o* protein *-uria* urinary condition	Albumin (a protein) in the urine. Also called **proteinuria** (pro teen NOOR ee ah).
Anuria A NOOR ee ah	*an-* without *-uria* urinary condition	Condition of no urine. Also called anuresis.
Azoturia a zoh TOOR ee ah	*azot/o* nitrogen *-uria* urinary condition	Excessive nitrogenous compounds, including urea, in the urine.
Bacteriuria back tur ee YOOR ee ah	*bacteri/o* bacteria *-uria* urinary condition	Bacteria in the urine.

Continued

Terms Related to Urinary Conditions Ending in -uria—cont'd

TERM	WORD ORIGIN	DEFINITION
Dysuria dis YOOR ee ah	*dys-* painful, abnormal *-uria* urinary condition	Condition of painful urination.
Glycosuria gly kohs YOOR ee ah	*glyc/o* sugar *-uria* urinary condition	Sugar in the urine.
Hematuria hee mah TOOR ee ah	*hemat/o* blood *-uria* urinary condition	Blood in the urine.
Nocturia nock TOOR ee ah	*noct/i* night *-uria* urinary condition	Condition of excessive urination at night.
Oliguria ah lig GYOOR ee ah	*olig/o* scanty, few *-uria* urinary condition	Condition of scanty urination.
Polyuria pah lee YOOR ee ah	*poly-* profuse, excessive *-uria* urinary condition	Condition of excessive urination.
Pyuria pye YOOR ee ah	*py/o* pus *-uria* urinary condition	Pus in the urine.

Terms Related to Urinary Signs

TERM	WORD ORIGIN	DEFINITION
Abscess AB ses		Cavity containing pus and surrounded by inflamed tissue.
Azotemia a zoh TEE mee ah	*azot/o* nitrogen *-emia* blood condition	Condition of excessive urea in the blood. Also called uremia.
Diuresis dye yoor EE sis	*di-* through, complete *ur/o* urine *-esis* state of	Condition of increased formation and excretion of urine, of large volumes of urine. Caffeine and alcohol are **diuretics** (dye yoor RET icks)—that is, they increase the amount of urine produced.
Edema eh DEE mah		Accumulation of fluid in the tissues; can result from kidney failure.
Enuresis en yoor EE sis	*en-* in *ur/o* urine *-esis* state of	Also commonly known as "bed-wetting," enuresis can be **nocturnal** (at night) or **diurnal** (during the day).
Hypertension hye pur TEN shun	*hyper-* excessive	Condition of high blood pressure.
Incontinence in KON tih nense		Inability to hold urine.
Polydipsia pah lee DIP see ah	*poly-* excessive, many *-dipsia* thirst	Condition of excessive thirst (usually accompanied by polyuria).
Retention		Inability to release urine.
Urgency		Intense sensation of the need to urinate immediately.

Exercise 3-3: URINARY CONDITIONS AND SIGNS

Matching.

_____ 1. pus in the urine   _____ 6. excessive urea in the urine

_____ 2. no urine   _____ 7. scanty urine

_____ 3. blood in the urine   _____ 8. protein in the urine

_____ 4. profuse urine   _____ 9. painful urination

_____ 5. bacteria in the urine   _____ 10. sugar in the urine

A. dysuria
B. polyuria
C. oliguria
D. glycosuria
E. azoturia
F. pyuria
G. albuminuria
H. hematuria
I. anuria
J. bacteriuria

⌧ BE CAREFUL!

Py/o means pus, and *pyel/o* means renal pelvis. A dilation of the renal pelvis caused by an accumulation of pus would be pyopyelectasis.

Circle the correct term.

11. Urinary *(incontinence, retention)* is the inability to release urine.
12. If a patient complains of an accumulation of fluid around her ankles, she may be exhibiting *(urgency, edema)*.
13. A patient with a renal *(abscess, diuresis)* has a cavity containing pus and surrounded by inflamed tissue in the kidneys.
14. A sign of kidney failure may be excessive urea in the blood, called *(anuria, azotemia)*.
15. A concerned parent calls in to discuss her 4-year-old son's inability to remain dry during the night. This bed-wetting may be diagnosed as *(oliguria, enuresis)*.
16. Caffeine and alcohol are substances that cause an increase in the volume of fluids excreted from the body. They effect a/an *(enuresis, diuresis)*.
17. A feeling of a need to urinate immediately is called *(urgency, incontinence)*.
18. The elderly gentleman was seen by his physician because he was unable to control his urination. He was suffering from urinary *(incontinence, retention)*.

DID YOU KNOW?

The term *diabetes* comes from the Greek word meaning to pass through, and an excessive production of urine is a symptom in both forms of diabetes. Insipidus refers to the "tasteless" nature of the urine of people with this disorder. Mellitus comes from the Latin word for honey.

Terms Related to Urinary System Disorders, Stones, and Diabetes

TERM	WORD ORIGIN	DEFINITION
Diabetes insipidus (DI) dye ah BEE teez in SIP ih dus	See **Did You Know?** box	Deficiency of antidiuretic (ADH) hormone, which causes the patient to excrete large quantities of urine **(polyuria)** and exhibit excessive thirst **(polydipsia)**.
Diabetes mellitus (DM) dye ah BEE teez meh LYE tus	See **Did You Know?** box	Metabolic disease caused by an absolute or relative deficiency of insulin and characterized by hyperglycemia, glycosuria, water and electrolyte loss, ketoacidosis, and possible eventual coma.
Polycystic kidney disease pah lee SIS tick	*poly-* many *cyst/o* sac *-ic* pertaining to	Inherited disorder characterized by an enlargement of the kidneys caused by many renal cysts bilaterally that reduce functioning of renal tissue (Fig. 3-5).

Continued

Terms Related to Urinary System Disorders, Stones, and Diabetes—cont'd

TERM	WORD ORIGIN	DEFINITION
Renal colic REE nul KAH lick	*ren/o* kidney *-al* pertaining to	Severe pain associated with stones lodged in the ureter.
Urolithiasis yoo roo lih THIGH uh sis	*ur/o* urine *lith/o* stones *-iasis* condition, presence of	Stones anywhere in the urinary tract, but usually in the renal pelvis or urinary bladder. Usually formed in patients with an excess of the mineral calcium. Also called **urinary calculi** (KAL kyoo lye) (Fig. 3-6).
Urinary tract infection (UTI)		Infection anywhere in the urinary system, caused most commonly by bacteria but also by parasites, yeast, and protozoa (*sing.* protozoon). Most frequently occurring disorder in the urinary system.

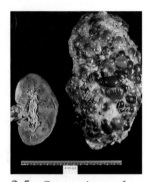

Fig. 3-5 Comparison of a polycystic kidney *(right)* with a normal kidney *(left)*. (*From Lewis SM: Medical-surgical nursing: assessment and management of clinical problems, ed 6, St Louis, 2005, Mosby.*)

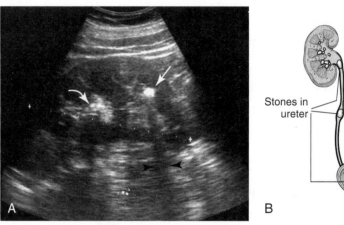

Fig. 3-6 A, Ultrasound of stones in the renal pelvis. **B,** Locations of ureteral calculi. (***A** from O'Neill WC: Atlas of renal ultrasonography, Philadelphia, 2001, Saunders; **B** from Frazier MS, Drzymkowski JW: Essentials of human diseases, ed 3, Philadelphia, 2004, Saunders.*)

◆ Exercise 3-4: URINARY DISORDERS, STONES, AND DIABETES

Matching.

_____ 1. inherited congenital disorder of the kidneys

_____ 2. pain caused by a stone lodged in the ureter

_____ 3. disease caused by deficiency of insulin

_____ 4. infection anywhere in the urinary system

_____ 5. deficiency of antidiuretic hormone

_____ 6. stones in the urinary tract

_____ 7. excessive thirst

A. urolithiasis
B. polydipsia
C. polycystic kidney disease
D. diabetes mellitus
E. urinary tract infection
F. renal colic
G. diabetes insipidus

8. Build terms for the following conditions:

A. stones in the kidney _____   C. stones in the bladder _____

B. stones in the ureter _____   D. stones in the urethra _____

Terms Related to Kidney Disorders

Term	Word Origin	Definition
Glomerulonephritis gloh MUR yoo loh neh FRY tis	*glomerul/o* glomerulus *nephr/o* kidney *-itis* inflammation	Inflammation of the glomeruli of the kidney characterized by proteinuria, hematuria, decreased urine production, and edema.
Hydronephrosis hye droh neh FROH sis	*hydro-* water *nephr/o* kidney *-osis* abnormal condition	Dilation of the renal pelvis and calices of one or both kidneys resulting from the obstruction of the flow of urine.
Nephritic syndrome neh FRIH tick	*nephr/o* kidney *-itic* pertaining to *syn-* together *-drome* to run	Group of signs and symptoms of a urinary tract disorder, including hematuria, hypertension, and renal failure.
Nephritis neh FRY tis	*nephr/o* kidney *-itis* inflammation	Inflammation of the kidney; a general term that does not specify the location of the inflammation or its cause.
Nephropathy neh FROP ah thee	*nephr/o* kidney *-pathy* disease	Disease of the kidneys; a general term that does not specify a disorder.
Nephroptosis neh frop TOH sis	*nephr/o* kidney *-ptosis* drooping, prolapse	Prolapse or sagging of the kidney.
Nephrotic syndrome neh FRAH tick	*nephr/o* kidney *-tic* pertaining to	Abnormal group of symptoms in the kidney, characterized by proteinuria, hypoalbuminemia, and edema; may occur in glomerular disease and as a complication of many systemic diseases (e.g., diabetes mellitus). Also called **nephrosis** (neh FROH sis).
Pyelonephritis pye uh loh neh FRY tis	*pyel/o* renal pelvis *nephr/o* kidney *-itis* inflammation	Infection of the renal pelvis and parenchyma of the kidney, usually the result of lower urinary tract infection.
Renal failure	*ren/o* kidney *-al* pertaining to	Inability of the kidneys to excrete wastes, concentrate urine, and conserve electrolytes. May be acute or chronic.
Acute renal failure (ARF)		Sudden inability of the kidneys to excrete wastes, resulting from hemorrhage, trauma, burns, toxic injury to the kidney, pyelonephritis or glomerulonephritis, or lower urinary tract obstruction. Characterized by oliguria and rapid azotemia.
Chronic renal failure (CRF)		Long-term inability of the kidney to excrete wastes.
Renal hypertension	*ren/o* kidney *-al* pertaining to *hyper-* excessive *-tension* pressure	High blood pressure secondary to kidney disease.
Renal sclerosis REE nul sklih ROH sis	*ren/o* kidney *-al* pertaining to *sclerosis* a hardening	Hardening of the arteries of the kidneys. Also known as **nephrosclerosis** (neh froh sklih ROH sis).

Terms Related to Bladder, Ureter, and Urethra Disorders

TERM	WORD ORIGIN	DEFINITION
Cystitis sis TYE tis	*cyst/o* urinary bladder *-itis* inflammation	Inflammation of the urinary bladder.
Cystocele SIS toh seel	*cyst/o* urinary bladder *-cele* herniation	Herniation of the urinary bladder (Fig. 3-7).
Ureterocele yoo REE tur oh seel	*ureter/o* ureter *-cele* herniation	Prolapse of the terminal end of the ureter into the bladder.
Urethral stenosis yoo REE thruhl sten NOH sis	*urethr/o* urethra *-al* pertaining to *stenosis* a narrowing	Narrowing of the urethra. Also called a **urethral stricture.**
Urethritis yoo ree THRY tis	*urethr/o* urethra *-itis* inflammation	Inflammation of the urethra.
Vesicoureteral reflux ves ih koh yoo REE tur ul REE flucks	*vesic/o* urinary bladder *ureter/o* ureter *-al* pertaining to *re-* back *-flux* flow	Abnormal backflow of urine from the bladder to the ureter.

DID YOU KNOW?

Secondary hypertension is hypertension caused by another disorder; if the hypertension is without known cause, then it is called essential hypertension.

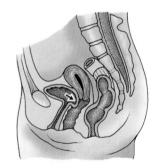

Fig. 3-7 Cystocele. The urinary bladder is displaced downward, which causes bulging of the anterior vaginal wall. *(From Ignatavicius DD, Workman ML:* Medical-surgical nursing: critical thinking for collaborative care, *ed 5, Philadelphia, 2005, Saunders.)*

◈ Exercise 3-5: KIDNEY, URETER, BLADDER, AND URETHRAL DISORDERS

Matching.

_____ 1. -ptosis

_____ 2. hydro-

_____ 3. acute

_____ 4. chronic

_____ 5. syndrome

_____ 6. -cele

A. group of signs/symptoms with a common cause
B. long term
C. prolapse
D. herniation
E. water
F. sudden, severe

Matching.

_____ 7. inability of the kidneys to excrete wastes

_____ 8. a hardening of the arteries of the kidneys

_____ 9. prolapse of the kidney

_____ 10. inflammation of the renal parenchyma and the renal pelvis

_____ 11. disease of the kidney

_____ 12. inflammation of the kidney

_____ 13. hypertension, renal failure, and hematuria characterize this syndrome

_____ 14. inflammation of the capillaries within the renal corpuscles

_____ 15. inflammation of the tube leading from the bladder to the outside of the body

_____ 16. inflammation of the bladder

_____ 17. herniation of the tube from the kidney to the bladder

_____ 18. backward flow of urine from the bladder toward the kidney

A. glomerulitis
B. cystitis
C. nephritis
D. nephroptosis

E. vesicoureteral reflux
F. urethritis
G. pyelonephritis
H. nephritic syndrome

I. nephrosclerosis
J. nephropathy
K. ureterocele
L. renal failure

Terms Related to Benign Neoplasms

TERM	WORD ORIGIN	DEFINITION
Renal adenoma	*ren/o* kidney *-al* pertaining to *aden/o* gland *-oma* tumor	Small, slow-growing noncancerous tumors of the kidney, usually found at autopsy.
Renal oncocytoma	*onc/o* tumor *cyt/o* cell *-oma* tumor	The most common benign solid renal tumor.
Transitional cell papilloma	*papill/o* nipple *-oma* tumor	Also referred to as bladder papilloma. Although this type of tumor is benign when found, recurrences are occasionally malignant.

Terms Related to Malignant Neoplasms

TERM	WORD ORIGIN	DEFINITION
Renal cell carcinoma	*ren/o* kidney *-al* pertaining to *carcin/o* cancerous tumor of epithelial origin *-oma* tumor	Also referred to as hypernephroma or adenocarcinoma of the kidney, this is the tenth most common cancer. Although the cause is unknown, risk factors include smoking and obesity.
Nephroblastoma	*nephr/o* kidney *blast/o* embryonic *-oma* tumor	Also called Wilms tumor, these tumors develop from kidney cells that did not develop fully before a child's birth. These cancerous tumors of the kidney occur mainly in children.
Transitional cell carcinoma (TCC) of the bladder	*carcin/o* cancerous tumor of epithelial origin *-oma* tumor	These malignant tumors account for approximately 90% of all bladder cancers and arise from the cells lining the bladder (Fig. 3-8).

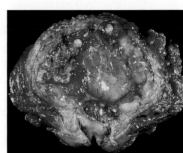

Fig. 3-8 Carcinoma of the bladder. *(From Damjanov I, Linder J: Anderson's pathology, ed 10, St Louis, 1996, Mosby.)*

◈ Exercise 3-6: NEOPLASMS

Fill in the blank.

1. What is the most common type of benign kidney tumor? _____

2. What is the eponym for nephroblastoma? _____

3. What is the most common type of bladder cancer? _____

4. What is a term for kidney cancer? (one of three) _____

St. Mary's Outpatient Clinic
999 Holyoke Drive
Boston, MA 01922

PROGRESS NOTE

Established patient arrives complaining of stress incontinence and some lower abdominal pain, and she feels her abdomen may have some slight swelling.

On pelvic examination, she does have a slight cystocele. Rectal is normal. Her abdomen may be a little distended, although I am not sure. I will schedule her for a barium enema, and we may need to do a CT scan. I suggested she develop a schedule for the bathroom on a regular basis to see if this controls her stress incontinence. If not, we will recommend urologic evaluation.

Urinalysis shows no signs of infection and no other symptoms apparent for her stress incontinence.

IMPRESSION: Stress incontinence
                    Abdominal pain, possibly caused by previous history of GI reflux

Maurice Doate, MD

◆ Exercise 3-7: PROGRESS NOTE

Using the progress report on p. 144, answer the following questions.

1. Aside from pain and possibly some swelling, what is this patient's main complaint?

_____

2. What type of herniation does she exhibit? _____

3. What tests is she scheduled for? _____

 Age Matters

Pediatrics

As a body system, the only significant disorder that occurs during the pediatric years for the urinary system is urinary tract infections. Other problems of fluid imbalances (which the kidneys help to control) are dehydration and electrolyte disorders. Examples would be hypernatremia and hyponatremia and hypokalemia and hyperkalemia.

Geriatrics

Urinary tract infections are also a problem with older adults. As with children, the problems of dehydration and electrolyte imbalances also affect this age group. Kidney function may decrease as individuals grow older, and as a result, blood pressure and blood levels of urea will increase. Senior citizens who lose kidney function are then in need of dialysis, if not a kidney transplant.

Overall general decreases in muscle tone may also cause problems with bladder function. As a result, stress incontinence in particular may become a concern.

DIAGNOSTIC PROCEDURES

Urinalysis

Urinalysis (UA) is the physical, chemical, and/or microscopic examination of urine. The following box gives examples of the constituents examined and the normal and abnormal findings with their possible interpretations.

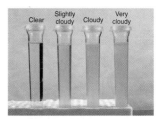

Fig. 3-9 Appearance of urine. *(From Bonewit-West K: Clinical procedures for medical assistants, ed 6, Philadelphia, 2004, Saunders.)*

URINALYSIS

Physical Examination
Appearance (Fig. 3-9)
Normal finding: Clear
Abnormal finding with interpretation: Cloudiness may indicate a UTI.

Color (Fig. 3-10)
Normal finding: Straw colored or light amber
Abnormal findings with interpretations: Lighter color may indicate diabetes insipidus or overhydration. Darker colors may indicate a concentrated urine caused by dehydration, drugs, or liver disease.

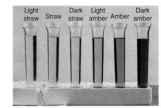

Fig. 3-10 Color of urine. *(From Bonewit-West K: Clinical procedures for medical assistants, ed 6, Philadelphia, 2004, Saunders.)*

Continued

URINALYSIS—cont'd

Physical Examination—cont'd

Quantity

Normal finding: Approximately 1½ L per day

Abnormal findings with interpretations: Profusion may indicate diabetes insipidus or a variety of other conditions precipitating diuresis. Smaller than normal amounts may be a result of dehydration, blockages, or strictures.

Specific Gravity (SG): Measures the ability of the kidneys to regulate the concentration of urine.

Normal finding: Normal is a reading of 1.015-1.025, which is slightly more dense than the weight of water.

Abnormal findings with interpretations: Diabetes or kidney damage may be the cause of a low specific gravity.

Chemical Examination

Bilirubin

Normal finding: Not present

Abnormal finding with interpretation: Presence may indicate liver disease or biliary obstruction.

Blood

Normal finding: Not present

Abnormal findings with interpretations: Red blood cells may indicate an inflammation or trauma in the urinary tract. White blood cells may indicate a UTI.

Creatinine

Normal finding: 1-2.5 mg/24 hr

Abnormal findings with interpretations: An increase may indicate infection. A decrease may indicate kidney disease.

Glucose

Normal finding: Not present

Abnormal finding with interpretation: Presence may indicate diabetes mellitus.

Ketones

Normal finding: Not present

Abnormal finding with interpretation: Diabetes mellitus or starvation may be the cause.

pH

Normal finding: 5.0-7.0; slightly acidic is normal.

Abnormal findings with interpretations: pH increases in alkalosis, decreases in high-protein diets.

Protein

Normal finding: Not present

Abnormal findings with interpretations: Increased amounts present in kidney disease; albumin present when glomeruli are damaged.

Microscopic Examination

Bacteria

Normal finding: Not present

Abnormal finding with interpretation: Urinary tract infection

Pus

Normal finding: Not present

Abnormal finding with interpretation: Pyelonephritis

Terms Related to Laboratory Tests

TERM	WORD ORIGIN	DEFINITION
Blood urea nitrogen (BUN) YOOR ee ah		Blood test that measures the amount of nitrogenous waste in the circulatory system; an increased level is an indicator of kidney dysfunction.
Creatinine clearance test kree AT ih nin		Test of kidney function that measures the rate at which nitrogenous waste is removed from the blood by comparing its concentration in the blood and urine over a 24-hour period.

Terms Related to Imaging

TERM	WORD ORIGIN	DEFINITION
Computed tomography (CT) scan toh MAH gruh fee	*tom/o* section *-graphy* recording	Computerized image that shows a "slice" of the body.
Intravenous urography (IVU) in truh VEE nus yoo RAH gruh fee	*intra-* within *ven/o* vein *-ous* pertaining to *ur/o* urine *-graphy* process of recording	Radiographic imaging of the kidneys, ureters, and bladder done with a contrast medium (Fig. 3-11). Also called **intravenous pyelography (IVP).**
Kidney, ureter, and bladder (KUB)		Radiographic imaging of the kidney, ureters, and bladder without a contrast medium.
Nephrotomography neh froh toh MAH gruh fee	*nephr/o* kidney *tom/o* section *-graphy* process of recording	Sectional radiographic exam of the kidneys.
Voiding cystourethrography (VCUG) VOY ding sis toh yoor ee THRAH gruh fee	*cyst/o* bladder *urethr/o* urethra *-graphy* process of recording	Radiographic imaging of the urinary bladder and urethra done with a contrast medium while patient is urinating (Fig. 3-12).

Pelvis of kidney

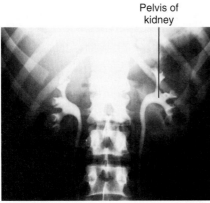

Fig. 3-11 Intravenous urogram (IVU). *(From Lewis SM: Medical-surgical nursing: assessment and management of clinical problems, ed 6, St Louis, 2005, Mosby.)*

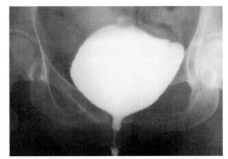

Fig. 3-12 Female voiding cystourethrogram (VCUG). *(From Bontrager KL: Textbook of radiographic positioning and related anatomy, ed 6, St Louis, 2005, Mosby.)*

Terms Related to Other Diagnostic Procedures

TERM	WORD ORIGIN	DEFINITION
Biopsy BYE op see	*bi/o* life, living -*opsy* viewing	Taking a piece of tissue for microscopic study. A **closed biopsy** is done by an endoscopy or aspiration (by suction through a fine needle). An **open biopsy** is done through an incision.
Cystoscopy sis TOSS koh pee	*cyst/o* bladder -*scopy* visual examination	Visual examination of the urinary bladder using a cystoscope (Fig. 3-13).

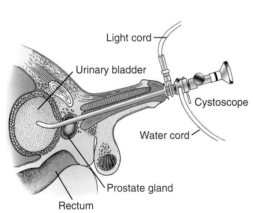

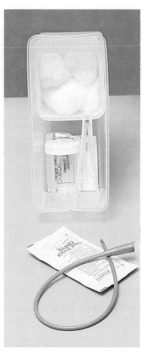

Fig. 3-13   Cystoscopy. *(From LaFleur Brooks M: Exploring medical terminology: a student-directed approach, ed 6, St Louis, 2005, Mosby.)*

Fig. 3-14   *Top*, indwelling catheter kit. *Bottom*, straight catheter. *(From Elkin MK, Perry AG, Potter PA: Nursing intervention and clinical skills, ed 3, St Louis, 2004, Mosby.)*

Terms Related to Instruments

TERM	WORD ORIGIN	DEFINITION
Catheter KATH uh tur		Hollow, flexible tube that can be inserted into a vessel, organ, or cavity of the body to withdraw or instill fluid, monitor types of various information, and visualize a vessel or cavity. Catheters can be inserted through the urethra into the bladder to drain urine (Fig. 3-14).
Cystoscope SIS toh skohp	*cyst/o* urinary bladder -*scope* instrument for visual examination	Instrument for visual examination of the inside of the bladder. (See Fig. 3-13 for a drawing of a cystoscope.)
Laparoscope LAP ur oh skohp	*lapar/o* abdomen -*scope* instrument for visual examination	Type of endoscope consisting of an illuminated tube with an optical system, inserted through the abdominal wall for examining the peritoneal cavity.

Terms Related to Instruments—cont'd

TERM	WORD ORIGIN	DEFINITION
Lithotrite LITH oh tryte	*lith/o* stone -*trite* instrument to crush stones	Instrument used to crush a calculus in the urinary bladder; fragments may then be expelled or washed out.
Nephroscope NEFF roh skohp	*nephr/o* kidney -*scope* instrument for visual examination	Fiberoptic instrument used specifically for the disintegration and removal of renal calculi; an ultrasonic probe emitting high-frequency sound waves breaks up the calculi, which are removed by suction through the scope.
Stent stehnt		Tubular device for supporting hollow structures during surgical anastomosis or for holding arteries open after angioplasty.
Urinometer yoor ih NOM meh tur	*urin/o* urine -*meter* instrument to measure	Type of hydrometer used to measure the specific gravity (SG) of a urine sample. Also known as a **urometer.**

◈ Exercise 3-8: DIAGNOSTIC PROCEDURES

Using the urinalysis box provided on pp. 145-146, answer the following.

If a urinalysis reveals:

1. a small amount of urine, then the patient may have _____.

2. pus in the urine, then the patient may have _____.

3. a low specific gravity, then the patient may have _____.

4. the presence of white blood cells, then the patient may have _____.

5. the presence of bacteria, then the patient may have _____.

6. the presence of ketones, then the patient may have _____.

Fill in the blanks.

7. Both the BUN and creatinine clearance tests measure the function of the _____ in their ability to remove waste from the blood.

8. BUN stands for _____.

9. X-rays of the urinary system may take many forms. A radiographic technique that images the kidneys, ureters, and bladder using a contrast medium is called _____.

10. A sectional radiographic exam of the kidney is called _____.

11. A radiographic technique that images the bladder and urethra while the patient is voiding is called _____.

12. Endoscopies are visual examinations of the interior of the body. Name a visual examination of the following:

A. kidney _____   C. bladder _____

B. ureters _____   D. urethra _____

13. If a biopsy is done through an incision, it is considered _____.

Matching.

_____ 14. a tube for supporting structures

_____ 15. an instrument to measure SG of urine

_____ 16. a tube to insert in an organ

_____ 17. an instrument to crush stones

_____ 18. an instrument to view the bladder

_____ 19. an instrument to view the kidney and crush stones within it

A.   catheter
B.   stent
C.   lithotrite
D.   urinometer
E.   nephroscope
F.   cystoscope

St. Mary's Outpatient Clinic
999 Holyoke Dr.
Boston, MA 01922

EMERGENCY ROOM NOTE

Patient is a 46-year-old who had hysterectomy performed approximately 1 week ago. She called our office this morning complaining of fever, nausea, and vomiting over the past 24 hours.

Upon arrival, the patient relates a 24-hour history of nausea, vomiting, and abdominal tenderness. Of note, the patient has an indwelling catheter, which was inserted postoperatively because of her inability to void. She was to return to the office postoperatively on the third postop day for possible removal of the catheter.

Urine sample taken from the catheter shows red and white blood cells. Urine culture is performed, and the patient is given antibiotics.

ASSESSMENT: Bladder infection caused by indwelling catheter

Maurice Doate, MD

◆ **Exercise 3-9: EMERGENCY ROOM NOTE**

Using the emergency room note above, answer the following questions.

1. Why did this patient have a catheter? _____

2. When was it inserted? _____

3. What types of tests were done to test for a bladder infection? _____

≋ THERAPEUTIC INTERVENTIONS

Terms Related to Therapeutic Interventions

TERM	WORD ORIGIN	DEFINITION
Ileal conduit ILL ee ul KON doo it	*ile/o* ileum *-al* pertaining to	Channel, pipe, or tube that guides urine from the ureters to the ileum in the digestive system to be excreted through the large intestine, when the bladder is no longer available for storing the urine and releasing it through the urethra. Also known as a **ureteroileostomy** (yoo ree tur oh ill ee AH stuh mee).
Lithotripsy LITH oh trip see	*lith/o* stone *-tripsy* crushing	Process of crushing stones either to prevent or clear an obstruction in the urinary system; crushing may be manual, by high-energy shock waves, or by pulsed dye laser. In each case, the fragments may be expelled naturally or washed out (Fig. 3-15). Use of shock waves is termed extracorporeal shock wave lithotripsy (ESWL).
Nephrectomy neh FRECK tuh mee	*nephr/o* kidney *-ectomy* removal	Resection of the kidney.
Nephrolithotomy neh froh lith AH tuh mee	*nephr/o* kidney *-lithotomy* removal of a stone	Incision of the kidney for removal of a kidney stone.
Nephropexy neh froh PECK see	*nephr/o* kidney *-pexy* suspension	Suspension or fixation of the kidney.
Nephrostolithotomy neh frah stoh lith AH tuh mee	*nephr/o* kidney *stom/o* opening *-lithotomy* removal of a stone	Removal of a stone from the kidney through a preexisting nephrostomy.
Nephrostomy neh FRAH stuh mee	*nephr/o* kidney *-stomy* new opening	Opening made in the kidney so that a catheter can be inserted.
Nephrotomy neh FRAH tuh mee	*nephr/o* kidney *-tomy* incision	Incision of the kidney.
Transurethral procedure trans yoo REE thrul	*trans-* through *urethr/o-* urethra *-al* pertaining to	Any procedure conducted through the urethra.
Urethrolysis yoo ree THRAH lih sis	*urethr/o* urethra *-lysis* destruction of adhesions	Destruction of adhesions of the urethra.
Vesicotomy vess ih KAH tuh mee	*vesic/o* bladder *-tomy* incision	Incision of the urinary bladder.

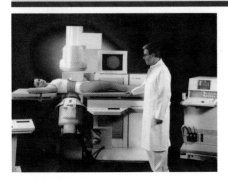

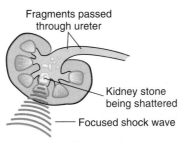

Fragments passed through ureter

Kidney stone being shattered

Focused shock wave

Fig. 3-15
Lithotripsy.

⊗ BE CAREFUL!

Do not confuse *ilium*, which is a pelvic bone, with *ileum*, which is a part of the small intestine.

Terms Related to Kidney Failure Treatment

TERM	WORD ORIGIN	DEFINITION
Continuous ambulatory peritoneal dialysis (CAPD) pair eh tuh NEE ul dye AL ih sis	*peritone/o* peritoneum *-al* pertaining to *dia-* through, complete *-lysis* separation, breakdown	Type of renal dialysis in which an indwelling catheter in the abdomen permits fluid to drain into and out of the peritoneal cavity to cleanse the blood.
Hemodialysis (HD) hee moh dye AL ih sis	*hem/o* blood *dia-* through, complete *-lysis* separation, breakdown	Type of renal dialysis that cleanses the blood by shunting it from the body through a machine for diffusion and ultrafiltration and then returning it to the patient's circulation (Fig. 3-16).
Renal dialysis dye AL ih sis	*ren/o* kidney *-al* pertaining to *dia-* through, complete *-lysis* separation, breakdown	Process of diffusing blood across a semipermeable membrane to remove substances that a healthy kidney would eliminate, including poisons, drugs, urea, uric acid, and creatinine.
Renal transplantation	*ren/o* kidney *-al* pertaining to *trans-* across *-plant* a sprout or shoot *-ation* a process	Surgical transfer of a complete kidney from a donor to a recipient (Fig. 3-17).

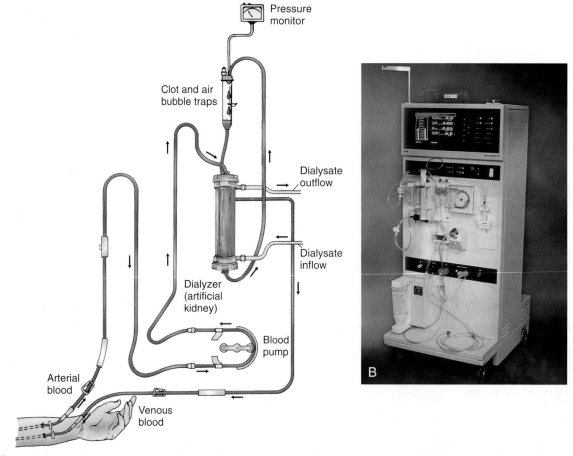

Fig. 3-16 **A,** A hemodialysis circuit. **B,** Hemodialysis machine. *(From Ignatavicius DD, Workman ML: Medical-surgical nursing: critical thinking for collaborative care, ed 5, Philadelphia, 2005, Saunders.)*

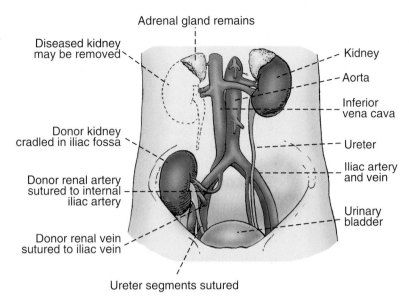

Adrenal gland remains

Diseased kidney may be removed

Kidney

Aorta

Inferior vena cava

Donor kidney cradled in iliac fossa

Ureter

Iliac artery and vein

Donor renal artery sutured to internal iliac artery

Urinary bladder

Donor renal vein sutured to iliac vein

Ureter segments sutured

Fig. 3-17 Kidney transplant. *(From Black JM, Hawks JH, Keene A: Medical-surgical nursing: clinical management for positive outcomes, ed 7, Philadelphia, 2005, Saunders.)*

◆ Exercise 3-10: URINARY THERAPEUTIC INTERVENTIONS

Matching.

_____ 1. excision of a kidney

_____ 2. incision of a kidney

_____ 3. removal of a renal calculus

_____ 4. fixation of a kidney

_____ 5. new opening of a kidney

_____ 6. removal of a stone from the kidney through a preexisting opening

A. nephrostolithotomy
B. nephrolithotomy
C. nephrectomy
D. nephrostomy
E. nephrotomy
F. nephropexy

Fill in the blank with one of the following choices.

lithotripsy, renal transplant, ileal conduit, urethrolysis, dialysis procedures

7. What is the health care term for the destruction of adhesions in the urethra?

   _____

8. What is another term for a ureteroileostomy? _____

9. The patient with renal calculi was a candidate for a procedure in which the stones were crushed. This

   is called _____.

10. What do CAPD and HD have in common? _____

11. Roger experienced kidney failure and required the surgical transplantation of a complete kidney from

    a donor. This procedure is called a(n) _____.

≋ PHARMACOLOGY

Acidifiers: Drugs that decrease the pH of the urine to help prevent kidney stones. Use of urinary acidifiers may be seen more commonly in animals. Examples include methionine and aluminum chloride.

Alkalinizers: Drugs that increase the pH of the urine to treat acidosis or to promote excretion of some drugs and toxins. Sodium bicarbonate is the most commonly agent used in these serious conditions.

Anticholinergics: Drugs that help control urinary incontinence by blocking nerves that control bladder and sphincter muscles. Examples include atropine, tolterodine (Detrol), and solifenacin (VESIcare). The latter two drugs specifically antagonize muscarinic receptors to treat incontinence more exclusively than other general anticholinergics.

Antidiuretics: Drugs that suppress the urine formation. Examples include vasopressin (also known as antidiuretic hormone, ADH) and desmopressin (DDAVP).

Antiinfectives: Drugs that fight infection in the urinary system, such as antibiotics, antiseptics, and antifungals. Nitrofurantoin (Macrobid), sulfamethoxazole/trimethoprim (Septra, Bactrim), and levofloxacin (Levaquin) are common examples.

Antispasmodics: Drugs that help prevent muscle spasms in the bladder in the treatment of incontinence. Examples include flavoxate (Urispas) and oxybutynin (Ditropan).

Diuretics: Drugs that increase the formation of the urine by promoting excretion of water and sodium. These drugs are often used to treat high blood pressure, congestive heart failure, and peripheral edema. Examples include hydrochlorothiazide (Hydro-Diuril, also found in many combinations), furosemide (Lasix), and triamterene (Dyrenium, also found in many combinations).

◆ Exercise 3-11: PHARMACOLOGY

Matching.

_____ 1. diuretic

_____ 2. antispasmodic

_____ 3. antiinfective

_____ 4. alkalinizer

_____ 5. anticholinergic

_____ 6. acidifier

_____ 7. antidiuretic

A. increases the pH of urine
B. suppresses urine formation
C. prevents muscle spasms
D. decreases the pH of urine
E. increases formation of urine
F. antibiotics, antifungals, antiseptics
G. helps control urinary incontinence

Abbreviations

Abbreviation	Definition	Abbreviation	Definition
ADH	Antidiuretic hormone	HD	Hemodialysis
ARF	Acute renal failure	IVU	Intravenous urography
BUN	Blood urea nitrogen	K	Potassium
CAPD	Continuous ambulatory peritoneal dialysis	KUB	Kidney, ureter, and bladder
		L	Liter
CRF	Chronic renal failure	mg	Milligram
Cl	Chloride	Na	Sodium
CT	Computed tomography	pH	Acidity/alkalinity
cysto	Cystoscopy	SG	Specific gravity
DI	Diabetes insipidus	STD	Sexually transmitted disease
DM	Diabetes mellitus	UA	Urinalysis
ESRD	End-stage renal disease	UTI	Urinary tract infection
ESWL	Extracorporeal shock wave lithotripsy	VCUG	Voiding cystourethrography

◆ **Exercise 3-12: ABBREVIATIONS**

Write the meanings of the abbreviations.

1. The patient with DM had produced 3.0 L of urine in the last 24 hours.

_____

2. The patient with CRF was treated with HD.

_____

3. Ellen's UA noted a low SG. The diagnosis was DI.

_____

4. Antonia was treated for a UTI.

_____

5. A VCUG helped to confirm the patient's diagnosis of hydronephrosis.

_____

Careers

Triage Nurse

Although many people would run from the possibility, some individuals crave the excitement of a career that demands decision making, often under tremendous pressure. One setting for that type of work is the emergency department (ED). Numerous television shows have drawn attention to the types of situations that employees may face in that kind of setting.

One potential career path to explore is that of triage nurse. The term *triage* is derived from an Old French term meaning *to sift*. The triage nurse sorts ED patients according to the urgency of their complaints and determines the order in which they will be seen by the physicians. The triage nurse is also responsible for an initial assessment, noting all pertinent information necessary for further evaluation and treatment of the patient.

Related to the ED triage nurse is the telephone triage nurse, a position that allows patients to be "sorted" over the phone as to the severity of their disorders. These nurses work in a specialty area that has grown in response to increasing health care costs and overcrowded emergency departments.

Ideally, both the triage nurse and the telephone triage nurse would have experience in med-surg nursing practices dealing with a wide variety of patient disorders. The American Nurses Association has a series of links to specialty sites that include the Emergency Nurses Association (ENA) and Trauma Information Pages. The website is http://nursingworld.org/mindex/snphtm. The ENA site has information on certification for this vocation.

Careers Related to the Urinary System

Hemodialysis Technician

Hemodialysis or renal dialysis technicians work under the direction of physicians or nurses to assist patients undergoing dialysis treatment. They assemble the supplies necessary for dialysis, obtain patient vital signs, measure and adjust blood flow rates, and monitor patients and equipment throughout the procedure. Training may be on the job, in a vocational school, or in a community college. There are three credentialing programs for hemodialysis technicians, each one suggesting a minimum of 6 months to 1 year of experience before sitting for the exam. The National Association of Nephrology Technicians/Technologists provides information at http://www.dialysistech.org/news/position.htm.

Urologist

Urologists are medical doctors who diagnose and treat disorders of both the male and female urinary tracts. They are required to have a 4-year undergraduate degree, 4 years of medical school, and 5 years of residency training. Specialties may include renal transplants, urinary tract stones, and pediatric or female urology. Urologists who specialize in male disorders may choose to treat male infertility and erectile dysfunction. Board certification may be obtained through the American Board of Urology. For more information on this career, visit http://www.ama-assn.org/ama/pub/category/2320.html.

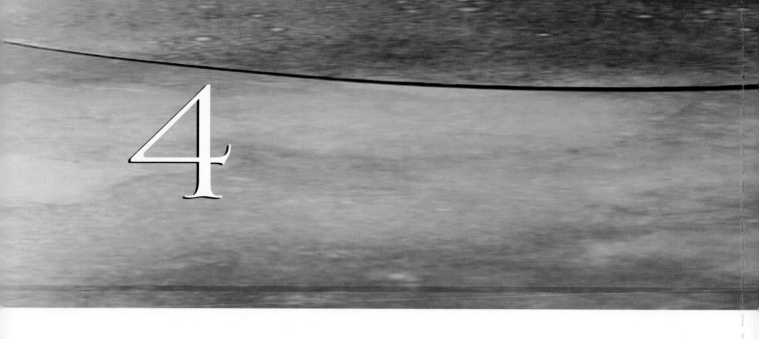

4

OBJECTIVES

You will be able to do the following after completing this chapter:

Key Terms
1. Define, appropriately use, and spell all the Key Terms for this chapter.

Major Functions of the Urinary System
2. State the five major functions of the urinary system.

Urinary System Structure
3. Identify and locate the four major structures in the urinary system.
4. Describe the structure and main functions of the kidneys.
5. Explain the purpose of urine and describe urine formation.
6. Explain the structure of a nephron and its function in the kidney.
7. Describe the structure and function of the ureters.
8. Describe the structure and function of the urinary bladder.
9. Describe the structure and function of the urethra.

Diseases and Disorders of the Urinary System
10. List 13 common signs and symptoms of urinary system disorders.
11. List seven common diagnostic tests for urinary disease and describe the use of each.
12. List six urinary diseases and disorders and briefly describe the etiology, signs and symptoms, diagnosis, therapy, and interventions for each.
13. Explain the purpose of dialysis and list two types.

Patient-Centered Professionalism
14. Analyze a realistic medical office situation and apply your understanding of the urinary system to determine the best course of action.
15. Describe the impact on patient care when medical assistants have a solid understanding of the structure and function of the urinary system.

ANATOMY AND PHYSIOLOGY OF THE URINARY SYSTEM

KEY TERMS

The Key Terms for this chapter have been organized into sections so that you can easily see the terminology associated with each aspect of the urinary system.

Major Functions of the Urinary System

azotemia Nitrogenous waste, especially urea, accumulating in the blood.

erythropoietin Hormone responsible for red blood cell production.

excretory system Urinary system; body system that separates and eliminates waste from blood, tissues, and organs.

renin Hormone responsible for blood pressure control.

uremia Azotemia; accumulation of toxins, such as urea, in the blood.

urinary system Body system that eliminates waste in the body and maintains water and chemical balance.

Structure of the Urinary System

Kidneys

aldosterone Hormone responsible for increased sodium reabsorption.

antidiuretic hormone (ADH) Hormone responsible for reducing urine production.

Bowman's capsule C-shaped structure surrounding the glomerulus.

calyces Cuplike edges of the renal pelvis that collect urine.

capsule Container; something that holds; in the urinary tract—Bowman's capsule.

cortex Outer layer, such as the outer layer of the kidney.

filtration Process by which substances are removed by passing through a membrane or other partial barrier.

glomerulus Group of capillaries responsible for filtering blood in the nephrons of the kidney.

hilum Depression where blood vessels, nerves, and the ureter enter and exit the kidney; plural *hila.*

kidney Organ of the urinary system that produces urine.

Loop of Henle Part of the tubular collection system in the nephron.

medulla Inner portion of an organ such as the kidney.

nephron Functioning unit of the kidney.

pyramids Triangular shapes; sections within the kidneys that contain the tubules.

renal artery Artery that takes blood into the kidney.

renal pelvis Collecting area for urine at the proximal end of the ureter.

retroperitoneal Located behind the peritoneum.

solute Substance dissolved in a liquid or semisolid substance.

urea Nitrogen waste product excreted in the urine.

urine Liquid and dissolved substances excreted by the kidneys.

Ureters

renal calculi Kidney stones made of mineral salts.

ureters Pair of muscular tubes that carry urine from the kidneys to the bladder.

urinary reflux Backflow of urine from the bladder into the ureters during urination.

Urinary Bladder

micturition Urination; voiding.

micturition reflex Nerve stimulation that allows the expelling of urine from the bladder.

rugae Muscular folds that allow organs such as the bladder to expand.

trigone Triangular area in the bladder formed by the entrance of ureters and exit of the urethra.

urinary bladder Hollow muscular organ that holds urine before it is excreted from the body.

KEY TERMS—cont'd

urination Process of excreting urine; micturition; voiding.
voiding Urination, or micturition.

Urethra

meatus Opening to the outside of the body, as in the urethra.
semen Fluid of the male reproductive system that contains spermatozoa.
urethra Membranous canal that transports urine from the bladder to the outside of the body.

Diseases and Disorders of the Urinary System

Signs and Symptoms

albuminuria Presence of large amounts of serum albumin and other proteins in the urine; usually a sign of renal disease or heart failure; also called *proteinuria.*
anuresis Condition of no urine production or having a urine output of less than 100 mL per day. Also called *anuria.*
bacteriuria Bacteria in the urine.
diuresis Increased urine production.
dysuria Painful or difficult urination.
enuresis Involuntary discharge of urine at an age after bladder control should be achieved; bedwetting.
frequency Increase in number of times urination occurs over a short time.
glycosuria Presence of glucose in the urine.
hematuria Presence of blood in the urine.
incontinence Inability to retain urine or feces because of a loss of sphincter control.
ketonuria Presence of ketones in the urine.
nocturia Excessive urination at night.
oliguria Diminished urine output.
polydipsia Excessive thirst.
polyuria Excretion of abnormally large amounts of urine.
proteinuria Presence of excess serum protein in the urine; also called *albuminuria.*
pyuria Presence of pus in the urine.
retention Inability to empty the bladder fully.
urgency Feeling of the need to urinate immediately.

Diagnostic Tests and Procedures

blood urea nitrogen (BUN) Blood test that measures the amount of nitrogenous waste in the circulatory system.
creatinine clearance test Test that measures the rate at which nitrogenous waste is removed from the blood by comparing its concentration in the blood and urine over a 24-hour period.
cystoscopy Visual examination of the urinary bladder using a cystoscope.
intravenous pyelography (IVP) Imaging of the kidneys, ureters, and bladder with a contrast medium. Also called *intravenous urography (IVU).*
kidneys, ureters, and bladder (KUB) Imaging of the kidneys, ureters, and bladder without a contrast medium.
nephrologist Specialist who is concerned with kidneys and their structure and function.
renal computed tomography Imaging that shows a transverse view of the kidney.
urinalysis Physical, chemical, and microscopic examination of the urine.
urologist Specialist in the treatment of diseases of the kidneys, urinary tract, and male reproductive organs.

Diseases and Disorders

acute renal failure (ARF) Renal failure occurring suddenly from trauma or any condition that impairs blood flow to the kidneys.
chronic renal failure (CRF) Renal failure resulting from long-term inability to excrete waste products.
cystitis Inflammation of the urinary bladder.
dialysis Process used to clean the blood of toxins.
diuretics Medication that causes increased urine excretion.
glomerulonephritis Inflammation of the glomeruli of the nephron.
hemodialysis Process in which an artificial kidney machine filters a patient's blood and returns filtered blood back to the patient.
kidney transplant Donor kidney replaces the kidney of a person with a malfunctioning kidney to function as a kidney for the recipient.
peritoneal dialysis Process in which a solution is passed through the patient's peritoneal cavity and drained to remove waste products that the kidney cannot excrete.
polycystic kidney Replacement of kidney tissue with marble-like cysts.
pyelonephritis Inflammation of the renal pelvis and nephron, including connective tissue of the kidneys.
renal failure Progressive loss of nephrons, resulting in loss of renal function.

What Would You Do?

Read the following scenario and keep it in mind as you learn about the urinary system in this chapter.

Juanita is a regular patient in the medical office and has been in good health most of her life. At her office visit, she is complaining of pain in the flanks of her legs, in her lower abdomen, and in her back under her ribs. She also says that she has had burning and frequency of urination that has become progressively worse over 2 weeks. Furthermore, she says when she has to go to the bathroom, she has to hurry or she will not make it. The burning is not on the perineum but occurs as she starts the flow of urine. These symptoms have only made her incontinence worse, and she now has nocturia.

When asked if she can pinpoint anything new in her hygiene routine, Juanita states that she has been using a new perfumed soap on a regular basis to take her bath. On obtaining a urinalysis, hematuria is present. In addition, white blood cells are found on the microscopic examination. The physician has prescribed medications for treating what he has diagnosed as "urinary cystitis." Juanita would like to talk to the medical assistant to ask some questions.

Would you be able to answer Juanita's questions?

The urinary system eliminates waste in our bodies and also maintains water and chemical balance, keeping our bodies in homeostasis. The urinary system depends on the other body systems to carry out its functions. For example, when you need to urinate, your bladder sends a message to the brain, letting it know of this need; thus the brain controls urination. Also, the digestive system creates fluid waste products that need to be eliminated by the urinary system, and muscles contract and relax to move waste products through the body and allow urine to exit the body.

Actually, as with the other body systems, the urinary system interacts in some way with all the body's other systems. Knowing the structure and function of all body systems, including the urinary system, will help medical assistants to understand the disease process. Their patients will receive the benefits of this understanding.

≋ MAJOR FUNCTIONS OF THE URINARY SYSTEM

The **urinary system,** an **excretory system** ("excrete" means to separate and eliminate waste from the blood, tissues, and organs), performs five major functions. An easy way to remember these functions is with the acronym "FREPS," as follows:

1. **F**iltration filters toxic wastes out of the bloodstream for removal from the body (products of cell metabolism, excess salts, urea).
2. **R**eabsorption (resorption) retains essential elements (water, sugar, salts) that the body needs to maintain pH and homeostasis.

3. **E**xcretion excretes the waste products outside the body by way of the urethra.
4. **P**roduction of **erythropoietin** (a hormone that stimulates red blood cell production in the red bone marrow) is activated when the kidneys do not receive enough oxygen.
5. **S**ecretion of **renin** (enzyme needed for blood pressure regulation). If a person's blood pressure is insufficient to allow filtration in the glomerulus, renin is released into the blood and activates the blood protein *angiotensin,* which raises the blood pressure by causing the blood vessels to constrict.

Maintaining the proper water and electrolyte balance within the body is essential to good body homeostasis. Water, salts, and other substances are lost through urination, perspiration, digestion, and the respiratory process. If the body is to function properly, a normal balance of water and electrolytes must be maintained.

The pH scale ranges from 0 (very acidic) to 14 (very alkaline). The normal pH of urine is 6.5, or slightly acidic. When this system does not work as it should, toxins and nitrogen-containing waste materials build up in the bloodstream, and **uremia** or **azotemia** may occur.

PATIENT-CENTERED PROFESSIONALISM

- Why is it important for the medical assistant to understand all the functions of the urinary system?

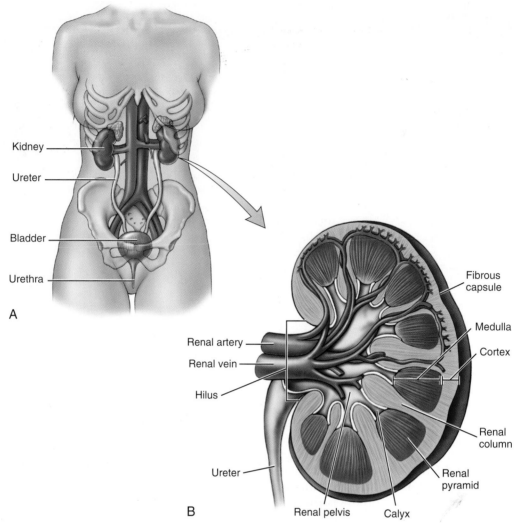

Fig. 4-1   The urinary system. **A,** Main organs of the urinary system. **B,** Structure of the kidney. *(From Herlihy B, Maebius NK: The human body in health and illness, ed 2, Philadelphia, 2003, Saunders.)*

STRUCTURE OF THE URINARY SYSTEM

The urinary organs consist of a pair of kidneys that secrete urine and two ureters that transport the urine from each kidney to the urinary bladder, where urine is stored until the urethra carries it to the outside of the body (Fig. 4-1).

Kidneys

The **kidneys** are main organs of the urinary system and are crucial to the proper functioning of our bodies.

Location

The kidneys are located in the dorsal aspect of the body **(retroperitoneal),** about 1½ to 2 inches above the waist in the lumbar area on either side of the spinal column and are protected by the ribs. To find your kidneys, try the following:

- Stand up and put your hands on your hips (with your thumbs pointing toward your back).
- Move your hands up until you can feel your ribs.
- Your thumbs should be located at your kidneys.

Located on top of each kidney is an adrenal gland. The adrenal glands release **aldosterone,** a hormone that maintains the balance of sodium and chloride ions in the blood. The right kidney is positioned slightly lower than the left kidney because the liver pushes the right kidney downward. The kidneys are held in place by bands of connective tissue and cushioned by fat deposits. A condition known as *renal ptosis* (sagging or prolapse of the kidney) occurs in very thin people as a result of inadequate fatty cushions.

Function

Metabolic wastes are excreted mainly by the kidneys, but the lungs, skin, and digestive tract also dispose

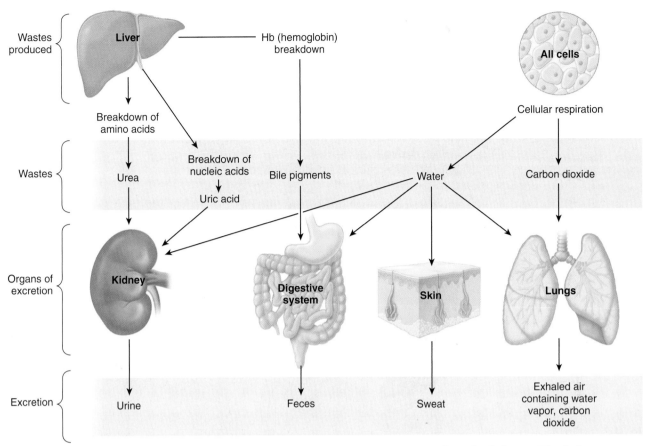

Fig. 4-2 Wastes containing nitrogen are produced by the liver and transported to the kidneys. The kidneys excrete these wastes in the urine. *(Modified from Solomon EP:* Introduction to human anatomy and physiology, *ed 2, Philadelphia, 2003, Saunders.)*

of metabolic wastes (Fig. 4-2). The kidneys also regulate the water-salt balance of the body fluids and maintain the body's pH.

The main function of the kidneys is to filter **urea** and other waste products from the blood. This process allows for the production of **urine.** Urine is composed of 95% water and 5% solid wastes. These wastes include nitrogenous wastes and some electrolytes (e.g., sodium, potassium). Daily production of urine is 1.5 to 2.5 liters. Kidney failure, or **renal failure,** occurs if the kidneys produce less than 30 mL of urine per hour.

URINE COMPOSITION

Urine concentration and volume are controlled by actions of the following factors:

- *Renin.* When the filtration process of the kidneys declines, specialized cells within the kidneys release renin. Renin is an enzyme that reacts with a blood protein to form a substance that stimulates the adrenal gland to secrete aldosterone.

- *Aldosterone.* The release of aldosterone causes increased sodium reabsorption and concentrated urine.
- **Antidiuretic hormone (ADH).** A drop in blood pressure causes the posterior pituitary gland to secrete ADH, which causes increased water reabsorption. This process results in urine that is concentrated because of decreased urination and increased blood pressure (because more fluid is found in blood vessels).

URINE FORMATION

Urine formation occurs in the nephron when blood enters the kidney. Blood enters through the **renal artery,** which subdivides into smaller branches (arterioles) that take blood to Bowman's capsule and circulate it through the **glomerulus,** a cluster of capillaries that allows for filtration of fluids. Blood pressure forces small molecules (e.g., water, electrolytes, nutrients, waste materials) out of the blood, through the glomerulus, and into the renal tubule. This process is called **filtration.** Within the renal tubules, water, electrolytes, and nutrients needed by the body are reabsorbed by the cells and

TABLE 4-1	Urine Formation Process	
Pressure	**Process**	**Types of Molecules**
Filtration	Blood pressure forces small molecules from glomerulus into Bowman's capsule	Water, glucose, proteins, salts, urea, creatinine, uric acid
Reabsorption (resorption)	Selective molecules are returned to blood	Water, glucose, proteins, salts
Secretion of toxins	Molecules continue through nephrons to collecting ducts	Uric acid, creatinine, ammonia, salts
Reabsorption of water	Water and salts return to nephrons to be excreted	Water, salts
Excretion	Wastes are excreted into collecting ducts in the form of urine	Water, salts, urea, uric acid, ammonia, salts, creatinine

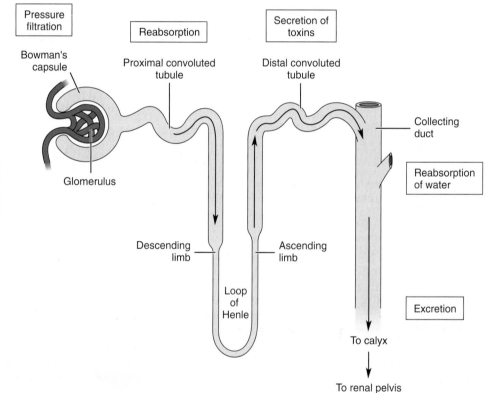

Fig. 4-3 Kidneys: regulation and excretion. *(Modified from Herlihy B, Maebius NK: The human body in health and illness, ed 2, Philadelphia, 2003, Saunders.)*

returned to the blood. Toxins are then carried out with the remaining fluid, and urine is formed (Table 4-1 and Fig. 4-3).

Structure
It is important to understand the external, internal, and microscopic structure of the kidney.

EXTERNAL STRUCTURE
If you have ever seen a kidney bean, or a bean-shaped swimming pool, you have a good idea of the shape of a kidney. It is about 5 cm (2 inches) wide and 10 cm (4 inches) long, with a thickness of 2.5 cm (1 inch)—about the size of a fist. Each kidney

is held in a fibrous **capsule.** The median side of each kidney has a depression called the **hilum,** or *hilus*, where the blood vessels, ureter, and nerves enter and exit the kidney.

INTERNAL STRUCTURE
The kidney has three main areas: the cortex, medulla, and renal pelvis.

- The **cortex** is the outer layer. It is located next to the fibrous capsule (forms the outside of the kidney) and appears granular because it contains filters.

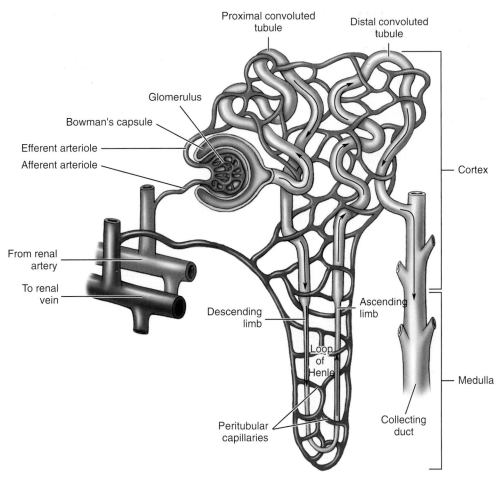

Fig. 4-4 The nephron unit. *(From Herlihy B, Maebius NK:* The human body in health and illness, *ed 2, Philadelphia, 2003, Saunders.)*

- The **medulla** is the inner layer. It is divided into sections shaped like triangles, called **pyramids.** The pyramids have collecting tubules that empty into the renal pelvis, the main collecting area for urine. The cuplike edges of the renal pelvis closest to the pyramids (called the **calyces**) collect urine formed in the kidneys.
- The **renal pelvis** narrows to form the ureter, which empties into the bladder.

MICROSCOPIC STRUCTURE

The main functioning units of the kidney are the **nephrons** (Fig. 4-4). Each kidney consists of about 1 million nephrons. A nephron is a microscopic unit responsible for filtering waste products from the blood. The nephrons are funnel shaped, with a single coiled tube that twists into various shapes. At the beginning of the tube is a cup-shaped (or C-shaped) capsule called **Bowman's capsule.** This structure surrounds the glomerulus, a group of capillaries responsible for filtering the blood. The filtered blood enters a series of tubules and ends with the collecting tubule, which empties into the renal

pelvis that empties urine into the bladder. It is through this tubular system that nutrients and electrolytes are reabsorbed into the blood. The **Loop of Henle** is an important part of this tubular collection system, reabsorbing **solutes** (especially sodium), and diluting the urine by osmosis (see Fig. 4-3). The peritubular capillaries around the tubule are important in the resorption of fluids around the nephrons.

Ureters

There are two **ureters.** Each is about 25 cm (10 inches) long and carries urine from the renal pelvis to the urinary bladder by peristalsis. The ureters are muscular tubes, so even if a person is lying down, urine can travel through the ureters to the bladder. The bladder compresses against the ureter opening, which prevents urine from backing up into the ureters.

When the urine flows from the bladder back into the ureter during urination, this is known as **urinary reflux.** This abnormal condition may result from a congenital defect, obstruction within

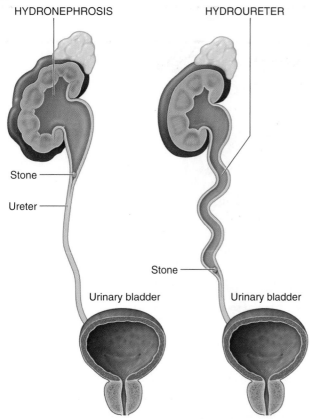

HYDRONEPHROSIS   HYDROURETER

Stone

Ureter

Stone

Urinary bladder   Urinary bladder

Fig. 4-5 Hydronephrosis caused by a stone in the upper part of the ureter, and hydroureter by a stone in the lower part of the ureter. *(Modified from Chabner DE: The language of medicine, ed 7, Philadelphia, 2004, Saunders.)*

the bladder, or a urinary infection. Because of the solutes in urine, some people tend to form kidney stones, or **renal calculi.** The calculi are washed into the ureter by urine. When a calculus or urolith is too large, it cannot pass through the ureter, causing obstruction (Fig. 4-5). This causes severe pain in the flank and into the groin.

Urinary Bladder

The **urinary bladder** is a hollow muscular sac shaped like a balloon. The bladder wall is arranged in folds called **rugae** that allow the bladder to stretch as it fills. The bladder is located in the ventral area of the pelvic cavity, just behind the pelvic bone. Its main function is to store urine until a reflex contraction causes urine to exit the body through the urethra.

The process of excreting urine is called **urination, micturition,** or **voiding.** This process occurs when the two sphincters (ring-shaped muscles) open and allow urine to leave the bladder. The upper sphincter muscle located below the bladder works involuntarily. The lower sphincter is under conscious control. The **micturition reflex**

occurs when the stretch receptors located in the wall of the bladder transmit a nerve impulse and initiate the urge to expel urine. The **trigone** is the triangular area within the bladder that is formed by the entrance site of the ureters and the exit site of the urethra.

Urethra

The **urethra** extends from the bladder to the outside of the body. The urethral opening to the outside of the body is the **meatus.** The male urethra is longer (about 8 inches) than the female urethra and expels both urine and **semen** from the body. The female urethra excretes only urine. The fact that the female's urethra is shorter (about 1½ inches long) and is closer to the vagina and anus explains why women have more lower urinary tract infections (UTIs) than males.

FOR YOUR INFORMATION

Ureter versus Urethra
- There are two ureters; an easy way to remember this is to note that there are two "e"s in the word "ureter."
- There is one urethra; an easy way to remember this is to note that there is only one "e" in "urethra."

PATIENT-CENTERED PROFESSIONALISM

- Why would it be important for the medical assistant to ask a patient with renal disease about daily input and output of fluids?

DISEASES AND DISORDERS OF THE URINARY SYSTEM

Diseases and disorders of the urinary system may be caused by infections, malignant and benign tumors, or congenital abnormalities. Cardiac (e.g., hypertension) and endocrine (e.g., diabetes) problems, stones in the urinary tract, and trauma to the urinary system can also lead to urinary disorders. A **urologist** treats diseases and disorders of the urinary system. A **nephrologist** treats diseases of the kidneys.

Drugs may be prescribed to treat urinary problems (Table 4-2). As a medical assistant, you need to be able to recognize the common signs and symptoms of and diagnostic tests for the

TABLE 4-2 Urinary Drug Classifications

Drug Classification	Common Generic (Brand) Drugs
Antihypertensives Reduce blood pressure	lisinopril (Zestril) clonidine (Catapres)
Antibacterials Combat microorganisms; first-line drugs in treatment of UTIs	sulfisoxazole (Gantrisin) trimethoprim-sulfamethoxazole (TMP-SMZ) (Septra DS)
Antiseptics Prophylaxis; second-line of defense for treatment of UTIs	cinoxacin (Cinobac) nitrofurantoin (Macrobid)
Diuretics Increase urination	furosemide (Lasix) chlorothiazide (Diuril)
Antispasmodics Genitourinary muscle relaxant	flavoxate (Urispas) oxybutynin (Ditropan)
Analgesics Provide anesthetic effect on lining of urinary tract	phenazopyridine (Pyridium) pentosan (Elmiron)

UTIs, Urinary tract infections.

BOX 4-1 Common Signs and Symptoms of Urinary Disease

Albuminuria	Presence of large amounts of protein; usually a sign of renal disease or heart failure; also called **proteinuria**
Anuresis	Stopping of urine production or output of less than 100 mL per day. Also called anuria.
Bacteriuria	Bacteria in urine
Diuresis	Increased urine production
Dysuria	Painful or difficult urination
Enuresis	Involuntary discharge of urine after the age when bladder control is expected, especially at night; bedwetting
Frequency	Need to urinate often, without increased daily output
Glycosuria	Presence of glucose in the urine
Hematuria	Presence of blood in the urine
Incontinence	Inability to retain urine because of the loss of sphincter control
Ketonuria	Presence of ketones in the urine
Nocturia	Excessive urination at night
Oliguria	Diminished amount of urine output
Polydipsia	Excessive thirst (often seen in diabetic patients)
Polyuria	Excretion of abnormally large amounts of urine
Pyuria	Presence of pus in the urine
Retention	Inability to empty the bladder fully
Uremia	Large amount of urea and other nitrogenous wastes in the blood
Urgency	Feeling of need to urinate immediately

different types of urinary system disorders and diseases.

- Study Box 4-1 to familiarize yourself with the common signs and symptoms.
- Study Box 4-2 to learn about common diagnostic tests.
- Study Table 4-3 to understand the diseases and disorders that affect the urinary system.
- Study Box 4-3 to learn about dialysis and kidney transplantation.

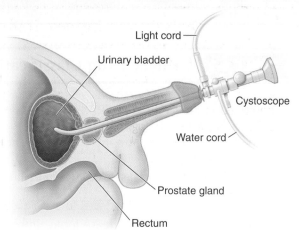

Fig. 4-6 Cystoscopy. *(Modified from Shiland BJ: Mastering healthcare terminology, St Louis, 2003, Mosby.)*

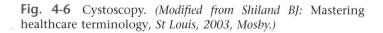

BOX 4-2	**Diagnostic Tests and Procedures for the Urinary System**

Blood urea nitrogen	BUN; measures amount of nitrogenous waste in the circulatory system
Creatinine clearance test	Measures rate at which nitrogenous waste is removed from the blood by comparing its concentration in the blood and urine over a 24-hour period
Urinalysis	Physical, chemical, and/or microscopic examination of the urine

Normal Values
  Glucose: Negative
  Bilirubin: Negative
  Ketones: Negative
  Specific gravity: 1.1 to 1.25 ± 0.05
  Blood: Negative
  pH: 4.5 to 8
  Protein: Negative
  Urobilinogen: 2 mg/dl
  Nitrites: Negative
  Leukocytes: Negative

Renal computed tomography	Imaging that shows a transverse view of the kidney
Intravenous pyelography	IVP; imaging of the kidneys, ureters, and bladder with a contrast medium
Kidneys, ureters, and bladder	KUB; imaging of the kidneys, ureters, and bladder without a contrast medium
Cystoscopy	Visual examination of the urinary bladder using a cystoscope (Fig. 4-6)

BOX 4-3	**Dialysis and Kidney Transplantation**

Dialysis

Dialysis is used to cleanse the blood of toxins brought on by acute renal disease or end-stage renal disease (ESRD). The process is continued until the problem is corrected or a kidney transplant can be performed. Dialysis can be used indefinitely, but it is not a cure. Dialysis allows the body to maintain the proper fluid, electrolyte, and acid-base balance. There are two methods used to clean the blood: **hemodialysis** and **peritoneal dialysis.**

Hemodialysis

A machine called an *artificial kidney* filters the patient's blood of impurities and returns the blood to the patient's body. A catheter is surgically implanted in the patient's artery, usually in the nondominant arm. The patient's blood passes through a semipermeable membrane in the machine. This procedure takes about 4 hours and must be done on an average of three times a week. The benefit of hemodialysis is that the patient is dialyzed by a professional, and the risk of infection is lower than with self-performed dialysis.

BOX 4-3 Dialysis and Kidney Transplantation—cont'd

Peritoneal Dialysis

Peritoneal dialysis can be done with minimal equipment and in the patient's home. A catheter is surgically implanted in the patient's peritoneal cavity. A dialyzing solution is passed through the peritoneum and later drained. The procedure takes about 30 minutes and is done four times a day, 7 days a week. It can also be done every night during sleep for patients meeting certain criteria. The benefit of peritoneal dialysis is that the patient does not need to travel to a dialysis center on a regular basis. However, this type of dialysis must be done daily.

Medical Assistant's Role in Dialysis

The role of the medical assistant in dialysis is twofold. First, the medical assistant is responsible for taking the patient's weight, obtaining vital signs, measuring the abdominal girth of the patient, recording any patient concerns since his or her last visit, and making certain all current laboratory work is available for the physician's review. Second, following hand hygiene protocol and observing for signs of adverse affects during the procedures is critical. While not directly involved in the instillation of the dialysis fluid, the medical assistant's observation and listening skills are of value to the medical team.

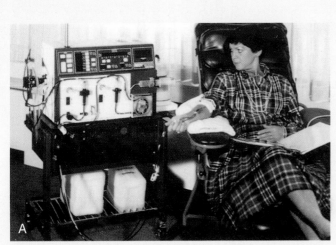
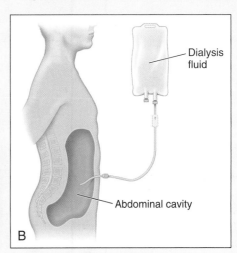

A, Hemodialysis. **B,** Peritoneal dialysis. *(From Thibodeau GA, Patton KT: The human body in health and disease, ed 3, St Louis, 2002, Mosby.)*

Kidney Transplantation

A person with ESRD can have a **kidney transplant** if a suitable donor is found. Blood and tissue typing must be done carefully to avoid rejection of the donated organ. A transplant is having a donor's kidney surgically implanted in the patient (recipient). The recipient requires lifelong *immunosuppressive* medication to prevent organ rejection and antibiotics to prevent infection.

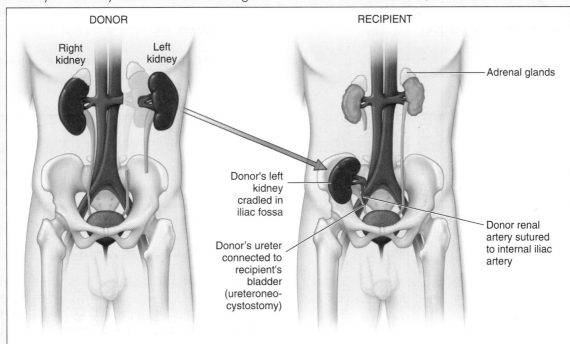

(Modified from Chabner DE: The language of medicine, ed 7, Philadelphia, 2004, Saunders.)

TABLE 4-3 Diseases and Disorders of the Urinary System

Disease and Description	Etiology	Signs and Symptoms	Diagnosis	Therapy	Interventions
Glomerulonephritis Inflammation of glomeruli	Can be idiopathic or following group A beta hemolytic streptococcus infection	Decreased urine output, protein in urine (proteinuria), hematuria, back pain, edema, increased blood pressure	Clinical examination, urinalysis, and blood tests showing elevated BUN; x-rays to include KUB	Antibiotic therapy, rest, sodium restrictions, and **diuretics** to control edema (swelling)	Interventions depend on the cause of the condition
Renal failure Progressive loss of nephrons resulting in loss of renal function **Acute renal failure (ARF)** occurs suddenly from trauma (any condition that damages the kidneys) **Chronic renal failure (CRF)** occurs with long-term inability to excrete waste products	Decreased blood flow to kidney caused by obstruction of urine flow, toxins, or prior kidney disease	Urine reduction, lethargy, weakness, increased blood pressure	Blood studies to include increased BUN, creatinine, and potassium levels; hemoglobin and hematocrit decreased; radiographic studies to include IVP and sonograms of kidney	Monitoring fluids, sodium, and potassium intake to prevent system overload; nutritional therapy to provide for protein replacement; dialysis and possible kidney transplant (see Box 4-3)	Encourage support by family to maintain diet and fluid restrictions
Pyelonephritis Inflammation of renal pelvis and nephrons including connective tissue of kidneys	Bacterial infection from bladder travels through one or both ureters to kidney	Rapid onset of fever, chills, nausea, and vomiting; lower back pain	Urine specimen has a strong odor, blood, and pus; x-rays show enlarged kidneys	Antibiotic therapy with increased fluid intake and bedrest	Encourage follow-up evaluations after initial episode treated to evaluate renal function

Condition	Description	Cause	Signs and Symptoms	Diagnosis	Treatment	Nursing Care
Renal calculi	Kidney stones made of mineral salts found in urinary tract. Stones may move into ureters	Unknown cause, although excessive amounts of calcium and uric acid in blood have been attributed to stone formation	Onset of sudden and severe pain in lower back accompanied by urinary frequency; patient may complain of nausea, vomiting, hematuria, fever, and chills	Family history, urinalysis, KUB, IVP, urogram	Remove calculi through lithotripsy (Fig. 4-7) or surgery if it does not pass; provide medications for discomfort and infection; diet modifications and increased fluid intake; straining urine to catch the stone and analyze its composition	Encourage patient to avoid causative factors in diet
Polycystic kidney	Kidney tissue is replaced with marble-like cysts (Fig. 4-8)	Hereditary disease that presents itself in late adolescence or adulthood	Patient has impaired renal function with complaints of lower back pain, hematuria, and high blood pressure	Clinical presentation with positive results for blood, protein, and pus; x-rays show enlarged kidneys	Dialysis and/or kidney transplant; management of urinary tract infections and hypertension	Maintain follow-up care
Cystitis	Inflammation of urinary bladder	*Females:* Entry of bacteria via urinary meatus to urethra, caused by fecal contamination, and effects of sexual intercourse. *Males:* Obstructive causes (e.g., strictures, enlarged prostate)	Dysuria, frequency, urgency, nocturia; also, suprapubic pain	Urine culture to detect presence of bacteria and sensitivity testing to determine correct antimicrobial drug	Antibiotic therapy, antispasmodics, and increased fluid consumption	Encourage patient to finish antibiotic therapy and to drink fluids to promote renal blood flow and to flush out bacteria in the urinary tract; also encourage patient to urinate frequently (every 2-3 hours) and to empty bladder completely on urination

BUN, Blood urea nitrogen; *IVP,* intravenous pyelogram; *KUB,* kidneys, ureters, and bladder.

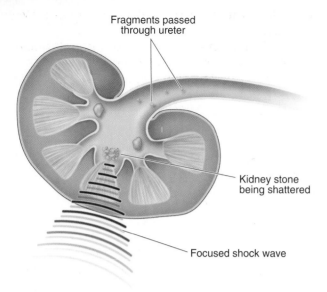

Fig. 4-7 Lithotripsy. *(Modified from LaFleur Brooks M: Exploring medical terminology: a student-directed approach, ed 5, St Louis, 2000, Mosby.)*

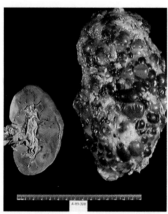

Fig. 4-8 Polycystic kidney *(right)* and normal kidney *(left). (From Lewis SM: Medical-surgical nursing: assessment and management of clinical problems, ed 5, St Louis, 2000, Mosby.)*

PATIENT-CENTERED PROFESSIONALISM

- What are the benefits to patients when medical assistants understand the diseases and disorders that affect the urinary system?
- How does understanding the signs and symptoms and diagnostic tests associated with urinary disease allow the medical assistant to provide better care to patients?

CONCLUSION

The urinary system maintains the homeostatic balance of the body's fluids by removing unwanted wastes from the blood, maintaining fluid balance, and regulating pH. The other structures of the urinary system either transport or store urine once it is formed.

The nephrons play a key role in the function of the urinary system. Your blood passes through your kidneys approximately 300 times each day. As it passes through, the nephrons "clean" all your blood in about 45 minutes, and they send about 6 cups of urine to the bladder every day. It is amazing to consider that less than half of one kidney is capable of doing all the work usually done by two kidneys.

With a solid understanding of the urinary system, medical assistants can help patients follow their treatment plans and maintain homeostasis.

SUMMARY

Reinforce your understanding of the material in this chapter by reviewing the curriculum objectives and key content points below.

1. Define, appropriately use, and spell all the Key Terms for this chapter.
   - Review the Key Terms if necessary.
2. State the five major functions of the urinary system.
   - Filters toxins from the blood.
   - Reabsorbs essential substances the body needs.
   - Excretes waste products from the body.
   - Produces erythropoietin.
   - Secretes renin.
3. Identify and locate the four major structures in the urinary system.
   - The structure of the urinary system includes two kidneys, two ureters, a urinary bladder, and a urethra.
   - The two kidneys are retroperitoneal in the lumbar area protected by the ribs. A ureter exits each kidney and enters the bladder. The urethra exits the bladder and carries urine outside the body.
4. Describe the structure and main functions of the kidneys.
   - The kidney is a main organ of the urinary system.
   - The kidneys clean the blood by filtering out nitrogenous wastes and reabsorbing nutrients and water.
   - The kidney is enclosed in a capsule and has an outer layer (cortex), inner layer (medulla), and a collection site (renal pelvis).
5. Explain the purpose of urine and describe urine formation.
   - Urine is produced in the kidneys and carries waste products out of the body.

- Blood enters the kidney through the renal artery, enters Bowman's capsule, and flows through the glomerulus, where the blood is filtered.
- The filtered blood enters the renal tubules, where needed nutrients and water are reabsorbed by the cells.
- From the renal tubules, urine enters the renal pelvis for collection and further transport to the ureters for eventual exit from the body.

6. Explain the structure of a nephron and its function in the kidney.
   - The nephron is the basic filtering unit of the kidney.
   - Review Figs. 4-3 and 4-4 for the pathway of the filtering process.

7. Describe the structure and function of the ureters.
   - The ureters are tubes leading from each kidney to the bladder.
   - Ureters force urine into the bladder with peristaltic movements of their muscular walls.

8. Describe the structure and function of the urinary bladder.
   - The urinary bladder is an expandable reservoir and holds urine until it can be released.
   - Sphincter muscles of the bladder work under conscious and unconscious control.

9. Describe the structure and function of the urethra.
   - The urethra is a single tube leading from the bladder to the outside of the body.
   - The male urethra is longer than the female urethra and is used for urine excretion and reproductive purposes.
   - The female urethra is shorter than the male urethra and only secretes urine.

10. List 13 common signs and symptoms of urinary system disorders.
    - Refer to Box 4-1.

11. List seven common diagnostic tests for urinary disease and describe the use of each.
    - Refer to Box 4-2.

12. List six urinary diseases and disorders and briefly describe the etiology, signs and symptoms, diagnosis, therapy, and interventions for each.
    - Refer to Table 4-3.

13. Explain the purpose of dialysis and list two types.
    - Dialysis cleanses the blood of toxins brought on by acute or end-stage renal disease.
    - Hemodialysis uses an artificial kidney machine to filter the patient's blood.
    - Peritoneal dialysis passes a special solution through the patient's peritoneum to cleanse the blood.

14. Analyze a realistic medical office situation and apply your understanding of the urinary system to determine the best course of action.
    - Knowledge of the urinary system and its terminology and processes can help medical assistants address patient concerns and support the physician's instructions.

15. Describe the impact on patient care when medical assistants have a solid understanding of the structure and function of the urinary system.
    - Medical assistants who understand the urinary system are better able to communicate with patients concerning problems and treatment of the urinary system and why it is so important to follow the physician's prescribed treatment plan.

For Further Exploration

Diseases that affect the kidney are numerous. To be effective with patient teaching, the medical assistant needs to be aware of causes, treatments, and medications available.

Research kidney disease to better understand the disease process, underlying causes, medications, complications, and treatments.

Keywords: Use the following keywords in your search: kidney disease, chronic kidney disease, kidney failure, dialysis, Medline.

WORD PARTS: URINARY SYSTEM

Urinary Tract
Combining Forms

cyst/o	bladder
noct/i	night
olig/o	scanty
ureter/o	ureter
urethr/o	urethra
vesic/o	bladder

Kidney
Combining Forms

azot/o	urea; nitrogen
cali/o, calic/o	calyx
cortic/o	cortex
glomerul/o	glomerulus
nephr/o	kidney
medull/o	medulla; middle
pyel/o	renal pelvis
ren/o	kidney
ur/o	urine; urinary tract

Abbreviations: Urinary System

ADH	antidiuretic hormone
ARF	acute renal failure
BUN	blood urea nitrogen
C&S	culture and sensitivity
CRF	chronic renal failure
HD	hemodialysis
IVP	intravenous pyelogram
KUB	kidneys, ureters, and bladder
UA	urinalysis
UTI	urinary tract infection

MEDICAL TERMINOLOGY OF THE BLOOD, LYMPHATIC, AND IMMUNE SYSTEMS

CHAPTER AT A GLANCE

ANATOMY AND PHYSIOLOGY

acquired immunity	basophils	homeostasis	natural immunity	spleen
agglutination	blood	immunity	neutrophils	stem cells
agglutinin	coagulation	immunoglobulins	nonspecific immunity	T cells
agglutinogens	cytokines	leukocytes	plasma	thymus
antibody	eosinophils	lymph	platelets	tonsil
antigen	erythrocytes	lymph nodes	Rh factor	
appendix	hemoglobin	lymph organs	serum	
B cells	hemostasis	lymph vessels	specific immunity	

KEY WORD PARTS

PREFIXES	SUFFIXES	COMBINING FORMS
anti-	-apheresis	aden/o
auto-	-cytosis	bas/o
inter-	-edema	eosino/o
pan-	-emia	erythr/o
poly-	-lysis	hem/o, hemat/o
trans-	-penia	home/o
	-phil	leuk/o
	-philia	lymph/o, lymphat/o
	-stasis	neutr/o
		thrombocyt/o

KEY TERMS

AIDS	blood cultures	hemophilia	mononucleosis
allergy	bone transplant	hemorrhage	pancytopenia
anaphylaxis	complete blood count	hypovolemia	purpura
anemia	dyscrasia	leukemia	splenectomy
apheresis	edema	leukocytosis	thrombocytopenia
autoimmunity	hematocrit	lymphadenopathy	
blood transfusion	hemoglobin	lymphangiography	

FUNCTIONS OF THE BLOOD, LYMPHATIC, AND IMMUNE SYSTEMS

Homeostasis (hoh mee oh STAY sis), or a "steady state," is a continual balancing act of the body systems to provide an internal environment that is compatible with life. The two liquid tissues of the body, the **blood** and **lymph** (limf), have separate but interrelated functions in maintaining this balance. They combine with a third system, the **immune** (ih MYOON) system, to protect the body against **pathogens** (PATH oh jenz) that could threaten the organism's viability.

The **blood** is responsible for the following:

- Transportation of gases (oxygen [O_2] and carbon dioxide [CO_2]), chemical substances (hormones, nutrients, salts), and cells that defend the body.
- Regulation of the body's fluid and electrolyte balance, acid-base balance, and body temperature.
- Protection of the body from infection.
- Protection of the body from loss of blood by the action of clotting.

The **lymph system** is responsible for the following:

- Cleansing the cellular environment.
- Returning proteins and tissue fluids to the blood (drainage).
- Providing a pathway for the absorption of fats and fat-soluble vitamins into the bloodstream.
- Defending the body against disease.

The **immune system** is responsible for the following:

- Defending the body against disease via the immune response.

Fig. 5-1 is a Venn diagram of the interrelationship between the three systems, with the shared goals of homeostasis and protection at the intersection of the three circles.

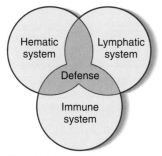

Fig. 5-1 Diagram of interrelationship between the hematic, lymphatic, and immune systems.

◇ Exercise 5-1: FUNCTIONS OF THE BLOOD, LYMPHATIC, AND IMMUNE SYSTEMS

1. What is the term for the process of maintaining a "steady state" within the body?

_____

2. Sort the following functions into their respective systems by writing the name of the system *(blood, lymphatic, or immune)* responsible for each.

_____ A. cleansing the cellular environment

_____ B. defending the body via the immune response

_____ C. protection of the body from infection

_____ D. transportation of substances throughout the body

_____ E. providing a pathway for absorption of substances into the bloodstream

_____ F. regulation of body temperature, fluids, and acid-base balance

_____ G. returning proteins and tissue fluids to the blood

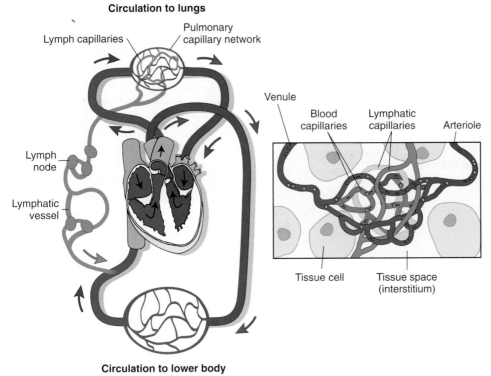

Fig. 5-2 Relationship of the lymphatic vessels to the circulatory system.

_____ H. protecting the body from blood loss by clotting

_____ I. defending the body against disease

ANATOMY AND PHYSIOLOGY

The **hematic** (hem AT ick) and **lymphatic** (lihm FAT ick) systems flow through separate yet interconnected and interdependent channels. Both are systems composed of vessels and the liquids that flow through them. The **immune** system, a very complex set of levels of protection for the body, includes blood and lymph cells.

Fig. 5-2 shows the relationship of the lymphatic vessels to the circulatory system. Note the close relationship between the distribution of the lymphatic vessels and the venous blood vessels. Tissue fluid is drained by the lymphatic capillaries and transported by a series of larger lymphatic vessels toward the heart.

The clearest path to understanding the interconnected roles of these three systems is to look at the hematic system first.

Hematic System

The hematic system is composed of blood and the vessels that carry the blood throughout the body. Because blood can be an extremely important part of the diagnostic process, students need to understand its normal composition. Blood is composed of a solid portion that consists of formed elements, or **cells,** and a liquid portion called **plasma** (PLAZ muh). Blood cells make up 45% of the total blood volume, and plasma makes up the other 55% (Fig. 5-3).

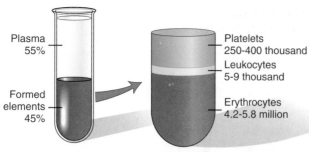

Fig. 5-3   Composition of blood.

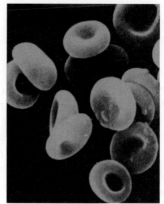

Fig. 5-4   Erythrocytes, or red blood cells. *(From Thibodeau GA, Patton KT:* Anatomy and physiology, *ed 5, St Louis, 2002, Mosby.)*

(Whole) Blood = Blood Cells (45%) + Plasma (55%)

The solid portion of blood is composed of three different types of cells:

1. **Erythrocytes** (eh RITH roh sites), also called red blood cells **(RBCs).**
2. **Leukocytes** (LOO koh sites), also called white blood cells **(WBCs).**
3. **Thrombocytes** (THROM boh sites), also called clotting cells, cell fragments, or **platelets** (PLATE lets).

In a milliliter of blood, there are 4.2 to 5.8 million RBCs, 250,000 to 400,000 platelets, and 5000 to 9000 WBCs. These cells together account for approximately 8% of body volume. Converted to more familiar liquid measure, there are about 10.5 pt (5 L) of blood in a 150-lb (68-kg) person.

Components of Blood

Erythrocytes (Red Blood Cells)

The erythrocytes (which are normally present in the millions) have the important function of transporting O_2 and CO_2 throughout the body (Fig. 5-4). The vehicle for this transportation is a protein-iron pigment called **hemoglobin** (HEE moh gloh bin).

The formation of RBCs in the bone marrow is stimulated by a hormone from the kidneys called **erythropoietin** (eh rith roh POY uh tin). RBCs have a life span of approximately 120 days, after which they decompose into **hemosiderin** (hee moh SID uh rin), an iron pigment resulting from **hemolysis** (heh MALL uh sis), and bilirubin. The iron is stored in the liver to be recycled into new RBCs, and the bile pigments are excreted via the liver.

Abnormal RBCs can be named by their **morphology** (more FALL uh jee), the study of shape or form. RBCs normally have a biconcave, disklike shape. (Although the center is depressed, there is not an actual hole.) Those that are shaped differently often have difficulty in carrying out their function.

For example, sickle cell anemia is a hereditary condition characterized by erythrocytes (RBCs) that are abnormally shaped. They resemble a crescent or sickle. An abnormal hemoglobin found inside these erythrocytes causes sickle-cell anemia in a number of Africans and African-Americans.

Leukocytes (White Blood Cells)

Although there are fewer leukocytes (thousands, not millions), there are different types with different functions. In general, WBCs protect the body from invasion by pathogens. The different types of cells provide this defense in a number of different ways. There are two main types of WBCs: granulocytes and agranulocytes.

GRANULOCYTES (POLYMORPHONUCLEOCYTES)

Named for their appearance, **granulocytes** (GRAN yoo loh sites), also called **polymorphonucleocytes** (pah lee morf oh NOO klee oh sites), have small grains within the cytoplasm and multilobed nuclei. Both names are used interchangeably.

There are three types of granulocytes, each with its own function. Each of them is named for the type of dye that it attracts.

1. **Eosinophils** (ee ah SIN oh fils) are cells that absorb an acidic dye, causing them to appear reddish. An increase in eosinophils is a response to a need for their function in defending the body against allergens and parasites.
2. **Neutrophils** (NOO troh fils) are cells that do not absorb either an acidic or basic dye and consequently are a purplish color. They are also called **phagocytes** (FAG oh sites) because they specialize in **phagocytosis** (fag oh sye TOH sis) and generally combat bacteria in pyogenic infections. This means that these cells are drawn to the site of a pathogenic "invasion," where they consume the enemy and remove the debris resulting from the battle.
3. **Basophils** (BAY soh fils) are cells that absorb a basic (or alkaline) dye and stain a bluish color. Especially effective in combating parasites, they release histamine (a substance that initiates an inflammatory response) and heparin (an **anticoagulant** [an tee koh AGG yoo lunt]), both of which are instrumental in healing damaged tissue.

AGRANULOCYTES (MONONUCLEAR LEUKOCYTES)

Agranulocytes (a GRAN yoo loh sites) are cells named for their lack of granules. The alternative name, **mononuclear leukocytes,** is so given because they have one nucleus. Both names are used interchangeably. Although these cells originate in the bone marrow, they mature after entering the lymphatic system. There are two types of these WBCs:

1. **Monocytes** (MON oh sites): These cells, named for their single, large nucleus, transform into **macrophages** (MACK roh fay jehs), which eat pathogens (phagocytosis) and are effective against severe infections.
2. **Lymphocytes** (LIM foh sites): These cells are key in what is called the **immune response,** which involves the "recognition" of dangerous, foreign (viral) substances, and the manufacture of their neutralizers. The foreign substances are called **antigens** (AN tih juns), and the neutralizers are called **antibodies** (AN tih bod ees).

Thrombocytes (Platelets)

Platelets (also known as *thrombocytes*) have a round or oval shape and are so named because they look like small plates. Platelets aid in the process of **coagulation** (koh agg yoo LAY shun), the process of changing a liquid to a solid. When blood cells escape their normal vessels, they **agglutinate** (ah GLOO tih nate), or clump together, by the following process: First, they release **factor X** (formerly called *thrombokinase*), which, in the presence of calcium, reacts with the blood protein, **prothrombin** (proh THROM bin), to form **thrombin.** Thrombin then converts another blood protein, **fibrinogen** (fye BRIN ah jen), to **fibrin** (FYE brin), which eventually forms a meshlike fibrin clot (blood clot), achieving **hemostasis** (hee moh STAY sis) (control of blood flow; that is, stopping the bleeding). See Fig. 5-5 for a visual explanation of the clotting process.

⊗ BE CAREFUL!

Whereas granulocytes are also known as *polymorphonucleocytes,* abbreviated *PMNs* or *polys,* the matter is further confused in that neutrophils are commonly referred to as *polymorphs (PMNs, polys)* because they have the greatest degree of nuclear polymorphism, in addition to being the most common type of leukocyte.

⊗ BE CAREFUL!

Don't confuse *cyt/o,* meaning cell, with *cyst/o,* meaning a bladder or a sac.

DID YOU KNOW?

The process of blood formation is called **hematopoiesis** (hee muh toh poy EE sis). All blood cells originate from a single type of cell called **a stem cell.** Hematopoietic stem cell research is currently an exciting area of health care investigation. The National Institutes of Health has a website that keeps an updated list of news links titled "NIH Stem Cell Information" at http://stemcells.nih.gov

Plasma

Plasma, the liquid portion of blood, is composed of the following:

1. Water, or H_2O (90%)
2. Inorganic substances (calcium, potassium, sodium)
3. Organic substances (glucose, amino acids, fats, cholesterol, hormones)
4. Waste products (urea, uric acid, ammonia, creatinine)
5. Plasma proteins (serum albumin, serum globulin, and two clotting proteins: fibrinogen and prothrombin)

   Serum (SEER um) (*pl.* sera) is plasma minus the clotting proteins. Serology is the branch of laboratory medicine that studies blood serum for evidence of infection by evaluating antigen-antibody reactions in vitro.

Serum = Plasma − (Prothrombin + Fibrinogen)

COMBINING FORMS FOR THE HEMATIC SYSTEM

MEANING	COMBINING FORM	MEANING	COMBINING FORM
alkaline, basic	bas/o	neutral	neutr/o
blood	hem/o, hemat/o	nucleus	nucle/o
cell	cyt/o	red	erythr/o
clotting	thromb/o	rosy, acidic	eosin/o
clumping	agglutin/o	safety, protection	immun/o
eat, swallow	phag/o	serum	ser/o
fiber	fibr/o	shape	morph/o
fibrin	fibrin/o	small grain	granul/o
iron	sider/o	white	Leuk/o
lymph	lymph/o, lymphat/o		

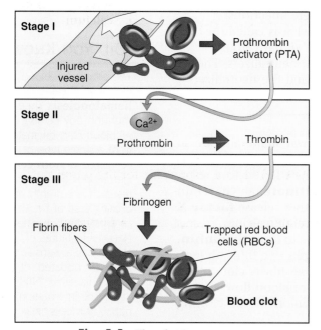

Stage I

Injured vessel → Prothrombin activator (PTA)

Stage II

Ca^{2+}

Prothrombin → Thrombin

Stage III

Fibrinogen

Fibrin fibers   Trapped red blood cells (RBCs)

Blood clot

Fig. 5-5 The clotting process.

PREFIXES AND SUFFIXES FOR HEMATIC ANATOMY AND PHYSIOLOGY

PREFIX, SUFFIX	MEANING
a-	without
-gen	producing, produced by
macro-	large
mono-	one, singular
pro-	before, in front of
-stasis	stopping, controlling

Exercise 5-2: HEMATIC SYSTEM

Circle the correct answer.

1. Whole blood is composed of *(blood cells and lymph, blood cells and plasma)*.
2. An average-size person has about *(25, 11)* pints of blood in his or her body.
3. RBCs are called *(leukocytes, erythrocytes)* and are responsible for transporting *(O_2 and CO_2, Ca and K)* through the use of *(hemosiderin, hemoglobin)*.
4. A normal RBC count should be in the *(thousands, millions, billions)*.
5. RBCs decompose in a process called *(hemostasis, hemolysis)*.
6. WBCs are called *(leukocytes, leukemia)* and generally *(defend the body against disease, regulate the body's fluid balance)*.
7. A normal WBC count should be in the *(thousands, millions, billions)*.
8. *(Agranulocytes, Granulocytes)* are so named because they have grains within their cytoplasm. The alternative name is *(mononuclear leukocytes, polymorphonucleocytes)*.
9. One type of WBC is named for its one-lobed nucleus *(mononuclear leukocyte, polymorphonucleocyte)* and its alternate name *(agranulocyte, granulocyte)*, for its lack of tiny grains in its nucleus.

Fill in the blank with the correct term from the following list.

neutrophils, eosinophils, basophils

10. Cells that absorb an acidic dye and defend against allergens and parasites. _____

11. Cells that absorb an alkaline dye, combat parasites, and release histamine and heparin.

_____

12. Cells that absorb a neutral dye and specialize in phagocytosis. _____

Match the types of plasma components with examples of each.

_____ 13. plasma protein   _____ 15. organic substance   A. urea
                                                                       B. cholesterol
_____ 14. inorganic substance   _____ 16. waste product   C. serum albumin
                                                                       D. calcium

Fill in the blanks.

17. Plasma is the _____ part of blood.

18. What is the principal component of plasma? _____

19. Plasma becomes serum when which two substances are removed? _____

20. Clotting cells are called _____cytes or platelets. They are responsible for the process of *(phagocytosis, coagulation)* (circle one).

21. Cut → _____ → release of Ca^+ and prothrombin → _____ → fibrinogen →

_____ → hemostasis.

Match the following combining forms, prefixes, and suffixes with their meanings.

_____ 22. hem/o, hemat/o	_____ 35. mon/o	A.	safety, protection
_____ 23. erythr/o	_____ 36. -stasis	B.	rosy, acidic
_____ 24. leuk/o	_____ 37. nucle/o	C.	stopping, controlling
_____ 25. thromb/o	_____ 38. fibr/o	D.	iron
_____ 26. lymph/o, lymphat/o	_____ 39. pro-	E.	before, in front of
_____ 27. immun/o	_____ 40. ser/o	F.	producing, produced by
_____ 28. morph/o	_____ 41. granul/o	G.	blood
_____ 29. cyt/o	_____ 42. -gen	H.	small grain
_____ 30. sider/o	_____ 43. agglutin/o	I.	eat, swallow
_____ 31. bas/o	_____ 44. macro-	J.	nucleus
_____ 32. eosin/o	_____ 45. fibrin/o	K.	fiber
_____ 33. neutr/o	_____ 46. a-	L.	red
_____ 34. phag/o		M.	large

N. serum
O. lymph
P. without
Q. clotting
R. neutral
S. fibrin
T. cell
U. clumping
V. alkaline, basic
W. white
X. one, singular
Y. shape

Blood Groups

Human blood is divided into four major different types: A, B, AB, and O. See Fig. 5-6 for a table of blood types, agglutinogens, and agglutinins. The differences are due to antigens present on the surface of the red blood cells. **Antigens** (ANN tih jens) are substances that produce an immune reaction by their nature of being perceived as foreign to the body. In response, the body produces substances called **antibodies** that nullify or neutralize the antigens. In blood, these

Blood Type	Antigen (RBC membrane)	Antibody (plasma)	Can receive blood from	Can donate blood to
A (40%)	A antigen	Anti-B antibodies	A, O	A, AB
B (10%)	B antigen	Anti-A antibodies	B, O	B, AB
AB (4%)	A antigen, B antigen	No antibodies	A, B, AB, O	AB
O (46%)	No antigen	Both Anti-A and Anti-B antibodies	O	O, A, B, AB

Fig. 5-6 ABO blood groups. *(From Herlihy B, Maebius, NK: The human body in health and illness, ed 2, Philadelphia, 2003, Saunders.)*

antigens are called **agglutinogens** (ah gloo TIN oh jens) because their presence can cause the blood to clot. The antibody is termed an **agglutinin** (ah GLOO tin nin). For example, type A blood has A antigen, type B has B antigen, type AB has both A and B antigens, and type O has neither A nor B antigens. If an individual with type A blood is transfused with type B blood, the A antigens will form anti-B antibodies because they perceive B blood as being foreign. Following the logic of each of these antigen-antibody reactions, an individual with type AB blood is a **universal recipient,** and an individual with type O blood is a **universal donor.**

Another antigen, the **Rh factor,** is important in pregnancy because a mismatch between the fetus and the mother can cause erythroblastosis fetalis, or **hemolytic** (hee moh LIT ick) disease of the newborn (HDN). In this disorder, a mother with a negative Rh factor will develop antibodies to an Rh+ fetus during the first pregnancy. If another pregnancy occurs with an Rh+ fetus, the antibodies will destroy the fetal blood cells.

◆ Exercise 5-3: BLOOD GROUPS

1. The four blood types are _____.

2. Not all blood types are interchangeable because of

_____.

3. A person with type A blood can donate blood to people with which blood type?

_____

4. Type O blood type is the *(universal donor, universal recipient),* whereas type AB is the *(universal donor, universal recipient)* (circle one).

5. HDN is an example of an antigen-antibody reaction of what blood factor?

_____

Lymphatic System

The lymphatic system is responsible for the following:

- Cleansing the cellular environment
- Returning proteins and tissue fluids to the blood
- Providing a pathway for the absorption of fats into the bloodstream
- Defending the body against disease

The lymphatic system (Fig. 5-7) is composed of **lymph** (or **interstitial fluid**), **lymph vessels, lymph nodes,** lymph organs (e.g., tonsils, adenoids, appendix, spleen, thymus gland, and patches of tissue in the intestines called *Peyer patches*), and lymphoid tissue. Monocytes and lymphocytes pass from the bloodstream through the blood capillary walls into the spaces between the cells in body tissue. When they pass into this lymph or interstitial fluid that surrounds cells, they perform their protective functions. Monocytes change into **macrophages** (MACK roh fay jehs), destroy pathogens, and collect debris from damaged cells. Lymphocytes are much more complicated and are essential to the immune response, so they are discussed in the next section. Once monocytes and lymphocytes pass into the lymphatic capillaries, the fluid is termed *lymph* or *lymphatic fluid.*

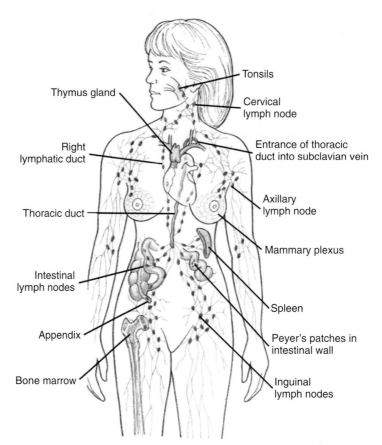

Fig. 5-7 The lymphatic system. *(From Thibodeau GA, Patton KT:* Anatomy and physiology, *ed 5, St Louis, 2002, Mosby.)*

Lymph moves in one direction to prevent pathogens from flowing through the entire body. The system filters out the microorganisms as the lymph passes through the various capillaries, vessels, and nodes. Lymph travels in the following sequence:

1. From the interstitial spaces between the cells, then
2. Toward the heart through lymphatic capillaries
3. To lymphatic vessels that carry lymph using a valvular system
4. To the lymphatic nodes, which are also called **lymph glands,** that filter the debris that has been collected through the use of macrophages. These nodes can become enlarged when pathogens are present. Note the major lymph nodes in Fig. 5-7, including the cervical, axillary, inguinal, and mediastinal nodes
5. Then to either the **right lymphatic duct** or the **thoracic duct,** both of which empty into the large subclavian veins in the neck
6. Once in the venous blood, the lymph is then recycled through the body through the circulatory system

The organs in the lymphatic system are the spleen, the thymus gland, the tonsils, the appendix, and Peyer's patches. The spleen is located in the upper left quadrant and serves to filter, store, and produce blood cells; remove RBCs; and activate B lymphocytes. The thymus gland is located in the mediastinum and is instrumental in the development of T lymphocytes (T cells). The tonsils are lymphatic tissue (lingual, pharyngeal, and palatine) that helps protect the entrance to the respiratory and digestive systems. The vermiform appendix and Peyer patches are lymphoid tissue in the intestines.

⊠ BE CAREFUL!

Don't confuse *thym/o,* which means thymus, with *thyr/o,* which means thyroid.

COMBINING FORMS FOR THE LYMPHATIC SYSTEM

MEANING	COMBINING FORM	MEANING	COMBINING FORM
armpit	axill/o	neck	cervic/o
groin	inguin/o	space between	interstit/o
lymph gland	lymphaden/o	spleen	splen/o
lymph vessel	lymphangi/o	thymus	thym/o
mediastinum	mediastin/o	tonsil	tonsill/o

◆ **Exercise 5-4: LYMPHATIC SYSTEM**

Fill in the blanks.

1. What are the two types of cells found in lymph? _____

2. How do these cells become part of lymphatic fluid?

    _____

3. What are the names of the two ducts that drain lymph back into the circulatory system?

    _____

Circle the correct answer.

4. The *(thymus, spleen)* changes lymphocytes into T lymphocytes.
5. The *(thymus, spleen)* activates B lymphocytes.
6. Macrophages develop from *(monocytes, lymphocytes)*.
7. The *(tonsils, spleen, appendix)* protect(s) the entrances to the digestive and respiratory systems.

Match the following combining forms with their meanings.

_____ 8. spleen   _____ 13. space between   A. lymphangi/o
                                                               B. thym/o
_____ 9. lymph vessel   _____ 14. lymph gland   C. interstit/o
                                                               D. splen/o
_____ 10. armpit   _____ 15. mediastinum   E. inguin/o
                                                               F. cervic/o
_____ 11. neck   _____ 16. thymus   G. mediastin/o
                                                               H. lymphaden/o
_____ 12. groin   I axill/o

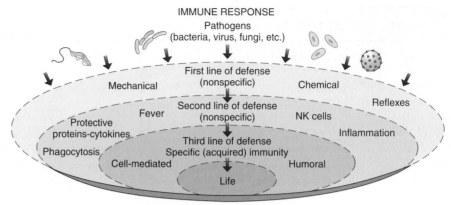

Fig. 5-8   The levels of defense.

Immune System

The immune system is composed of organs, tissues, cells, and chemical messengers that interact to protect the body from external invaders and its own internally altered cells. The chemical messengers are **cytokines** (SYE toh kynes), which are secreted by cells of the immune system that direct immune cellular interactions. Lymphocytes (leukocytes that are categorized as either **B cells** or **T cells**) secrete **lymphokines** (LIM foh kynes). Monocytes and macrophages secrete **monokines** (MAH noh kynes). **Interleukins** (in tur LOO kins) are a type of cytokine that sends messages among leukocytes to direct protective action.

The best way to understand this system is through the body's various levels of defense. The goal of pathogens is to breach these levels to enter the body, reproduce, and, subsequently, exploit healthy tissue, causing harm. The immune system's task is to stop them.

Fig. 5-8 illustrates the levels of defense. The two outside circles represent **nonspecific immunity** and its two levels of defense. The inner circle represents the various mechanisms of **specific immunity,** which can be **natural (genetic)** or **acquired** in four different ways. Most pathogens can be contained by the first two lines of nonspecific defense. However, some pathogens deserve a "special" means of protection, which is discussed under "Specific Immunity."

Nonspecific Immunity

This term refers to the various ways that the body protects itself from many types of pathogens, without having to "recognize" them. The *first line of defense* in nonspecific immunity (the outermost layer) consists of the following methods of protection:

- **Mechanical**—Examples include the skin, which acts as a barrier, and the sticky mucus on mucous membranes, which serves to trap pathogens.
- **Reflexes**—Examples include coughing, sneezing, vomiting, and diarrhea. Although not pleasant, these serve to expel pathogens that have gotten past the initial barriers.
- **Chemical**—Examples include tears, saliva, and perspiration. These have a slightly acidic nature that deters pathogens from entering the body while also washing them away. In addition, stomach acids and enzymes serve to kill germs.

The *second line of defense* in nonspecific immunity comes into play if the pathogens make it past the first line. Defensive measures include certain processes, proteins, and specialized cells.

Defensive processes include the following:

- **Phagocytosis** (fag oh sye TOH sis)—Pathogens that make it past the first line of defense and enter into the bloodstream may be consumed by neutrophils and monocytes.
- **Inflammation**—Acquiring its name from its properties, this is a protective response to irritation or injury. The characteristics (heat, swelling, redness, and pain) arise in response to an immediate vasoconstriction, followed by an increase in vascular permeability. These provide a good environment for healing. If caused by a pathogen, the inflammation is called an **infection.**
- **Pyrexia** (pye RECK see uh)—When infection is present, fever may serve a protective function by increasing the action of phagocytes and decreasing the viability of certain pathogens.

The **protective proteins** are part of the second line of defense. These include **interferons** (in tur FEER ons), which get their name from their ability to "interfere" with viral replication and limit a virus's ability to damage the body. A second protein type, the **complement proteins,** exist as inactive forms in blood circulation that become activated in the presence of bacteria, enabling them to lyse (destroy) the organisms.

Finally the last of the "team" in the second line of defense are the **natural killer (NK) cells.** This special kind of lymphocyte acts nonspecifically to kill cells that have been infected by certain viruses and cancer cells.

Specific Immunity

Specific immunity may be either **genetic**—an inherited ability to resist certain diseases because of one's species, race, sex, or individual genetics—or **acquired.** Specific immunity is dependent on the body's ability to identify a pathogen and prepare a specific response (antibody) to only that invader (antigen). Antibodies are also referred to as **immunoglobulins (Ig)** (ih myoo noh GLOB you lins). The acquired form can be further divided into natural and artificial forms, which in turn can each be either active or passive. After a description of the specific immune process, each of the four types is discussed.

Specific immunity is dependent on the agranulocytes (lymphocytes and monocytes) for its function. The monocytes metamorphose into macrophages, which dispose of foreign substances. The lymphocytes differentiate into either T lymphocytes (they mature in the thymus) or B lymphocytes (they mature in the bone marrow or fetal liver). Although both types of lymphocytes take part in specific immunity, they do it in different ways.

The T cells neutralize their enemies through a process of **cell-mediated immunity.** This means that they attack antigens directly. They are effective against fungi, cancer cells, protozoa, and, unfortunately, organ transplants. B cells use a process of **humoral immunity** (also called **antibody-mediated immunity**). This means that they secrete antibodies to "poison" their enemies.

Types of Acquired Immunity

Acquired immunity is categorized as *active* or *passive* and then is further subcategorized as *natural* or *artificial*. All describe ways that the body has acquired antibodies to specific diseases.

Active acquired immunity can take either of the following two forms:

1. **Natural:** Development of memory cells to protect the individual from a second exposure.
2. **Artificial:** Vaccination (immunization) that uses a greatly weakened form of the antigen, thus enabling the body to develop antibodies in response to this intentional exposure. Examples are the DTP and MMR vaccines.

DID YOU KNOW?

The word *humoral* in the term humoral immunity gets its name from the medieval term for body fluids—humors.

Passive acquired immunity can take either of the following two forms:

1. **Natural:** Passage of antibodies through the placenta or breast milk.
2. **Artificial:** Use of immunoglobulins harvested from a donor who developed resistance against specific antigens.

COMBINING FORMS FOR THE IMMUNE SYSTEM	
MEANING	COMBINING FORM
eat	phag/o
fever	pyr/o
flame	flamm/o
liquid	humor/o
white	leuk/o

PREFIXES AND SUFFIXES FOR THE IMMUNE SYSTEM	
PREFIX, SUFFIX	MEANING
inter-	between
non-	not
-kine	movement

 Exercise 5-5: IMMUNE SYSTEM

1. How do nonspecific and specific immunity differ?

   _____

2. Name examples of first-line defenses.

   _____

3. Name examples of second-line defenses.

   _____

4. What pathogens are neutralized by the following:

   A. interferons _____

   B. complement proteins _____

   C. NK cells _____

5. B cells get their name because they mature in the _____.

6. T cells are responsible for what type of immunity? _____

7. B cells are responsible for what type of immunity? _____

8. Monocytes change into _____.

Circle the correct answer.

9. *(Granulocyte, Agranulocyte)* cells participate in specific immunity.
10. T cells get their name because they mature in the *(thymus, thyroid)*.
11. If a patient has resistance to a disease because of heredity, this is called *(genetic, artificial)* immunity.

Choose from the following types of acquired immunity to fill in the blanks.

active natural, active artificial, passive natural, passive artificial

12. If a child has an immunization against measles, he/she has what type of immunity? _____

13. If an individual receives maternal antibodies, then this is a type of _____ immunity.

14. If an individual receives a mixture of antibodies from a donor, he or she has received

_____ immunity.

15. Acquiring a disease and producing memory cells for that disease is a type of _____ immunity.

Match the following word parts with their meanings.

_____ 16. fever	_____ 20. white	A. humor/o
_____ 17. eat	_____ 21. liquid	B. pyr/o
		C. leuk/o
_____ 18. flame	_____ 22. not	D. flamm/o
		E. inter-
_____ 19. between	_____ 23. movement	F. phag/o
		G. non-
		H. -kine

PATHOLOGY

Dyscrasia (dis KRAY zsa), a term that means *disease,* is used more specifically to describe only diseases of the blood or bone marrow. Many disorders of the blood have to do with too many or too few of certain types of blood cells. Many others have to do with abnormalities of their morphology or shape.

Terms Related to Blood Dyscrasias		
TERM	**WORD ORIGIN**	**DEFINITION**
Acute posthemorrhagic anemia	*post-* after *hem/o* blood *-rrhagia* burst forth *-ic* pertaining to *an-* no, not *-emia* blood condition	RBC deficiency caused by blood loss.
Anemia ah NEE mee ah	*an-* no, not *-emia* blood condition	Condition of lacking an adequate level of red blood cells for any of a variety of reasons.

Continued

Terms Related to Blood Dyscrasias—cont'd

TERM	WORD ORIGIN	DEFINITION
B₁₂ deficiency		Insufficient blood levels of cobalamin, also called vitamin B₁₂, which is essential for red blood cell maturation. Condition may be caused by inadequate dietary intake, as in some extreme vegetarian diets, or may result from absence of **intrinsic factor,** a substance in the gastrointestinal system essential to vitamin B₁₂ absorption.
Chronic blood loss		Long-term internal bleeding. May cause anemia.
Folate deficiency FOH late		Anemia as a result of a lack of folate from dietary, drug-induced, congenital, or other causes.
Hypovolemia hye poh voh LEE me ah	*hypo-* deficient *vol/o* volume *-emia* blood condition	Deficient volume of circulating blood.
Iron deficiency anemia	*an-* no, not *-emia* blood condition	Condition of having reduced numbers of RBCs because of chronic blood loss, inadequate iron intake, or unspecified causes. **Sideropenia** (sih dur roh PEE nee ah) is a type of iron deficiency anemia.
Pernicious anemia pur NIH shush	*an-* no, not *-emia* blood condition	Progressive anemia that results from a lack of intrinsic factor essential for the absorption of vitamin B₁₂.

Terms Related to Hemolytic Anemias

TERM	WORD ORIGIN	DEFINITION
Aplastic anemia a PLAS tick	*a-* no, not *plast/o* formation *-ic* pertaining to *an-* no, not *-emia* blood condition	Suppression of bone marrow function leading to a reduction of RBC production. Although causes of this often fatal type of anemia may be hepatitis, radiation, or cytotoxic agents, most causes are idiopathic. Also called **hypoplastic anemia.**
Autoimmune acquired hemolytic anemia hee moh LIT ick	*auto-* self *immune* safety, protection *hem/o* blood *-lytic* destruction *an-* no, not *-emia* blood condition	Anemia caused by the body's destruction of its own RBCs by serum antibodies.
Nonautoimmune acquired hemolytic anemia	*non-* not *hem/o* blood *-lytic* destruction *an-* no, not *-emia* blood condition	Anemia that may be drug induced or caused by an infectious disease.
Pancytopenia pan sye toh PEE nee ah	*pan-* all *cyt/o* cell *-penia* deficiency	Deficiency of all blood cells caused by dysfunctional stem cells.

Terms Related to Hemolytic Anemias—cont'd

TERM	WORD ORIGIN	DEFINITION
Sickle cell anemia	*an-* no, not *-emia* blood condition	Inherited anemia characterized by crescent-shaped RBCs. This abnormality in morphology causes RBCs to block small-diameter capillaries, thereby decreasing the oxygen supply to the cells (Fig. 5-9).
Thalassemia thal ah SEE mee ah	See **Did You Know?** box	Group of inherited disorders of people of Mediterranean, African, and Southeast Asian descent, in which the anemia is the result of a decrease in the synthesis of hemoglobin, resulting in the decreased production and increased destruction of RBCs.

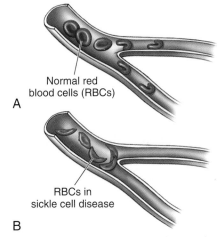

A

Normal red
blood cells (RBCs)

B

RBCs in
sickle cell disease

Fig. 5-9 A, Normal, donut-shaped red blood cells bend to fit through capillaries. **B,** Sickled red blood cells cannot bend and therefore block the flow of blood through the vessel. *(From Herlihy B, Maebius, NK: The human body in health and illness, ed 2, Philadelphia, 2003, Saunders.)*

DID YOU KNOW?

Sickle cell anemia is expressed only in individuals who inherit the gene from both parents. If only one gene is present, the patient is said to have the sickle cell trait but not the disease.

DID YOU KNOW?

The term *thalassemia* comes from the Greek word *thalassa,* meaning sea, especially the Mediterranean. Many people with thalassemia are of Mediterranean descent.

⬦ Exercise 5-6: DYSCRASIAS AND ANEMIAS

Matching.

_____ 1. -penia   _____ 6. post-

_____ 2. megal/o   _____ 7. -emia

_____ 3. sider/o   _____ 8. plast/o

_____ 4. -lytic   _____ 9. hypo-

_____ 5. a, an-   _____ 10. pan-

A. after
B. all
C. iron
D. deficiency (prefix)
E. pertaining to destruction

F. no, not, without
G. blood condition
H. formation
I. decrease (suffix)
J. large

Fill in the blank with one of the following terms.

pancytopenia, thalassemia, aplastic anemia, sickle cell anemia, autoimmune acquired hemolytic anemia, pernicious anemia, acute hemorrhagic anemia

11. What type of inherited anemia has misshapen blood cells that block blood vessels, causing oxygen

    deprivation to the cells? _____

12. What type of anemia is caused by the body destroying its own blood cells? _____

13. What type of inherited anemia may affect people of Mediterranean, African, and Southeast Asian

    descent? _____

14. What type of anemia is caused by bone marrow suppression? _____

15. Deficiency of all types of blood cells caused by dysfunctional stem cells is called _____.

16. Lack of intrinsic factor causes this type of progressive anemia. _____

17. Anemia caused by sudden blood loss is called _____.

Terms Related to Coagulation Disorders

TERM	WORD ORIGIN	DEFINITION
Hemophilia hee moh FEE lee ah	*hem/o* blood *-philia* tendency	Group of inherited bleeding disorders characterized by a deficiency of one of the factors necessary for the coagulation of the blood.
Polycythemia vera pah lee sye THEE mee ah VARE ah	*poly-* many *cyt/o* cell *-emia* blood condition *vera* true	Chronic increase in the number of RBCs and the concentration of hemoglobin. "Vera" signifies that this is not a sequela of another condition.
Purpura PURR purr uh	See **Did You Know?** box	Bleeding disorder characterized by hemorrhage into the tissues (Fig. 5-10).
Thrombocytopenia throm boh sye toh PEE nee ah	*thromb/o* clot *cyt/o* cell *-penia* deficiency	Deficiency of platelets causing an inability of the blood to clot. The most common cause of bleeding disorders.

DID YOU KNOW?

In the term *hemophilia*, the *-philia* suffix means a tendency; in this case, to bleed.

DID YOU KNOW?

Purpura comes from the Latin word for purple.

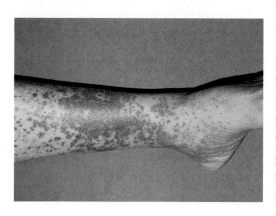

Fig. 5-10 Purpura. *(From Stevens A, Lowe J:* Pathology illustrated review in color, *ed 2, St Louis, 2000, Mosby.)*

Terms Related to Leukocytic Disorders

Term	Word Origin	Definition
Leukemia loo KEE mee ah	*leuk/o* white (blood cell) *-emia* blood condition	Any of a group of hematologic malignancies that manifest with the increase of immature WBCs at the expense of normal blood cells. (See pp. 223-224 for more information on leukemias.)
Leukocytosis loo koh sye TOH sis	*leuk/o* white (blood cell) *-cytosis* abnormal increase of cells	Abnormal increase in WBCs. Abnormal increases in each type of granulocyte are termed **eosinophilia, basophilia,** or **neutrophilia,** where the suffix *-philia* denotes *a slight increase.* Abnormal increases in the number of each type of agranulocyte are termed **lymphocytosis** or **monocytosis.**
Leukopenia loo koh PEE nee ah	*leuk/o* white (blood cell) *-penia* deficiency	Abnormal decrease in WBCs. Specific deficiencies are termed **neutropenia, eosinopenia, monocytopenia,** and **lymphocytopenia.**

◆ Exercise 5-7: COAGULATION AND WBC DISORDERS

Matching.

_____ 1. leukemia

_____ 2. hemophilia

_____ 3. purpura

_____ 4. polycythemia

_____ 5. leukopenia

_____ 6. leukocytosis

_____ 7. thrombocytopenia

A. platelet deficiency
B. slight increase of WBCs
C. hereditary bleeding disorder
D. deficiency of WBCs
E. excessive RBCs
F. hematological malignancy
G. hemorrhagic bleeding disorder of tissues

Terms Related to Lymphatic Disorders

Term	Word Origin	Definition
Edema eh DEE muh		Abnormal accumulation of fluid in the interstitial spaces of tissues.
Hypersplenism hye purr SPLEE niz um	*hyper-* excessive *splen/o* spleen *-ism* condition	Increased function of the spleen, resulting in hemolysis.
Lymphadenitis lim fad uh NYE tis	*lymphaden/o* lymph gland *-itis* inflammation	Inflammation of a lymph node.
Lymphadenopathy lim fad uh NOP puh thee	*lymphaden/o* lymph gland *-pathy* disease	Disease of the lymph nodes or vessels that may be localized or generalized.

Continued

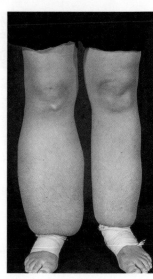

Fig. 5-11 Lymphedema. The patient had to bind her feet so that she could wear shoes. *(From Black JM, Hawks JH, Keene A: Medical-surgical nursing clinical management for positive outcomes, ed 7, Philadelphia, 2005, Saunders.)*

Terms Related to Lymphatic Disorders—cont'd

TERM	WORD ORIGIN	DEFINITION
Lymphangitis lim fan JYE tis	*lymphangi/o* lymph vessel *-itis* inflammation	Inflammation of lymph vessels.
Lymphedema lim fuh DEE muh	*lymph/o* lymph *-edema* swelling	Accumulation of lymphatic fluid and resultant swelling caused by obstruction, removal, or hypoplasia of lymph vessels (Fig. 5-11).
Lymphocytopenia lim foh sye toh PEE nee ah	*lymphocyt/o* lymphocyte *-penia* deficiency	Deficiency of lymphocytes caused by infectious mononucleosis, malignancy, nutritional deficiency, or a hematological disorder.
Lymphocytosis lim foh sye TOH sis	*lymph/o* lymph *-cytosis* increase of cells	Abnormal increase in lymphocytes.
Mononucleosis mah noh noo klee OH sis	*mono-* single, one *nucle/o* nucleus *-osis* abnormal condition	Increase in the number of mononuclear cells (monocytes and lymphocytes) in the blood caused by the Epstein-Barr virus. Can result in **splenomegaly** (enlarged spleen).

Terms Related to Immune Disorders

TERM	WORD ORIGIN	DEFINITION
Acquired immuno-deficiency syndrome (AIDS)		Syndrome caused by the human immunodeficiency virus (HIV) and transmitted through body fluids via sexual contact or intravenous exposure. HIV attacks the helper T cells, which diminishes the immune response (Fig. 5-12).
Allergy		Immune system's overreaction to irritants that are perceived as antigens. The substance that causes the irritation is called an **allergen.** Also called **hypersensitivity.**

Terms Related to Immune Disorders—cont'd

TERM	WORD ORIGIN	DEFINITION
Anaphylaxis an uh fuh LACK sis	*ana-* again, up, apart *-phylaxis* protection	Extreme form of allergic response in which the patient suffers severely decreased blood pressure and constriction of the airways.
Autoimmunity	*auto-* self *immunity* protection	Condition in which a person's T cells attack his/her own cells, causing extensive tissue damage and organ dysfunction. Examples of resultant **autoimmune diseases** include myasthenia gravis, rheumatoid arthritis, systemic lupus erythematosus, and multiple sclerosis.
Delayed allergy		Immune system hypersensitivity caused by activated T cells that respond to an exposure of the skin to a chemical irritant up to 2 days later. Examples are poison ivy and nickel. The resulting rash is called *contact dermatitis.*
Immediate allergy		Hypersensitivity of the immune system caused by IgE. Examples are insect bites and tree or grass pollens.

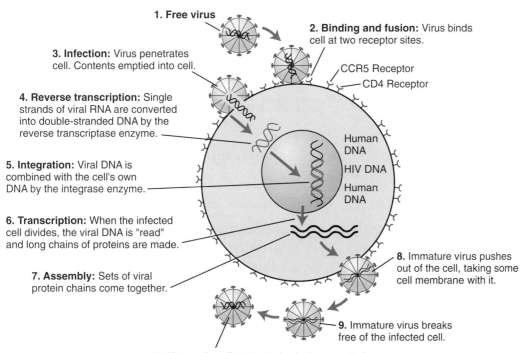

1. Free virus

2. Binding and fusion: Virus binds cell at two receptor sites.

3. Infection: Virus penetrates cell. Contents emptied into cell.

CCR5 Receptor
CD4 Receptor

4. Reverse transcription: Single strands of viral RNA are converted into double-stranded DNA by the reverse transcriptase enzyme.

Human DNA
HIV DNA
Human DNA

5. Integration: Viral DNA is combined with the cell's own DNA by the integrase enzyme.

6. Transcription: When the infected cell divides, the viral DNA is "read" and long chains of proteins are made.

7. Assembly: Sets of viral protein chains come together.

8. Immature virus pushes out of the cell, taking some cell membrane with it.

9. Immature virus breaks free of the infected cell.

10. Maturation: Protein chains in the new viral particle are cut by the protease into individual proteins that combine to make a working virus.

Fig. 5-12   HIV life cycle.

DID YOU KNOW?

Although **organ rejection** may not be viewed as an abnormal response, it is certainly an undesired one. The immune system recognizes any foreign tissue as such and responds to it with its characteristic search-and-destroy techniques. To inhibit this reaction to an organ transplant, immunosuppressant drugs are used.

DID YOU KNOW?

The term *anaphylaxis* is a misnomer. Early physiologists thought that the phenomenon was a lack of protection, not, as we know now, an exaggerated allergic response.

FIGHTING FUTURE DISEASES

The National Institute of Allergy and Infectious Diseases (NIAID) is one of the branches of the National Institutes of Health (NIH). Because its mission is to conduct and support research on immunological and infectious diseases, students may be interested in visiting its website and reading about its plans to combat emerging infectious diseases in the 21st century at http://www.niaid.nih.gov/strategicplan2000/emerge.htm.

For those interested in a more global view, another site that may be of interest is that of the World Health Organization at http://www.who.int/home-page/. Links include "Disease Outbreaks," "Traveller's Health," a "Press Media Centre," and "Information Resources."

◆ Exercise 5-8: ABNORMAL IMMUNE RESPONSES

Fill in the blank with one of the following terms.

anaphylaxis, lymphadenitis, autoimmune, allergy, immunosuppressant, lymphocytopenia, mononucleosis, hypersplenism, lymphocytosis

1. Hypersensitivity to a substance that would not otherwise threaten the life of an organism is called a(n) _____.

2. If a person's immune system attacks its own cells, he has a(n) _____ disease.

3. What type of drug is used to inhibit the rejection of transplanted organs? _____

4. What is the health care term for an extremely severe allergic reaction resulting in restricted airways and decreased blood pressure? _____

5. An abnormal increase in cells caused by the Epstein-Barr virus is called _____.

6. A lack of lymphocytes is called _____.

7. Inflammation of a lymph gland is called _____.

8. Increased splenic function is called _____.

9. An abnormal increase in lymphatic cells is called _____.

Fill in the blanks.

10. AIDS is caused by _____, which attacks _____ cells, resulting in diminished

_____ response.

◈ Exercise 5-9: LYMPHATIC AND IMMUNE DISORDERS

Match the word part with the correct term.

_____ 1. -pathy   _____ 4. edema   A. disease
                                                            B. lymph vessel
_____ 2. lymphaden/o   _____ 5. -megaly   C. enlargement
                                                            D. lymph gland
_____ 3. lymphangi/o   E. swelling

Terms Related to Benign Neoplasms

TERM	WORD ORIGIN	DEFINITION
Thymoma	*thym/o* thymus gland *-oma* tumor	Noncancerous tumor of epithelial origin that is often associated with myasthenia gravis.

Terms Related to Malignant Neoplasms

TERM	WORD ORIGIN	DEFINITION
Acute lymphocytic leukemia (ALL)	*lymph/o* lymph *cyt/o* cell *-ic* pertaining to *leuk/o* white *-emia* blood condition	Also termed acute lymphoblastic leukemia, this cancer is characterized by the uncontrolled proliferation of immature lymphocytes. It is the most common type of leukemia for individuals under the age of 19 (Fig. 5-13).
Acute myelogenous leukemia (AML)	*myel/o* bone marrow *-genous* pertaining to originating from *leuk/o* white *-emia* blood condition	This rapidly progressive form of leukemia develops from immature bone marrow stem cells.
Chronic lymphocytic leukemia (CLL)	*lymph/o* lymph *cyt/o* cell *-ic* pertaining to *leuk/o* white *-emia* blood condition	A slowly progressing form of leukemia in which immature lymphocytes proliferate. Occurs most frequently in middle age (or older) adults, rarely in children.
Chronic myelogenous leukemia (CML)	*myel/o* bone marrow *-genous* pertaining to originating from *leuk/o* white *-emia* blood condition	A slowly progressing form of leukemia in which immature bone marrow cells proliferate. Like CLL, it occurs most frequently in middle age (or older) adults, rarely in children.

Continued

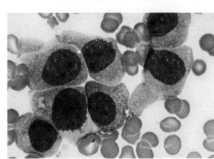

Fig. 5-13 Micrograph of leukemia. *(From Damjanov I, Linder J: Anderson's pathology, ed 10, St Louis, 1996, Mosby.)*

Terms Related to Benign Neoplasms—cont'd

TERM	WORD ORIGIN	DEFINITION
Hodgkin lymphoma	*lymph/o* lymph *-oma* tumor	Also termed *Hodgkin disease*, this cancer is diagnosed by the detection of a type of cell specific only to this disorder: Reed-Sternberg cells.
Myeloma, multiple	*myel/o* bone marrow *-oma* tumor	Also termed *plasma cell dyscrasia* or *myelomatosis*, this rare malignancy of the plasma cells is formed from B lymphocytes. It is called "multiple" myeloma because the tumors are found in many bones. If it occurs in only one bone, the tumor is referred to as a *plasmacytoma*.
Non-Hodgkin lymphoma	*lymph/o* lymph *-oma* tumor	A collection of all other lymphatic cancers but Hodgkin lymphomas. This type is the more numerous of the two lymphomas and is the sixth most common type of cancer in the United States.
Thymoma, malignant	*thym/o* thymus gland *-oma* tumor	Also termed *thymic carcinoma*, this rare malignancy of the thymus gland is particularly invasive and, unlike its benign form, is not associated with autoimmune disorders.

◈ Exercise 5-10: NEOPLASMS

Fill in the blank.

1. What is a noncancerous tumor of the thymus gland? _____

2. Which type of lymphoma is diagnosed by the detection of Reed-Sternberg cells? _____

3. Which is the most common type of leukemia in individuals under the age of 19? _____

4. Multiple myeloma is a malignancy of _____ cells.

Black Hawk Hospital
1400 Washington Ave.
Waterloo, IA 50707

PROGRESS NOTE

This 43-year-old female was seen as a result of having right ear pain for the last 3 to 4 days. She states the pain radiates to the side of her face and neck. Also complains of sore throat and increased pain to touch underneath her ear. No head pain, neck pain, no cough, cold, flu, no rhinorrhea, no congestion.

ALLERGIES: Codeine

MEDICATIONS: Calan SR 240 mg for HTN

FH/SH: Noncontributory

PHYSICAL EXAM:
Vital Signs: Temp 99.6, pulse 64, respirations 18, BP 128/74

HEENT: Ears show bilaterally clear tympanic membranes. Nose slightly congested. Throat clear. Only slight redness and injection of the peritonsillar region. Submental nodes are markedly tender on right side.

Neck: Supple, full ROM without any limitation

DIAGNOSIS: Right neck lymphadenopathy, early pharyngitis
Patient will be started on Amoxil 500 mg t.i.d.

Maurice Doate, MD

 Exercise 5-11: PROGRESS NOTE

Using the progress note above, answer the following questions.

1. What is the term for "disease of the lymph glands" in this report? _____

2. Where are these lymph glands located? _____

3. What lymphatic tissue is red and swollen (injected)? _____

Age Matters

Pediatrics

Childhood disorders of the blood, lymphatic, and immune systems range from hypersensitivities (allergies) to congenital disorders (hemolytic disease of the newborn) to acute lymphocytic leukemia.

Geriatrics

Unlike the children, seniors will have a host of diagnoses from this chapter on their charts. Anemias are common, along with a lack of blood volume (hypovolemia), which may be due to internal bleeding, trauma, or disease process. Cancers of these systems also appear in fairly significant numbers. Non-Hodgkin lymphoma and acute myelogenous leukemia account for thousands of hospitalizations every year.

DIAGNOSTIC PROCEDURES

Terms Related to Imaging

TERM	WORD ORIGIN	DEFINITION
Lymphadenography lim fad uh NAH gruh fee	*lymphaden/o* lymph gland *-graphy* process of recording	Radiographic visualization of the lymph gland after injection of a radiopaque substance. Also called **lymphography.**
Lymphangiography Lim FAN jee ah gruh fee	*lymphangi/o* lymph vessel *-graphy* process of recording	Radiographic visualization of a part of the lymphatic system after injection with a radiopaque substance (Fig. 5-14).
Splenic arteriography	*splen/o* spleen	Radiographic visualization of the spleen with the use of a contrast medium.

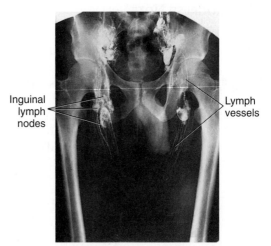

Inguinal lymph nodes

Lymph vessels

Fig. 5-14 Lymphangiogram of inguinal region and upper thighs. *(From Ballinger PW, Frank ED:* Merrill's atlas of radiographic positions and radiologic procedures, *ed 10, St Louis, 2003, Mosby.)*

Terms Related to Laboratory Tests

TERM	WORD ORIGIN	DEFINITION
AIDS tests—ELISA, Western blot		Tests to detect the presence of HIV types 1 and 2.
Allergy testing		Series of tests involving a patch, scratch, or intradermal injection of an attenuated amount of an allergen to test for hypersensitivity (Fig. 5-15).
Blood cultures		Blood samples are submitted to propagate microorganisms that may be present. Cultures may be indicated for bacteremia or septicemia, or to discover other pathogens (fungi, viruses, or parasites) (Fig. 5-16).
Complete blood cell count (CBC)		Twelve tests, including RBC (red blood cell count), WBC (white blood cell count), Hb (hemoglobin), Hct/PCV (hematocrit/packed-cell volume), and diff (WBC differential).
Coombs antiglobulin test koomz an tee GLOB yoo lin		Blood test to diagnose hemolytic disease of the newborn (HDN), acquired hemolytic anemia, or a transfusion reaction.
Diff count		Measure of the numbers of the different types of WBCs.
Erythrocyte sedimentation rate (ESR) eh RITH roh syte seh dih men TAY shun		Measurement of time for mature RBCs to settle out of a blood sample after an anticoagulant is added. An increased ESR indicates inflammation.
Hematocrit (Hct), packed-cell volume (PCV) hee MAT oh krit		Measure of the percentage of RBCs in the blood.

Continued

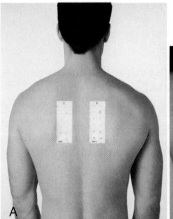
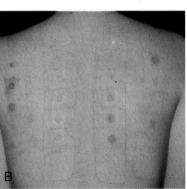

Fig. 5-15 **A,** Allergen patch test impregnated with individual allergens is applied to the back of the patient. **B,** Positive allergy reactions of varying intensity. *(From Habif TP: Clinical dermatology, ed 4, St Louis, 2004, Mosby.)*

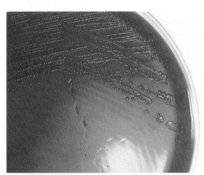

Fig. 5-16 Blood culture. *(From Bonewit-West K: Clinical procedures for medical assistants, ed 6, Philadelphia, 2004, Saunders.)*

Terms Related to Laboratory Tests—cont'd

TERM	WORD ORIGIN	DEFINITION
Hemoglobin (Hgb, Hb) HEE moh gloh bin		Iron-containing pigment of RBCs that carries oxygen to tissues.
Mean corpuscular hemoglobin (MCH) kor PUS kyoo lur		Test to measure the average weight of hemoglobin per RBC. Useful in diagnosing anemia.
Mean corpuscular hemoglobin concentration (MCHC)		Test to measure the concentration of hemoglobin in RBCs. This test is useful for measuring a patient's response to treatment for anemia.
Monospot MAH noh spot		Test for infectious mononucleosis.
Partial thromboplastin time (PTT) THROM boh plas tin		Test of blood plasma to detect coagulation defects of the intrinsic system; used to detect hemophilias.
Prothrombin time (PT) proh THROM bin		Test that measures the amount of time taken for clot formation. It is used to determine the cause of unexplained bleeding, to assess levels of anticoagulation in patients taking warfarin or with vitamin K deficiency, and to assess the ability of the liver to synthesize blood-clotting proteins.
Schilling test SHILL ing		Nuclear medicine test used to diagnose pernicious anemia and other metabolic disorders.
White blood cell count (WBC)		Measurement of the number of leukocytes in the blood. An increase may indicate the presence of an infection; a decrease may be caused by radiation or chemotherapy.

◆ Exercise 5-12: DIAGNOSTIC PROCEDURES

Matching. Some answers may be used more than once.

_____ 1. Coombs antiglobulin	_____ 9. Western blot	A. % RBCs
		B. if increased, inflammation indicated
_____ 2. Schilling test	_____ 10. Hct	C. anemia
		D. HIV
_____ 3. PTT	_____ 11. ELISA	E. response to anemia treatment
		F. determines cause of bleeding
_____ 4. PCV	_____ 12. MCH	G. hemophilia
		H. pernicious anemia
_____ 5. Monospot	_____ 13. MCHC	I. infectious mononucleosis
		J. hypersensitivity
_____ 6. ESR	_____ 14. allergy test	K. HDN, transfusion reaction
		L. microorganisms
_____ 7. blood culture	_____ 15. PT	M. prothrombin time
_____ 8. WBC		

Circle the correct answer.

16. Splenic arteriography is an x-ray *(record, process of recording)* of the spleen.
17. A lymphangiogram is a *(record, process of recording)* of a lymph *(gland, vessel)*.
18. Lymphadenography is an x-ray *(record, process of recording)* of a lymph *(gland, vessel)*.

≋ THERAPEUTIC INTERVENTIONS

Terms Related to Blood and Bone Marrow Interventions

TERM	WORD ORIGIN	DEFINITION
Apheresis aff ur EE sis	*apheresis* removal	Temporary removal of blood from a donor, in which one or more components are removed, and the rest of the blood is reinfused into the donor. Examples include **leukapheresis,** removal of WBCs; **plasmapheresis,** removal of plasma; and **plateletpheresis,** removal of thrombocytes.
Autologous bone transplant	*auto-* self *log/o* study *-ous* pertaining to	Harvesting of patient's own healthy bone marrow before treatment for reintroduction later.
Autologous transfusion ah TALL uh gus	*auto-* self *log/o* study *-ous* pertaining to *trans-* across *-fusion* pouring	Process in which the donor's own blood is removed and stored in anticipation of a future need (Fig. 5-17).
Autotransfusion	*auto-* self *trans-* across *-fusion* pouring	Process in which the donor is transfused with his or her own blood, after anticoagulation and filtration, from an active bleeding site in cases of major surgery or trauma.
Blood transfusion	*trans-* across *-fusion* pouring	Intravenous transfer of blood from a donor to a recipient, giving either whole blood or its components.
Homologous bone marrow transplant (BMT) hoh MALL uh gus	*homo-* same (species) *log/o* study *-ous* pertaining to	Transplantation of healthy bone marrow from a donor to a recipient to stimulate formation of new blood cells.

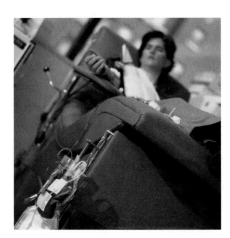

Fig. 5-17 Autologous blood transfusion.

⊠ BE CAREFUL!

Do not confuse *apheresis,* meaning removal of blood, with *poiesis,* which means formation.

DID YOU KNOW?

Apheresis is from a Greek word meaning removal. It may also be used as a suffix to create a term that means to remove blood constituents, such as *leukapheresis,* the removal of WBCs.

Terms Related to Lymphatic and Immune System Interventions

TERM	WORD ORIGIN	DEFINITION
Adenoidectomy ad eh noyd ECK tuh mee	*adenoid/o* adenoid *-ectomy* removal	Removal of the adenoids. Also called the **pharyngeal tonsils.**
Biopsy of lymphatic structures	*bi/o* living *-opsy* viewing *lymphat/o* lymph *-ic* pertaining to	Removal of the lymph nodes or lymphoid tissue to be examined for disease.
Lymphadenectomy lim fad uh NECK tuh mee	*lymphaden/o* lymph gland *-ectomy* removal	Removal of a lymph node.
Splenectomy spleh NECK tuh mee	*splen/o* spleen *-ectomy* removal	Removal of the spleen.

◇ Exercise 5-13: THERAPEUTIC INTERVENTIONS

Fill in the blanks with one of the following terms.

adenoidectomy, plasmapheresis, splenectomy, leukapheresis, autologous, homologous

1. Someone who has a transfusion of his/her own blood that has been stored in advance has what type

   of transfusion? _____

2. A patient who receives a bone marrow transplant from a donor has a(n) _____ bone marrow transplant.

3. A resection of the pharyngeal tonsils is called _____.

4. A separation of the white blood cells from the rest of the blood is called _____.

5. If plasma is separated from the rest of a unit of donated blood, the process is called _____.

6. Removal of the organ composed of lymphoid tissue in the upper left quadrant of the body is a(n)

   _____.

◇ Exercise 5-14: MEDICAL LETTER

Using the medical letter on the opposite page, answer the following questions.

1. How do you know that the patient had a slight fever? _____

2. On examination, what phrase might explain why her throat was sore? _____

3. Decode "cervical lymphadenopathy." _____

4. How do you know that the patient's spleen was enlarged? _____

5. What term tells you that test results showed an increase in the number of lymphocytes?

   _____

6. How do you know that she had been exposed to the Epstein-Barr virus? _____

Black Hawk Hospital
1400 Washington Ave.
Waterloo, IA 50707

MEDICAL LETTER

Sally C. Quinn, MD
Student Health Center
Black Hawk Hospital
1400 Washington Avenue
Waterloo, IA 50707

Allen B. Corwin, MD
River City Physician Practice
7777 S. Shore Dr.
Mason City, IA 50428

Re: Melissa Askins

Dear Dr. Quinn,

Please find the enclosed summary of treatment for Melissa R. Askins, date of birth 8/3/198x, a college student that I treated in my office last month. She requested that I forward this to you as her primary care physician in her home town, which I understand she will be returning home this summer.

This 19-year-old college student had a 2-week history of a sore throat, stiffness and tenderness of her neck, and extreme fatigue. On examination, she was mildly pyrexic with posterior cervical lymphadenopathy, palatal petechiae, and pharyngeal inflammation without an exudate. Abdominal examination showed marked splenomegaly. There was no evidence of a skin rash or jaundice.

The clinical diagnosis of infectious mononucleosis was confirmed on investigation with more than 50% of the lymphocytes showing atypical lymphocytosis. Her serum contained IgM antibodies to the Epstein-Barr viral antigen. Liver function test results were normal.

She was treated symptomatically and advised to avoid strenuous activity until her splenomegaly had completely resolved because of the danger of splenic rupture. She was also advised to abstain from alcohol for at least 6 months because many patients show clinical or biochemical evidence of liver involvement.

Sincerely,
Allen B. Corwin, MD

≋ PHARMACOLOGY

Circulatory Drugs

Anticoagulants: Drugs that prevent or delay the coagulation of the blood and the formation of thrombi. Examples include heparin, warfarin (Coumadin), enoxaparin (Lovenox), anisindione (Miradon), and lepirudin (Refludan).

Antiplatelets: Drugs that inhibit the function of platelets or destroy them. Examples include aspirin, clopidogrel (Plavix), dipyridamole (Persantine), ticlopidine (Ticlid), and abciximab (ReoPro).

Blood-flow modifiers: Drugs that promote blood flow by keeping platelets from clumping or decreasing blood viscosity. Examples include the prescription medications cilostazol (Pletal) and pentoxifylline (Trental) and the herbal product ginkgo biloba.

Colony-stimulating factors (CSF): Agents that stimulate the production of white blood cells in the bone marrow. The two kinds are granulocyte CSF (G-CSF) and granulocyte-macrophage CSF (GM-CSF). Available synthetic agents of each type are filgrastim (Neupogen) and sargramostim (Leukine), respectively.

Erythropoietic agents: Growth factors that increase production of RBCs by stimulating erythropoiesis. Two available agents are epoetin alfa (Epogen, Procrit) and darbepoetin alfa (Aranesp).

Hematinics (hee muh TUN icks): Drugs that increase the number of erythrocytes and/or hemoglobin concentration in the erythrocytes, usually to treat iron-deficient anemia. Examples are iron supplements and B-complex vitamins.

Hematopoietic (hem uh toh poy EH tick) agents: Drugs that stimulate blood cell production. Subdivisions of this class include colony-stimulating factors, erythropoietic agents, and thrombopoietic factors.

Hemostatics: Drugs that help stop the flow of blood. Examples include aminocaproic acid (Amicar) and tranexamic acid (Cyklokapron).

Thrombolytics: Drugs that aid in the dissolution of blood clots. "Clot busters" are used to treat obstructing thrombi (clots) especially in the case of myocardial infarction or pulmonary embolism. Examples are tissue plasminogen activator (tPA), streptokinase (Streptase), and alteplase (Activase).

Thrombopoietic factors: Agents that stimulate the production of thrombocytes or platelets. Oprelvekin (Neumega) is an available agent.

Lymphatic and Immune Drugs

Antihistamines: Drugs that block histamine (H_1) receptors to manage allergy symptoms. Examples include clemastine (Tavist), diphenhydramine (Benadryl), loratadine (Claritin), and fexofenadine (Allegra).

Anti-IgE (Immunoglobulin E) agents: Monoclonal antibodies that treat allergic asthma and allergic rhinitis. Omalizumab (Xolair) is the first available agent in this class.

Antineoplastics: Drugs used to treat cancer by preventing growth or promoting destruction of neoplastic (tumor) cells. There are numerous drugs that fall into this category, including methotrexate and rituximab (Rituxan).

Antiretrovirals: Drugs that manage the replication of HIV and its progression into AIDS. Examples include zidovudine or AZT (Retrovir) and efavirenz (Sustiva).

Corticosteroids: Drugs also known as "steroids" that suppress the immune system and reduce inflammation. Examples include fluticasone (Flovent, Flonase), hydrocortisone (Cortizone), and prednisone (Deltasone).

Cytotoxic agents: Drugs used as immunosuppressants or antineoplastics in order to damage or destroy cells.

Immunosuppressants: Drugs that reduce the immune response. Examples include azathioprine (Imuran), cyclophosphamide (Cytoxan), cyclosporine (Sandimmune), and tacrolimus (Prograf).

Leukotriene receptor antagonists: Drugs that block leukotrienes to manage later stages of allergic reactions; especially used to manage allergic asthma. The most popular agent in this class is montelukast (Singulair).

Protease (PRO tee aze) inhibitors: These drugs are a type of antiretroviral and used to treat HIV infection. By blocking the production of an essential enzyme called protease, these drugs keep the virus from replicating. Examples are indinavir (Crixivan), nelfinavir (Viracept), and saquinavir (Invirase).

Vaccines (immunizations): Substances administered to induce the immunity or reduce the pathological effects of a disease. Examples are the measles, mumps, rubella vaccine and the chicken pox vaccine.

◈ **Exercise 5-15: PHARMACOLOGY**

Match each drug group with its action.

_____ 1. thrombolytics

_____ 2. antiplatelets

_____ 3. hematopoietic agents

_____ 4. hematinics

_____ 5. anticoagulants

_____ 6. antihistamines

_____ 7. immunosuppressants

_____ 8. antineoplastics

_____ 9. hemostatics

_____ 10. vaccines

A. treat allergic reactions
B. delay clotting of blood
C. inhibit clotting, destroy thrombocytes
D. help induce immunity
E. increase WBCs
F. stop the flow of blood
G. decrease tumor cells
H. lesson the immune response
I. increase RBC or Hgb concentration
J. destroy clots

Abbreviations

Abbreviation	Definition	Abbreviation	Definition
A, B, AB, O	Blood types	HIV	Human immunodeficiency virus
AIDS	Acquired immunodeficiency syndrome	Ig	Immunoglobulin
		Lymphs	Lymphocytes
ANA	Antinuclear antibody	MCH	Mean corpuscular hemoglobin
Baso	Basophils	MCHC	Mean corpuscular hemoglobin concentration
BMT	Bone marrow transplant		
CBC	Complete blood cell count	Neut	Neutrophils
CO_2	Carbon dioxide	NK	Natural killer cells
Diff	Differential WBC count	O_2	Oxygen
EBL	Estimated blood loss	PCV	Packed-cell volume, hematocrit
EBV	Epstein-Barr virus	Plats	Platelets, thrombocytes
Eos	Eosinophils	PMNs, polys	Polymorphonucleocytes
ESR	Erythrocyte sedimentation rate	PT	Prothrombin time
Hb	Hemoglobin	PTT	Partial thromboplastin time
Hct, crit	Hematocrit, packed-cell volume	RBC	Red blood cell (count)
HDN	Hemolytic disease of the newborn	Rh	Rhesus
Hgb	Hemoglobin	WBC	White blood cell (count)

◈ Exercise 5-16: ABBREVIATIONS

Write out the term for the following abbreviations.

1. Karl was admitted with a Dx of EBV.

   _____

2. The patient's blood sample was tested for Hct and Hb.

   _____

3. The AIDS patient was HIV positive.

   _____

4. The patient left surgery with an EBL of 300 cc.

   _____

5. The patient was admitted for a BMT with his twin as the donor.

   _____

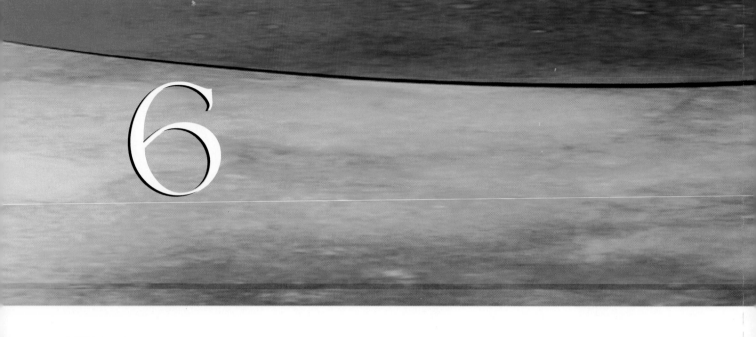

Objectives

You will be able to do the following after completing this chapter:

Key Terms
1. Define, appropriately use, and spell all the Key Terms for this chapter.

Blood
2. List the eight components of blood plasma.
3. List three types of blood cells and describe the function of each.
4. List the four blood types and explain the importance of compatibility.
5. Explain the importance of Rh factor as it relates to pregnancy and transfusions.
6. List nine diseases of the blood and describe the etiology, signs and symptoms, diagnosis, therapy, and interventions for each.

Lymphatic System
7. List the four divisions of the lymphatic system and describe the function of each.
8. List four diseases of the lymphatic system and describe the etiology, signs and symptoms, diagnosis, therapy, and interventions for each.

Immune System
9. List the immune system's three lines of defense and describe each.
10. Distinguish between *genetic* (inborn) immunity and *acquired* immunity and give an example of each.
11. List three diseases of the immune system and describe the etiology, signs and symptoms, diagnosis, therapy, and interventions for each.
12. Describe the considerations associated with the testing of AIDS patients.

Patient-Centered Professionalism
13. Analyze a realistic medical office situation and apply your understanding of the circulatory system to determine the best course of action.
14. Describe the impact on patient care when medical assistants have a solid understanding of the structure and function of the circulatory system.

ANATOMY AND PHYSIOLOGY OF THE BLOOD, LYMPHATIC, AND IMMUNE SYSTEMS

KEY TERMS

The Key Terms for this chapter have been organized into sections so that you can easily see the terminology associated with each aspect of the circulatory, lymphatic, and immune systems.

Blood

antibody Protein produced in response to the presence of an antigen.

erythrocyte Red blood cell (RBC).

formed elements Blood components (blood cells; e.g., RBCs, WBCs, platelets).

hematopoiesis Production of blood cells.

leukocyte White blood cell (WBC).

plasma Liquid matrix of the blood.

serum Liquid portion of the blood after blood clotting.

stem cell Main cell from which all cells develop.

thrombocyte Platelet.

Erythrocytes

biconcave Concave (depressed spheres) on both sides.

erythropoiesis Process of red blood cell formation.

erythropoietin Hormone that stimulates bone marrow to produce erythrocytes.

hemoglobin Iron-containing pigment found in red blood cells used to transport oxygen.

macrophage Cells responsible for destroying worn-out red blood cells and cellular debris; major phagocyte.

metabolism Energy production.

red blood cells (RBCs) Cells in the blood that transport oxygen and carbon dioxide to and from the tissues.

reticulocyte Immature red blood cell.

Leukocytes

agranulocytes White blood cells without granules in the cytoplasm.

basophils White blood cells that respond to allergic reactions.

differential count Laboratory blood test that determines the percentage of each type of white blood cell present in a blood sample.

eosinophils White blood cells that react to the release of histamine in the body.

granulocytes White blood cells containing granules in the cytoplasm.

lymphocyte Type of leukocyte that is agranular; also a lymph cell.

microorganism Organism (e.g., a bacterium) that can be seen only by using a microscope.

monocytes Granular white blood cells that assist with phagocytosis.

neutrophils Granular white blood cells that are the body's first response to an infection.

phagocytes White blood cells that engulf foreign material.

phagocytosis Process of engulfing and digesting foreign material.

white blood cells (WBCs) Cells in the blood that help provide protection against infection and disease.

Thrombocytes

coagulation Clotting.

coagulation factors Substances in plasma that are released to form clots.

fibrin Protein that forms a clot.

fibrinogen Clotting factor.

hemostasis Cessation of bleeding through a series of events: vasoconstriction, formation of a plug, and blood clotting.

platelet Cell fragment responsible for clotting; thrombocyte.

prothrombin Substance needed for clot formation.

thrombin Substance formed by the combination of prothrombin and calcium.

Blood Types and Rh Factor

ABO blood groups Blood types (A, B, AB, or O).

KEY TERMS—*cont'd*

agglutinate, agglutination Process of blood cells clumping together when the wrong blood type is transfused.

antigen Substance found in the body that marks cells as self or nonself and stimulates production of antibodies.

donor Person who gives blood.

hemolysis Breaking down of the membranes of red blood cells.

recipient Person who receives blood.

Rh factor Rhesus factor, an antigen factor in blood.

transfusion Process of taking blood from a donor and infusing it into a recipient.

type and crossmatch Process of determining a person's blood type and establishing compatibility of another's blood type for transfusions.

universal donor Blood type with neither type A nor type B antigens; type O blood.

universal recipient Blood type with A and B antigens; type AB blood.

Blood Diseases

ecchymosis Hemorrhagic (bruised) area of skin caused by trauma to a blood vessel; blue-black changing to greenish-brown.

petechiae Small purple or red spots appearing on the skin as a result of hemorrhages within the dermis.

protozoa Single-cell animal.

Lymphatic System

edema Abnormal tissue swelling.

interstitial fluid Fluid between the cells of tissue.

lymph Fluid transported in the lymphatic vessels.

lymph nodes Small oval-shaped bodies of lymphoid tissue that contain lymph and macrophages to fight infection.

lymphatic vessels Vessels that transport lymph from the body toward the subclavian vein for return to the blood.

lymphatics Larger vessels formed by lymph capillaries.

lymphoid organs Spleen, tonsils, thymus, and lymph vessels.

mastectomy Removal of breast tissue.

pharynx Throat.

spleen Organ that stores and destroys red blood cells and produces lymphocytes and monocytes.

T lymphocyte Lymphocyte that matures in the thymus gland and directly attacks foreign substances (e.g., viruses).

thymosin Hormone secreted by the thymus that helps to develop the T cells.

thymus gland Lymphatic organ located in the mediastinum and a primary site for T cell formation.

tonsils Lymphoid tissue located in the pharynx and the base of the tongue.

Immune System

acquired immunity Immunity achieved through the body's production of antibodies either from disease process or through vaccination (active or passive immunity).

active immunity Immunity provided by having the disease.

artificially acquired immunity Process of providing immunity by vaccination.

attenuated Altered; weakened, as in a vaccine.

B lymphocyte Lymphocyte that matures in lymphoid tissue and produces antibodies that react against the toxins produced by bacteria.

genetic immunity Natural (inborn) immunity.

immunity Defense against a specific disease.

interferons Proteins produced by T cells and cells infected with viruses that block the ability of a virus to reproduce.

natural acquired immunity Process of immunity in which the body produces its own antibodies through disease.

nonspecific immunity Process of immunity in which the body reacts to eliminate the effects of microorganisms.

passive immunity Immunity provided by antibodies being passed through the placenta or mother's milk or through gamma globulin.

pathogens Disease-producing bacteria.

resistance Ability of the body to fight off infection or disease.

specific immunity Selective immune response of the body against a particular microorganism.

vaccination Process of injecting antigens of a disease into the body to produce artificially acquired immunity.

What Would You Do?

Read the following scenario and keep it in mind as you learn about the blood, lymphatic, and immune systems in this chapter.

Pierce Fisher has come to the health clinic today to see Dr. Giffin for a routine physical examination. Pierce tells Lisa, the medical assistant, that he has been having episodes of dizziness and has some pain in his RLQ. Lisa notices that while Pierce's blood pressure is WNL, his temperature and pulse are elevated. Dr. Giffin exams Pierce and orders a stat CBC with a differential count as a way of ruling out a diagnosis of appendicitis. As Lisa is completing the blood draw, Pierce has several questions about his blood work and what it can tell the physician about his condition.

When Pierce's blood results come back, would you be able to tell what the results indicate?

In the cardiovascular chapter, you were able to trace the movement of blood through the heart, to the lungs, and out to the other body systems through a network of blood vessels that work together to sustain life. By understanding the function and composition of blood, you will begin to recognize what a complex transport medium blood is and how it performs vital pickup and delivery services for the body. In addition, this chapter introduces two other systems: the lymphatic system and the immune system. These two systems are not typically considered "body systems" because their functions are carried out by specific cells, tissues, and organs within the circulatory system. Their most important functions are to maintain fluid balance and immunity. Therefore they play an important role in sustaining human life.

≋ BLOOD

Another component of the circulatory system is the blood itself. The function of blood is to transport oxygen and nutrients throughout the body and carry off wastes. Blood is important to our bodies in the following ways:

1. Blood takes oxygen from the lungs and nutrients from the digestive system to the body tissue.
2. Blood carries waste products away from the cells and to the kidneys and lungs for excretion.
3. Blood aids in regulating body temperature.
4. Blood distributes various hormones and chemicals throughout the body.

An average adult has 4 to 6 liters of blood. The *pH* (degree of acidity or alkalinity of a substance) of blood is 7.4, or slightly alkaline. Whole blood is divided into two parts: the plasma (liquid matrix) and the formed elements (blood cells) (Fig. 6-1).

Blood is made up of approximately 55% plasma and 45% formed elements, depending on each individual. Understanding the normal structure and function of blood, as well as the different types of blood diseases, requires knowledge of these two components.

Plasma

A pale-yellow fluid, **plasma** is about 90% water. The remaining 10% is composed of nutrients, electrolytes, gases, clotting factors, **antibodies** (substances that produce an immunity), waste products, and hormones (Table 6-1).

TABLE 6-1	Substances Carried in the Blood
Category	**Substances**
Nutrients	Carbohydrates
	Proteins
	Fats
Electrolytes	Chloride (Cl)
	Potassium (K)
	Calcium (Ca)
	Sodium (Na)
	Bicarbonate (HCO_3^-)
	Phosphate (PO_4)
Gases	Carbon dioxide (CO_2)
	Oxygen (O_2)
Proteins	Globulins
	Albumin
Clotting factors	Fibrinogen
	Prothrombin
Waste	Urea
	Uric acid
	Amino acids
Other	Antibodies
	Hormones
	Enzymes

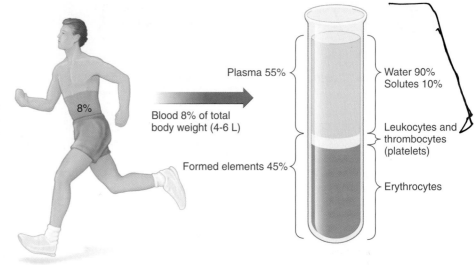

Fig. 6-1 Approximate components of blood. *(Modified from Applegate EJ:* The anatomy and physiology learning system, *ed 2, Philadelphia, 2000, Saunders.)*

Blood 8% of total body weight (4-6 L)

Plasma 55%

Water 90%
Solutes 10%

Leukocytes and thrombocytes (platelets)

Formed elements 45%

Erythrocytes

8%

BOX 6-1   **Stem Cell**

A stem cell has the ability to produce specialized cells for various tissues of the body (e.g., heart, brain, liver, etc.). There are two types:

Embryonic stem cell: Stem cells obtained from aborted fetuses or leftover fertilized eggs from in vitro fertilization.

Adult stem cell: Stem cells specific to blood, intestines, skin, and muscle; they are present in children as well as adults.

Stem cell research is controversial. You can learn more about the various sides of this issue by researching on the Internet.

Blood Cells

Blood is considered a tissue because it contains many types of cells. The blood cells are the **formed elements** of the blood and are composed of **erythrocytes** (red blood cells), **lymphocytes** (white blood cells), and **thrombocytes** (platelets) (Fig. 6-2). Blood cells are produced **(hematopoiesis)** in the bone marrow, found mostly in the flat and irregular bones and in lymphoid tissue (lymph nodes, spleen, thymus gland). All blood cells produced in the bone marrow originate from the same type of cell, the **stem cell** (Box 6-1). The stem cell differentiates into the erythrocyte, leukocyte, and platelet (Fig. 6-3).

Erythrocytes

Red blood cells (RBCs) are the most numerous of the blood cells. The human body has about 5 million RBCs per cubic millimeter of blood. RBCs

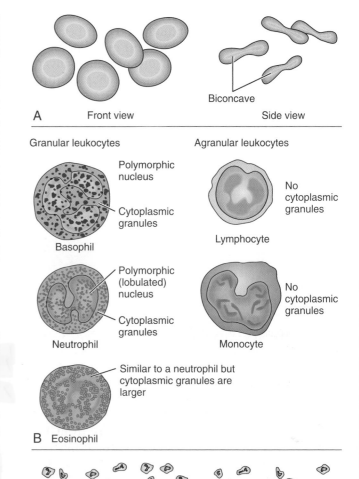

A   Front view   Biconcave   Side view

Granular leukocytes   Agranular leukocytes

Polymorphic nucleus

Cytoplasmic granules

Basophil

No cytoplasmic granules

Lymphocyte

Polymorphic (lobulated) nucleus

Cytoplasmic granules

Neutrophil

No cytoplasmic granules

Monocyte

Similar to a neutrophil but cytoplasmic granules are larger

B   Eosinophil

C

Fig. 6-2 Formed elements in blood: **A,** erythrocytes; **B,** leukocytes; **C,** platelets. *(Modified from Chester GA:* Modern medical assisting, *Philadelphia, 1999, Saunders.)*

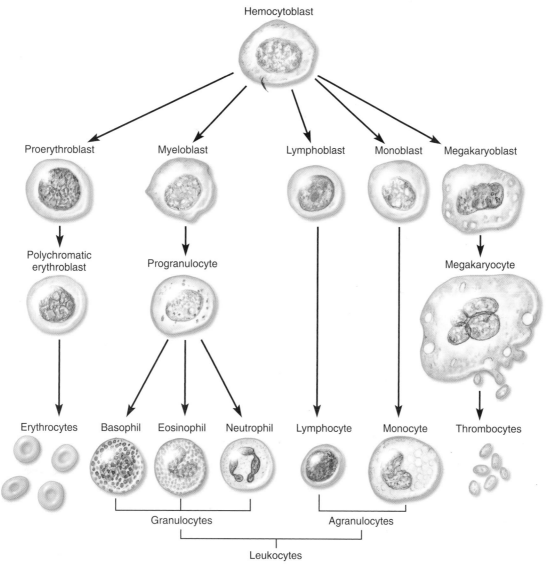

Fig. 6-3 Development of the formed elements in blood. *(Modified from Applegate EJ: The anatomy and physiology learning system, ed 2, Philadelphia, 2000, Saunders.)*

have a **biconcave** disk shape that makes it easier for them to "piggyback" oxygen. As blood flows through the body tissues, it releases the oxygen to be used in cellular **metabolism** (energy production).

RBCs contain **hemoglobin,** an iron-containing protein that carries both oxygen and carbon dioxide and provides the erythrocyte with its red color (Fig. 6-4). A healthy diet contains enough iron to ensure that adequate hemoglobin formation takes place. Vitamin B_{12} and folic acid are also necessary for normal RBC production.

Erythropoiesis is the process of RBC formation. This process begins in the bone marrow (Fig. 6-5). **Erythropoietin** (a hormone) is released from the kidney when the oxygen concentration is low in the blood. This stimulates the bone marrow to produce more erythrocytes. As the oxygen in the blood increases, this process subsides. An immature erythrocyte is referred to as a **reticulocyte.** As it matures, the RBC loses its nucleus, thus giving it more surface area to carry oxygen. The RBC erythrocyte count is normally between 4.5 and 5.5 million depending on gender. The life span of an RBC is 120 days. As the erythrocytes age and become fragile, their hemoglobin is recycled and the **macrophages** destroy them in the liver and spleen.

Leukocytes

White blood cells (WBCs) have a nucleus and are less numerous than erythrocytes. Leukocytes range from 4500 to 11,000 per cubic millimeter of blood. WBCs act as scavengers, and their numbers increase during an infection or allergic reaction. This process of engulfing and digesting foreign material is called **phagocytosis.**

Hemoglobin

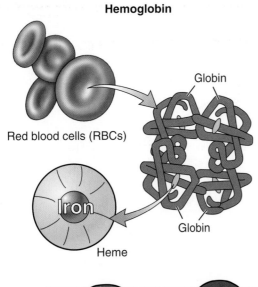

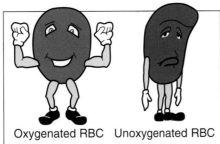

Fig. 6-4 Function of hemoglobin. *(From Herlihy B, Maebius NK: The human body in health and illness, ed 2, Philadelphia, 2003, Saunders.)*

There are five types of WBCs, which can be differentiated by their staining properties observed through the use of a microscope. Some WBCs **(neutrophils, basophils,** and **eosinophils)** have **granulocytes** in their cytoplasm. Other WBCs are **lymphocytes** and **monocytes,** which are **agranulocytes.** Table 6-2 compares the properties of the five leukocytes.

When a physician orders a **differential count** (diff), the physician wants to know what percentage of each type of WBC is present in the blood. An increase or decrease in differential cells is helpful to the physician in the diagnosis of disease.

Thrombocytes

Platelets are fragments of cells that vary in shape and size and do not have a nucleus. Their function is to stop bleeding by forming a clot to maintain **hemostasis** (prevention of blood loss) (Fig. 6-6). Thrombocytes range from 250,000 to 400,000 per cubic millimeter of blood.

An injury to a blood vessel causes a chain reaction that results in clot formation, as follows:

1. When a blood vessel is injured, the blood vessel constricts, and platelets release **coagulation factors** into the plasma that release prothrombin activator to begin the process of coagulation.
2. Platelet factors combine with **prothrombin** and calcium to form **thrombin,** which causes

Fig. 6-5 Regulation of red blood cell production by erythropoietin and oxygen (O_2). *(From Herlihy B, Maebius NK: The human body in health and illness, ed 2, Philadelphia, 2003, Saunders.)*

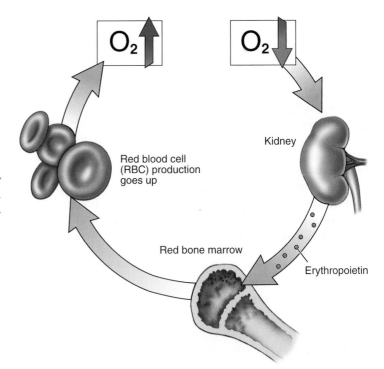

TABLE 6-2 Leukocytes

Cell Type and Description	Percent Present	Function	Size and Shape of Nucleus	Granule Staining Properties
Granulocyte *Neutrophils (also called segs)* Considered **phagocytes:** first responders to an acute infection or damaged site; engulf microbes by phagocytosis. Their numbers increase significantly during an acute infection. Diameter of 10-15 µm. ***NOTE: A band is an immature neutrophil whose nucleus has not segmented. Range 0%-5%***	55%-70%	Phagocytosis	3-5 lobes or segments	Pink
Eosinophils Protect the body by reacting to the release of histamine during an allergic reaction. They also provide a defense against parasitic worms. Diameter of 12-17 µm.	1%-3%	Allergic reactions	2 lobes or segments	Orange-red
Basophils Increase in response to allergic reactions. When basophils enter the tissue, they release histamine and heparin. Histamine dilates blood vessels to increase blood flow, and heparin inhibits the formation of blood clots. Diameter of 10-14 µm.	<1%	Allergic reaction Inflammatory response	2 lobes or U-shaped	Dark blue
Agranulocyte *Lymphocytes* Work to activate the immune system. As the body is invaded by a **microorganism** (bacteria/virus), the lymphocytes multiply and form a plasma cell that makes a specific antibody. The antibody trips the immune system into action. Diameter of 6-12 µm.	25%-30%	Immunity	Large, almost fills cells	Nucleus dark blue
Monocytes First line of defense in the inflammatory process. Enter damaged tissues and become macrophages that continue the process of digesting cellular debris that was begun by the neutrophils. Diameter of 12-20 µm.	3%-8%	Phagocytosis	U-shaped, surrounded by cytoplasm	Nucleus medium blue

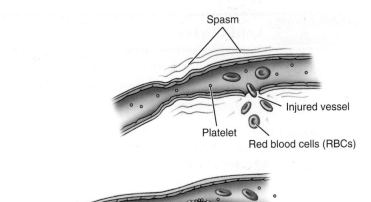

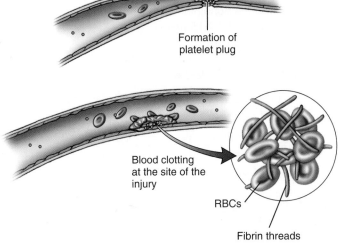

Fig. 6-6 Process of hemostasis. *(From Herlihy B, Maebius NK: The human body in health and illness, ed 2, Philadelphia, 2003, Saunders.)*

the platelets to become sticky and form a plug.

3. Thrombin reacts with **fibrinogen** to form a gel called **fibrin.**

4. RBCs become trapped in the fibrin threads, and a clot is formed.

Fig. 6-7 illustrates the stages of the **coagulation** (blood-clotting) process. Box 6-2 lists abbreviations for common blood terms.

Blood Types and Rh Factor

Blood can be grouped according to its inherited properties. Blood is grouped into the ABO blood groups as well as by its Rh factor.

Blood Types

Blood is classified using the **ABO blood group** system. ABO blood groups (blood types) are identified by the presence of or absence of genetically controlled proteins **(antigens)** on red blood cells. The four blood types are as follows:

- Type A
- Type B
- Type AB
- Type O

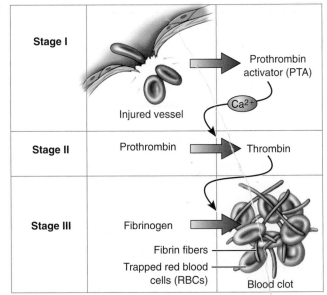

Fig. 6-7 Process of blood clotting. *(Modified from Herlihy B, Maebius NK: The human body in health and illness, ed 2, Philadelphia, 2003, Saunders.)*

Table 6-3 shows a person with type B blood born with type B antigens and anti-A antibodies on the RBC. Not all blood types are compatible. Care must be taken to give blood **transfusions** of the same blood type as the person receiving the transfusion.

Death for the **recipient** can result when antibodies in the recipient's blood plasma join to the antigens in the person's blood causing the RBCs of the **donor** to **agglutinate** (clump together). As Table 6-3 shows, a person with type B blood can receive blood from a person with B or O. People with type O blood have neither A nor B antigens that can cause agglutination with A or B antigens; therefore they are considered **universal donors.** A person with type AB blood can receive A, B, AB, and O; people in this group are considered **universal recipients** because these people have no antigens to combine with the antibodies. Compatible blood types are determined by performing a **type and crossmatch** on both the donor's and the recipient's blood.

Rh Factor

The **Rh factor** (rhesus factor) is another type of antigen that may be found on RBCs. If the Rh factor is found on the blood cells, this is recorded as Rh-positive (+). Failure to have the Rh antigen registers as Rh-negative (−).

Fig. 6-8 shows the dangers of a baby born to an Rh-negative mother and Rh-positive father. If the baby is Rh positive, the mother's RBCs will stimulate the mother's blood to form anti-Rh antibodies. The next pregnancy with an Rh-positive baby could cause **hemolysis** of the baby's RBCs (hemolytic disease of the newborn, or HDN).

Diseases of the Blood

As in the heart and blood vessels, diseases also affect the blood (Table 6-4). Some blood diseases are associated with one of the three types of blood cells;

BOX 6-2	**Abbreviations for Common Blood Terms**
Ab	antibody
Ag	antigen
CBC	complete blood count*
DIFF, diff	differential count
Hct, crit	hematocrit†
Hgb, Hb	hemoglobin; grams in 100 ml of blood
plat	platelet
PT	prothrombin time
PTT	partial thromboplastin time
RBC	red blood cell; RBC count
WBC	white blood cell; WBC count

*Number of RBCs, WBCs, and platelets per cubic millimeter of blood; Hct; Hgb; and cell volume measurements.
†Percentage of packed red blood cells in a given volume of blood expressed as a percentage.

TABLE 6-3	**Blood Types**				
Blood Type	**Antigen (RBC membrane)**	**Antibody (Plasma)**	**Can Receive Blood From**	**Can Donate Blood To**
A (40%)	A antigen	Anti–B antibodies	A, O	A, AB
B (10%)	B antigen	Anti–A antibodies	B, O	B, AB
AB* (4*)	A antigen, B antigen	No antibodies	A, B, AB, O	AB
O† (46%)	No antigen	Both anti–A and anti–B antibodies	O	O, A, B, AB

*Type AB: universal recipient.
†Type O: universal donor.

TABLE 6-4   Diseases of the Blood

Disease and Description	Etiology	Signs and Symptoms	Diagnosis	Therapy	Interventions
Diseases Related to Red Blood Cells (RBCs)					
Anemia: Disease diagnosed by certain elements missing in the blood.					
Iron deficiency anemia Low levels of iron in the blood	Chronic anemia with RBCs lacking sufficient iron for chronic blood loss Decreased iron intake Malabsorption	Pallor, fatigue, weakness	Laboratory tests show decrease in RBCs, Hgb, Hct Decreased serum iron and serum ferritin (**serum** is plasma minus clotting factors)	Diet with adequate iron-containing foods and correction of underlying cause (e.g., bleeding)	Reinforce the treatment plan and answer patient's questions
Pernicious anemia Megaloblastic anemia resulting in decrease of hydrochloric acid and deficiency of the intrinsic factor needed for vitamin B₁₂ absorption	Genetic predisposition	Complaints of weakness; beefy, red tongue; tingling or numbness in limbs	Laboratory tests to rule out other anemias; gastric analysis	Vitamin B₁₂ replacement and iron supplement	Encourage a well-balanced diet, including foods high in vitamin B₁₂
Malaria Caused by **protozoa** of the genus *Plasmodium*	Transmitted by an infected mosquito or blood products Mosquito injects spores into the wound, which settle in the liver	Chills, fever, headache, fatigue, sweating Signs of ruptured RBCs	Patient history of travel to the tropics, use of intravenous drugs, or recent blood transfusion Blood smear identifying parasite	Medication therapy for acute attacks	Eliminate breeding source for mosquitos Person should seek prophylactic treatment if traveling to known infested area
Septicemia Blood poisoning: systematic infection caused by a pathogenic organism	Complication of another infection	Patient's current complaints, including prior infections	Laboratory tests: positive blood cultures, CBC, BUN, PT, PTT	Antibiotic therapy for causative agent	Provide emotional support to family and patient; answer questions and explain course of treatment
Vitamin K deficiency Bleeding disorder caused by insufficient vitamin K (needed for blood to clot)	Inability to absorb vitamin K from foods	Poor blood coagulation	Laboratory tests, including PT	Vitamin K given parenterally	Diet high in vitamin K if malabsorption problem can be corrected

Polycythemia
Overproduction of RBCs by the bone marrow | Unknown; high incidence in Jewish men | Weakness and fatigue with complaints of headache, dizziness, and double vision | Blood tests show increased RBCs | Possible splenectomy or phlebotomy to reduce RBCs | Removal of a pint of blood

Diseases Related to White Blood Cells (WBCs)

Leukemia
Uncontrolled WBC (leukocyte) production interfering with normal blood cell production | Unknown | Fatigue, dyspnea on exertion, weight loss, and swollen cervical lymph nodes | Elevated WBCs; Decreased RBCs, Hgb, Hct; Tumor markers assist in determining type of leukemia | Medication therapy to induce remission (chemotherapy) | Assist patient with coping; encourage good nutrition and rest

Forms include *acute lymphocytic, chronic lymphocytic, acute myelogenous,* and *chronic myelogenous* leukemia

Diseases Related to Platelets

Thrombocytopenia
Decreased clotting capabilities of the blood | Idiopathic or secondary to another disease | **Petechiae** and **ecchymosis** on the skin; easy bruising; bleeding from nose and gums | Rule out other platelet disorders through blood tests | Medication to induce platelet production | Instruct patient in ways to reduce injury and bleeding

Diseases Related to Incompatibility

Erythroblastosis fetalis
Hemolytic disease of the newborn | Results from Rh incompatibility between mother and fetus | Cyanosis | Tests to confirm Rh compatibility (e.g., Coombs test, ABO typing) | Possible intrauterine transfusion; Immune globulin (RhoGAM) to mother to provide passive immunity in future pregnancies | Prenatal care; tests before delivery to determine compatibility of Rh between mother and father

BUN, Blood urea nitrogen; *CBC,* complete blood count; *Hct,* hematocrit; *Hgb,* Hemoglobin; *PT,* prothrombin time; *PTT,* partial thromboplastin time; *RBCs,* red blood cells; *WBCs,* white blood cells.

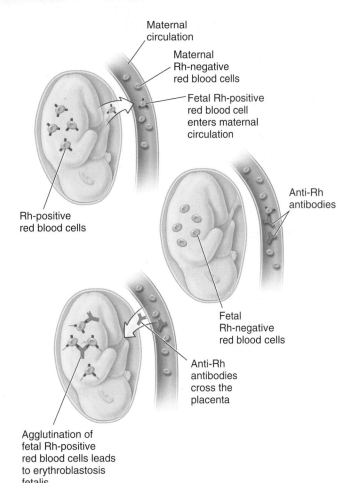

Fig. 6-8   Erythroblastosis fetalis. *(Modified from Thibodeau GA, Patton KT: Anatomy and physiology, ed 6, St Louis, 2003, Mosby.)*

others relate to incompatibility between blood types or Rh factors.

PATIENT-CENTERED PROFESSIONALISM

- Why is it necessary to understand the structure and function of each formed element of the blood? Explain the significance of each type of blood cell in a complete blood count (CBC).
- Explain the importance of knowing each parent's Rh factor before an infant's birth.
- How does blood typing affect a donor's and a recipient's ability to donate or receive blood?
- How is patient care affected by the medical assistant's understanding of blood cells, Rh factor, and blood typing?

LYMPHATIC SYSTEM

The final component of the circulatory system is the lymphatic system. The lymphatic system is an interconnected system of spaces and vessels between body tissues and organs. It filters out organisms that cause disease, produces certain white blood cells, and generates antibodies, all without the help of a pump (unlike the blood, which has the heart). The lymphatic system is also important for the distribution of fluids and nutrients in the body because it drains excess fluids and protein so that tissues do not swell. Understanding the structure and function of the lymphatic system will help you understand the diseases that affect this system.

Structure

The lymphatic system has four components: (1) the lymphatic vessels, (2) the lymphatic fluid, (3) the lymph nodes, and (4) the lymphoid organs.

Function

Lymph is formed when blood plasma filters out of the spaces between the cells of the tissue. Most of this tissue fluid **(interstitial fluid)** reenters the blood through the capillary walls.

The remaining tissue fluid enters the lymph capillaries and becomes lymph. The sole purpose of lymph is to return proteins, fats, hormones, and other needed substances back to the blood.

Lymphatic Vessels

The lymphatic system accomplishes the return of elements to the blood by way of four lymphatic vessels: (1) lymph capillaries, (2) lymphatics, (3) the thoracic duct, and (4) the right lymphatic duct.

Lymphatic vessels are found in all tissues and organs of the body that contain blood vessels.

- The lymph capillaries, like blood capillaries, unite to form larger vessels called **lymphatics,** which have valves to prevent backflow of lymph.
- The function of the lymphatics is to carry all materials not needed in the tissue spaces from the tissues through the vessels back to the subclavian veins.
- The lymphatics continue to spread out and form larger vessels (much like venules to veins) until they meet and form two main channels, the thoracic duct and the right lymphatic duct (Fig. 6-9).
- The *thoracic duct* receives lymph from the left side of the body, and the *right lymphatic duct* collects from the right side.

Lymph circulation, unlike blood circulation, flows only once through the lymphatic vessels and enters the blood (Fig. 6-10). Even though the drainage of lymph is continual, it is possible for fluid to accumulate in tissue spaces. When this happens, **edema** (swelling) results.

Lymph Nodes

Lymph nodes are small, oval-shaped bodies of lymphoid tissue. Lymph nodes vary in size from a

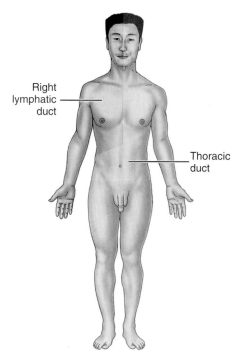

Fig. 6-9 Areas of the body that are drained by the main lymphatic ducts. *(From Herlihy B, Maebius NK: The human body in health and illness, ed 2, Philadelphia, 2003, Saunders.)*

pinhead to an almond and run along the course of the lymphatics. Nodes are usually found in groups or chains at the sides of the larger blood vessels, although they can stand alone. Lymph nodes contain lymphocytes and macrophages that serve as filters to kill foreign materials such as microorganisms or abnormal cells.

The function of the lymph nodes is twofold: (1) produce lymphocytes and monocytes and (2) serve as filters guarding against the spread of infection.

Lymphoid Organs

The **lymphoid organs** consist of the spleen, tonsils, and the thymus gland (Fig. 6-11).

Spleen

The **spleen,** located in the upper left quadrant, has the following three functions:

1. Storage of red blood cells until needed
2. Destruction and removal of worn out erythrocytes and platelets
3. Production of lymphocytes and monocytes by the spleen's lymphoid tissue

The spleen is a blood reservoir and can store about a pint of blood and release it quickly back into circulation when needed, such as after strenuous exercise or a hemorrhage. If the spleen is removed as a result of trauma (e.g., motor vehicle accident, injury), other internal organs will compensate for its function.

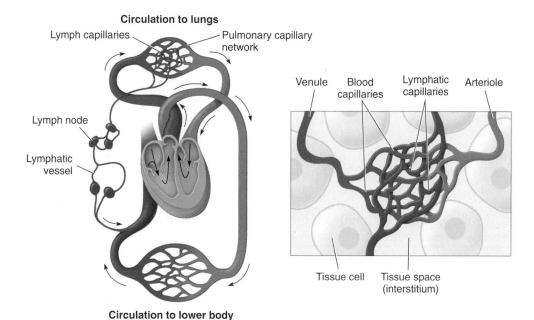

Fig. 6-10 Relationship of the lymphatic vessels to the circulatory system. *(Modified from Shiland BJ: Mastering healthcare terminology, St Louis, 2003, Mosby.)*

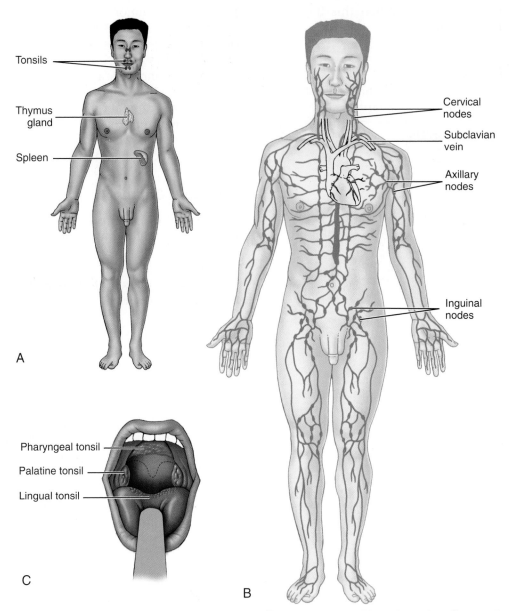

Fig. 6-11   Lymphoid tissue locations. **A**, Lymphoid organs. **B**, Distribution of lymph nodes. **C**, Tonsils. *(From Herlihy B, Maebius NK: The human body in health and illness, ed 2, Philadelphia, 2003, Saunders.)*

Tonsils

Tonsils are lymph nodes located in the **pharynx** (throat), nasal cavity, and at the back of the tongue. They are responsible for preventing bacteria from entering the body through the throat and for filtering tissue fluids in the mouth and nasal cavities. These often increase in size with throat and ear infections.

Thymus Gland

The **thymus gland** is located behind the sternum and just below the thyroid gland. The thymus gland is most active in the first few months after birth to establish the infant's immune system. The thymus secretes a hormone called **thymosin** that helps with the development of **T lymphocytes** (responsible for attacking viruses). After puberty the thymus gland gradually atrophies (decreases in size) and is replaced with fat and connective tissue. This event makes the body defense system more vulnerable to infection as a person ages.

Diseases of the Lymphatic System

Diseases of the lymphatic system relate to the drainage of lymph as well as the drainage of lymph nodes and the tissue itself (Table 6-5).

TABLE 6-5   Diseases of the Lymphatic System

Disease and Description	Etiology	Signs and Symptoms	Diagnosis	Therapy	Interventions
Diseases Related to Lymph Drainage					
Lymphedema Caused by inadequacy or inability of lymph to drain from limbs (Fig. 6-12) Complication after **mastectomy** if lymphatics are removed	Obstruction or removal of lymph nodes	Affected limb swollen	Patient history; examination and lymph-angiography to confirm site of blockage; history of surgical removal of lymphatics	Elevation of affected part	Encourage patient to wear prescribed elastic support garments
Lymphomas					
Hodgkin disease Chronic, progressive cancer of lymphoid tissue	Unknown	Swelling in cervical lymph nodes; fever, night sweats, weight loss	Lymph node biopsy	Radiation therapy in conjunction with chemotherapy	During treatment, encourage nutrition and provide support
Non-Hodgkin lymphoma Neoplasm disease of lymphoid tissue	Unknown	Painless lymphadenopathy Complaints of fatigue, malaise, fever, and night sweats	Lymph node biopsy	Radiation to primary site combined with chemotherapy drugs	During treatment, follow through with procedures and maintain nutrition
Infectious mononucleosis A viral infection involving lymphatic tissue, usually in cervical region	Epstein-Barr virus (EBV); transmitted through saliva	Fatigue, fever, sore throat, lymphadenopathy	Clinical presentation, mono laboratory tests CBC with differential: lymphocytes and monocytes <50%; elevated titer for EBV (monospot)	Based on symptoms Increased fluids during fever; antipyretic medications and antibiotics and steroids for secondary infections	Encourage good nutrition and rest

CBC, Complete blood count.

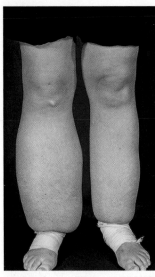

Fig. 6-12 Lymphedema. This patient had bound her feet so that she could wear shoes. *(From Black JM et al: Medical-surgical nursing: clinical management for positive outcomes, ed 6, Philadelphia, 2001, Saunders.)*

PATIENT-CENTERED PROFESSIONALISM

- Why do medical assistants need to understand the function of the lymphatics?
- How is the lymphatic system important to the healthy functioning of the human body?

IMMUNE SYSTEM

The lymphatic system plays an important role in protecting our bodies from diseases. Another system, the immune system, aids in fighting the diseases that occur in the body. Daily, our bodies are exposed to harmful disease-producing bacteria **(pathogens)**. The immune system provides **immunity,** the ability to counteract the toxic effects of many microorganisms.

Lines of Defense

The immune system has three lines of defense to resist the effects of microorganisms on the body: (1) physical and chemical barriers, (2) nonspecific immunity, and (3) specific immunity.

Physical and Chemical Barriers
Barriers prevent microorganisms from entering the body and include the following types:

- *Physical:* Skin and the membranes lining body passages
- *Chemical:* Sweat, tears, saliva, mucus

Nonspecific Immunity
Nonspecific immunity is a response from cells that surround and digest microorganisms, as well as from chemicals (e.g., histamine, certain antibodies) that help to destroy bacteria. Furthermore, **interferons** are produced by cells infected with a virus, and T cells block the virus' ability to reproduce. Nonspecific immunity depends on intact skin and mucous membranes, chemical barriers produced by the body, and reflex actions (Fig. 6-13).

The process of acquiring nonspecific immunity consists of the following:

1. Swelling, redness, warmth, and fever stimulate phagocytosis
2. Pain occurs in the area of an infection
3. An increased blood flow attracts white blood cells to the infected area
4. Phagocytes destroy invading bacteria (infection)
5. Nonspecific immunity is produced

Specific Immunity
Specific immunity is selective for a particular type of disease or microorganism. It comes from two types of lymphocytes. The T lymphocytes (T cells) attack the foreign body directly. The **B lymphocytes** (B cells) multiply rapidly when an antigen is introduced, resulting in the production of antibodies. These antibodies remain in the blood and provide long-term immunity.

The process of acquiring specific immunity is as follows:

1. The immune system recognizes, attacks, destroys, and "remembers" each type of microorganism that enters the body.
2. Antibodies and specialized cells are produced that bind to and inactivate microorganisms when the body is attacked again.

Types of Immunity

There are two main types of immunity: genetic (inborn) immunity and acquired immunity (Fig. 6-14).

Genetic Immunity
Genetic immunity, or natural (inborn) immunity, occurs when a person is born with a **resistance** to a specific disease (e.g., foot-and-mouth disease). This is species specific.

Acquired Immunity
Acquired immunity occurs either through a natural process of having a disease or an artificial process such as vaccination (Fig. 6-15).

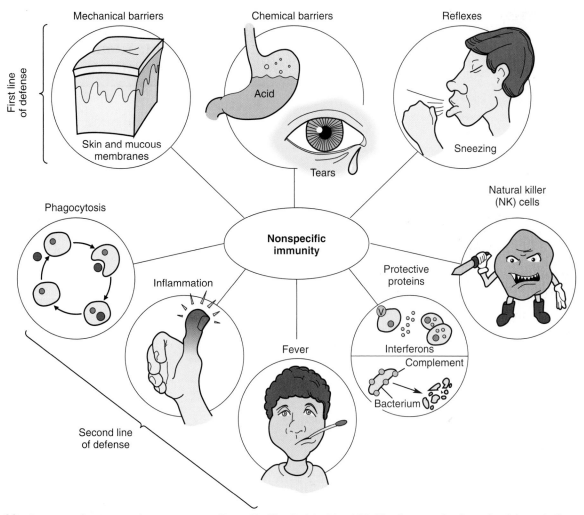

Fig. 6-13 Process of nonspecific immunity. *(From Herlihy B, Maebius NK:* The human body in health and illness, *ed 2, Philadelphia, 2003, Saunders.)*

Natural acquired immunity occurs when the body produces its own antibodies after having the disease **(active immunity)** (e.g., chickenpox) or after the antibodies pass through the placenta or mother's milk and provide immunity **(passive immunity).**

Artificially acquired immunity is considered active when a person is immunized or given a **vaccination,** which is a sample of the disease in a weakened **attenuated** state (e.g., measles, mumps). In response the body produces antibodies that fight off the disease when exposed. Passive artificial immunity occurs when antibodies developed in one organism are injected into another organism (e.g., rabies, tetanus), as with giving gamma globulin.

Diseases of the Immune System

Even though the immune system defends the body against disease, it is also susceptible to disease (Table 6-6). The body can also produce antibodies (immunity) against its own *(auto)* normal tissue. Two auto-

immune diseases are *rheumatoid arthritis* and *lupus erythematosus.* Varied symptoms can occur, such as joint pain, skin rash, and fever.

Special Considerations for AIDS Patients

Acquired immunodeficiency syndrome (AIDS) is a disease that has affected millions of people worldwide. AIDS patients are prone to opportunistic infections that arise because of the weakened immune system. Box 6-3 lists some common illnesses of the AIDS patient.

A patient must give consent before having the *human immunodeficiency virus* (HIV) antibody test. Most states require HIV counseling both before and after the test is given. Most also require that the test results be given in person (e.g., never leave a message), whether the results are negative or positive. The responsibility of this counseling lies with the physician or a trained HIV counselor.

A patient's medical record cannot be marked or coded in any manner on the outside to identify that an HIV test was performed. All results are privileged

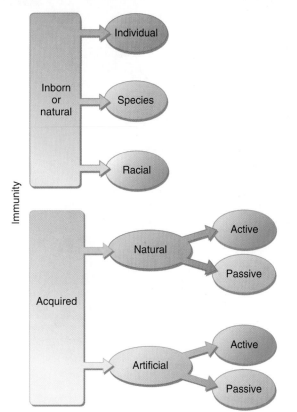

Fig. 6-14 Different types of immunity. *(Modified from Chester GA:* Modern medical assisting, *Philadelphia, 1999, Saunders.)*

BOX 6-3   Diseases and Infectious Agents Common to AIDS Patients

Bacterial
Pneumocystis carinii pneumonia
Mycobacterium tuberculosis

Parasitic
Toxoplasma gondii (brain lesions)
Cryptosporidium
Microsporidia

Viral
Cytomegalovirus (retinitis)
Herpes zoster (shingles)
Herpes simplex

Fungal
Thrush *(Candida albicans)*
Cryptococcal meningitis
Histoplasmosis
Coccidioidomycosis

Miscellaneous
Kaposi sarcoma
Lymphomas

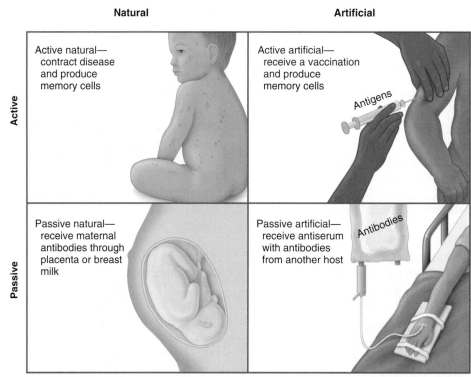

Fig. 6-15 Types of acquired immunity. *(Modified from Applegate EJ:* The anatomy and physiology learning system, *ed 2, Philadelphia, 2000, Saunders.)*

TABLE 6-6 Diseases of the Immune System

Disease and Description	Etiology	Signs and Symptoms	Diagnosis	Therapy	Interventions
Chronic fatigue syndrome Chronic disease that appears to be viral in nature and affects the entire body	Unknown	Impairment of short-term memory or concentration; sore throat; tender cervical or axillary nodes; pain without stiffness or redness; fatigue unrelated to exertion	History; patient complains of four or more symptoms for 6 months or longer	Gradual exercise program to increase over time; rest when fatigue is at its worst	Emotional support
Lupus erythematosus Chronic inflammatory disorder that affects the connective tissues in various parts of the body	Autoimmune reaction (body produces antibodies) against own cells, which suppresses the body's natural immunity and damages tissues	Anorexia, weight loss, malaise, abdominal pain, rash, polyarthralgia (arthralgia of multiple joints)	Patient history and rash; CBC with differential; erythrocyte sedimentation rate, serum electrophoresis; C-reactive protein	Reduce stress; avoid sunlight Nonsteroidal drug therapy, with short-term use of corticosteroids during acute episodes	Encourage use of sunscreen and stress reduction
Acquired immuno-deficiency syndrome (AIDS) Caused by virus that attacks entire immune system; transmitted through body fluids	Human immunodeficiency virus (HIV) (Fig. 6-16) attacks helper T cells, which interferes with immune system's ability to protect body from infection	Persistent cough; weight loss, oral lesions; appearance of lesions on face and upper torso (Kaposi sarcoma)	Patient history, positive HIV blood test; *Pneumocystis carinii* infection, candidiasis, or biopsy of lesion	Medications for opportunistic infections; antiviral therapy	Nutritional and emotional support

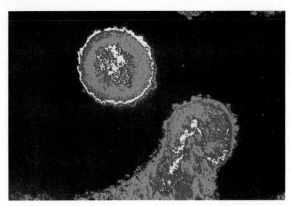

Fig. 6-16 The human immunodeficiency virus (HIV). *(From Shiland BJ:* Mastering healthcare terminology, *St Louis, 2003, Mosby.)*

and may not be disclosed except as provided by law. Currently, all 50 states require reporting of AIDS cases, without the patient's consent, to the Centers for Disease Control and Prevention (CDC) or to the state's health department. Because each state has its own reporting requirements, it is best to check in your particular state for information. Patients with HIV infection or AIDS have the same rights as people with other life-threatening illnesses and should be treated with dignity and respect.

PATIENT-CENTERED PROFESSIONALISM

- How does genetic or natural immunity differ from acquired immunity, and why do medical assistants need to understand this?
- When a person is HIV positive, they may not develop AIDS. Why is it important to understand the disease and how it can be transmitted?
- How can medical assistants improve the care they provide to AIDS patients?

CONCLUSION

The cardiovascular system is responsible for moving blood and lymph throughout the body. The condition of the blood and lymph is crucial to the body to maintain homeostasis. Blood tissue contains both plasma and formed elements—the blood cells and platelets. The red blood cells transport oxygen, nutrients, and carbon dioxide. The white blood cells help the body resist infections and clean up injured tissues. Platelets provide a means for the body to prevent a loss of essential body fluids.

The lymphatic system acts to balance fluids by collecting lymph from the bloodstream, removing contaminants, and returning the cleaned lymph back into the bloodstream, thus preventing the spread of disease. The immune system is made up of many cells and tissues contained within the body's network of systems. It plays an important role in defending the body against disease.

Medical assistants need to understand the structure and function of the entire cardiovascular system so they can understand the related disease processes. Providing the best patient care means knowing first the normal, and then the abnormal, condition of the body's systems.

SUMMARY

Reinforce your understanding of the material in this chapter by reviewing the curriculum objectives and key content points below.

1. Define, appropriately use, and spell all the Key Terms for this chapter.
   - Review the Key Terms if necessary.
2. List the eight components of blood plasma.
   - Blood plasma is the liquid portion of the blood.
   - Water, nutrients, electrolytes, gases, clotting factors, antibodies, waste products, and hormones are all components of blood plasma.
   - Blood is approximately 55% plasma and 45% formed elements (RBCs, WBCs, platelets).
3. List three types of blood cells and describe the function of each.
   - Erythrocytes are red blood cells (RBCs); they are the most numerous and contain hemoglobin, which carries oxygen.
   - Leukocytes are white blood cells (WBCs); they help fight disease.
   - Thrombocytes are platelets; they help stop bleeding by forming clots.
4. List the four blood types and explain the importance of compatibility.
   - Blood types are A, B, AB, or O; a person cannot receive blood that has a different antigen than the recipient's blood has.
   - A type and crossmatch must be performed to ensure compatibility of the donor's and the recipient's blood.
   - A transfusion of incompatible blood causes agglutination, and death can result for the recipient.
5. Explain the importance of Rh factor as it relates to pregnancy and transfusions.
   - Care must be taken in a pregnancy if the mother is Rh negative and the father is Rh positive.
   - A blood incompatibility results if people are exposed to a different Rh factor or blood group than their own. A mother will form antibodies against a fetus if the baby's blood

is Rh positive and the mother is Rh negative.

6. List nine diseases of the blood and describe the etiology, signs and symptoms, diagnosis, therapy, and interventions for each.
   - Diseases of the blood affect all three types of blood cells. Blood incompatibility will cause life-threatening medical situations.
   - Refer to Table 6-4.

7. List the four divisions of the lymphatic system and describe the function of each.
   - Lymph is formed when blood plasma filters out of the spaces between the tissue cells.
   - The lymphatic vessels carry substances from the tissues not needed by the body.
   - The lymph nodes produce lymphocytes and monocytes and filter out harmful and unwanted substances.
   - The lymphoid organs function to filter, produce blood cells, and store red blood cells until needed.

8. List four diseases of the lymphatic system and describe the etiology, signs and symptoms, diagnosis, therapy, and interventions for each.
   - Cancer can affect the lymphatic system and provide a means for cancer to metastasize.
   - Refer to Table 6-5.

9. List the immune system's three lines of defense and describe each.
   - Physical barriers include the skin and membranes, and chemical barriers include body fluids (sweat, tears, saliva, mucus).
   - Nonspecific immunity is the body reacting to eliminate the effects of microorganisms and other toxic substances.
   - Specific immunity is the body producing antibodies for long-term immunity against a particular microorganism or disease.

10. Distinguish between genetic (inborn) immunity and acquired immunity and give an example of each.
    - Genetic immunity occurs when a person is born with a resistance to a specific disease (e.g., foot-and-mouth disease).
    - Acquired immunity occurs either naturally (e.g., having measles) or artificially (e.g., vaccination) to protect the body against a specific disease.

11. List three diseases of the immune system and describe the etiology, signs and symptoms, diagnosis, therapy, and interventions for each.

- A compromised immune system allows opportunistic infections to occur.
- Refer to Table 6-6.

12. Describe the considerations associated with the testing of AIDS patients.
    - Counseling before and after testing is required.
    - Results of the test must be given in person.
    - There must be no special marking on the outside of the patient chart, and the confidentiality of the patient must be respected.

13. Analyze a realistic medical office situation and apply your understanding of the circulatory system to determine the best course of action.
    - Understanding the normal physiology of the circulatory system will help you understand how a disease process affects this system.

14. Describe the impact on patient care when medical assistants have a solid understanding of the structure and function of the circulatory system.
    - Medical assistants who understand the physiology of the circulatory system will be better prepared to assist with medical procedures, communicate clearly to patients, and perform effective patient teaching.

FOR FURTHER EXPLORATION

1. **Research current facts about blood and blood banking.** There are many myths about blood donation and receiving blood. It is important for the medical assistant to be knowledgeable about key facts concerning transfusions and donation.
   Keywords: Use the following keywords in your search: American Association of Blood Banks, transfusion, blood donation.

2. **Research the incidence of anemia in the United States.** People who suffer from certain diseases are more likely to develop anemia. In addition, specific groups of people who are not suffering from disease may also be at risk. Medical assistants need to understand the incidence of anemia to provide better care to patients.
   Keywords: Use the following keywords in your search: anemia, National Center for Health Statistics, incidence of anemia.

WORD PARTS: BLOOD, LYMPHATIC, AND IMMUNE SYSTEMS

BLOOD
Combining Forms

bas/o	Base
coagul/o	Clotting
cyt/o	Cell
eosin/o	Rosy, red
erythr/o	Red
granul/o	Granules
hem/o	Blood
hemat/o	Blood
hemoglobin/o	Hemoglobin
leuk/o	White
phag/o	Eat
thromb/o	Clot

Suffixes

-cytosis	Abnormal condition of cells
-emia	Blood condition
-globin	Protein
-lytic	Pertaining to destruction
-osis	Abnormal condition
-penia	Deficiency
-phage	Eat
-poiesis	Formation

LYMPHATIC AND IMMUNE SYSTEMS
Combining Forms

imnun/o	Protection
lymph/o	Lymph
spleen/o	Spleen
thym/o	Thymus gland

Prefixes

ana-	Again, up, apart
inter-	Between

Abbreviations: Lymphatic and Immune Systems

AIDS	Acquired immunodeficiency syndrome
ELISA	Enzyme-linked immunosorbent assay—test to detect anti-HIV antibodies
HD	Hodgkin disease
HISTO	Histoplasmosis-fungal infection seen in AIDS patients
HIV	Human immunodeficiency virus—causes AIDS
HSV	Herpes simplex virus
KS	Kaposi sarcoma

MEDICAL TERMINOLOGY OF ONCOLOGY

CHAPTER AT A GLANCE

KEY WORD PARTS

PREFIXES	SUFFIXES	COMBINING FORMS
ana-	-ectomy	bi/o
apo-	-genesis	carcin/o
brachy-	-oma	chem/o
dys-	-opsy	immun/o
ecto-	-plasia	radi/o
endo-	-plasm	sarc/o
hyper-	-ptosis	
meta-	-sarcoma	
muta-	-stasis	
neo-	-therapy	

KEY TERMS

anaplasia	grading	neoplasm
benign	immunotherapy	nodes
biopsy	leukemia	radiotherapy
BMT	lymphoma	sarcoma
brachytherapy	malignant	sentinel node
carcinoma	mammogram	staging
chemotherapy	metastasis	tumor marker
carcinoma in situ (CIS)	mixed tumor	
dedifferentiation	myeloma	

Where there is life, there is cancer. Although the types of cancer and their incidence (the number of new types diagnosed each year) may vary by geography, sex, race, age, and ethnicity, cancer exists in every population and has since ancient times. Archeologists have found evidence of cancer in dinosaur bones and human mummies. Written descriptions of cancer treatment have been discovered dating back to 1600 BC. The name itself comes from the Greek word for *crab*, used by Hippocrates to describe the appearance of the most common type of cancer, carcinoma.

CARCINOGENESIS

Cancer is not *one* disease but a group of hundreds of diseases with similar characteristics. The shared characteristics are uncontrolled cell growth and a spread of altered cells. Different types of cancers have different occurrence rates and different causes.

Current research suggests that there is no single cause of cancer. Radiation, bacteria, viruses, genetics, diet, smoking (or exposure to tobacco smoke), alcohol, and other factors all contribute to the development of cancer. Each of these factors is instrumental in disrupting the normal balance of cell growth and destruction within the body by causing a mutation in the DNA of cells (Fig. 7-1). Once this mutation takes place, a process of uncontrolled cell growth may begin. It is important to note that the cancer cells that replace normal cells no longer function to keep the body working. The only mission of cancer cells is to reproduce. Fig. 7-2 illustrates the process of **apoptosis** (ah pop TOH sis), the body's normal restraining function to keep cell growth in check. Fig. 7-3 shows the progression from normally functioning skin tissue to hyperplasia, to dysplasia, and finally to carcinoma in situ (CIS). Cancer is a continuum—from tissue made up of normally functioning cells fulfilling their role to keep the body

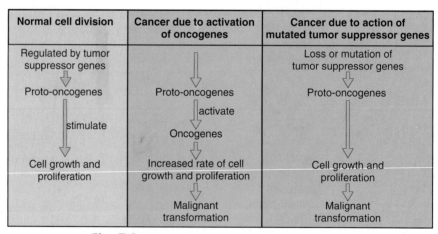

Normal cell division	Cancer due to activation of oncogenes	Cancer due to action of mutated tumor suppressor genes
Regulated by tumor suppressor genes		Loss or mutation of tumor suppressor genes
Proto-oncogenes	Proto-oncogenes	Proto-oncogenes
stimulate	activate	
	Oncogenes	
Cell growth and proliferation	Increased rate of cell growth and proliferation	Cell growth and proliferation
	Malignant transformation	Malignant transformation

Fig. 7-1   Normal cell growth vs. oncogenesis.

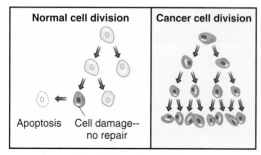

Fig. 7-2   Apoptosis.

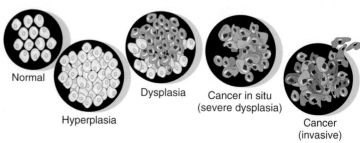

Fig. 7-3   Progression of skin cancer from hyperplasia to cancer.

healthy, to tissue replaced by cancerous cells that no longer perform the work of the tissue and now perform only the function of reproducing themselves. Cancers are capable of destroying not only the tissue in which they originate (the primary site) but also other tissues, through the process of **metastasis.** This spread of the cancer can occur by direct extension to contiguous organs and tissues or to distant sites through blood (Fig. 7-4) or lymphatic involvement.

NAMING MALIGNANT TUMORS

Oncology is the study of tumors, or neoplasms. All cancers are neoplasms (new growths), but not all neoplasms are cancerous. Cancerous tumors are termed *malignant*, whereas noncancerous tumors are termed *benign*.

Although the hundreds of known types of malignant tumors commonly share the characteristics listed previously, the names that they are given reflect their differences. All tissues (and hence organs) are derived from the progression of three embryonic germ layers that differentiate into specific tissues and organs. Tumors are generally divided into two broad categories and a varying number of other categories, based on their embryonic origin. Fig. 7-5 illustrates the different types of cancers and where they occur.

- **Carcinomas:** Approximately 80% to 90% of malignant tumors are derived from the outer (ectodermal) and inner (endodermal) layers of the embryo that develop into epithelial tissue that either covers or lines the surfaces of

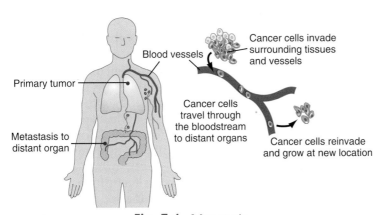

Fig. 7-4   Metastasis.

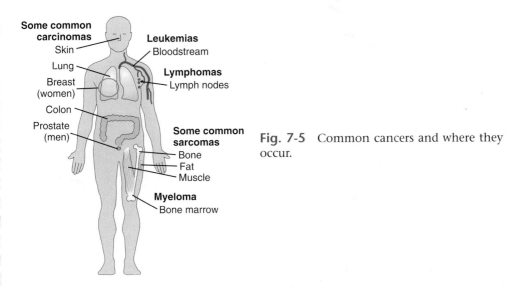

Fig. 7-5   Common cancers and where they occur.

the body. This category of cancer is divided into two main types. If derived from an organ or gland, it is an adenocarcinoma; if derived from squamous epithelium, it is a squamous cell carcinoma. Examples include gastric adenocarcinoma and squamous cell carcinoma of the lung.

- **Sarcomas** are derived from the middle (mesodermal) layer that becomes connective tissue (bones, muscle, cartilage, blood vessels, and fat). Most end in the suffix -*sarcoma*. Examples include osteosarcoma, chondrosarcoma, hemangiosarcoma, mesothelioma, and glioma.
- **Lymphomas** develop in lymphatic tissue (vessels, nodes, and organs, including the spleen, tonsils, and thymus gland). Lymphomas are solid cancers and may also appear outside of the sites of lymphatic organs in the stomach, breast, or brain; these are called *extranodal lymphomas*. All lymphomas may be divided into two categories: Hodgkin lymphoma and non-Hodgkin lymphoma.
- **Leukemia** is cancer of the bone marrow. An example is acute myelocytic leukemia.
- **Myelomas** arise from the plasma cells in the bone marrow. An example is multiple myeloma.
- **Mixed tumors** are a combination of cells from within one category or between two cancer categories. An example is teratocarcinoma.

STAGING AND GRADING

To treat cancer, the treating physician must determine the severity of the cancer, the grade, and its stage, or size and spread. Cancers at different grades and stages react differently to various treatments.

Grading is a means of affixing a value to a clinical opinion of the degree of **dedifferentiation (anaplasia)** of the cancer cells, or how much the cells appear different from their original form. Healthy cells are well differentiated; cancer cells are poorly differentiated. The pathologist determines this difference and assigns a grade ranging from I to IV. The higher the grade, the more cancerous, or dedifferentiated, the tissue sample. Grading is a measure of the cancer's *severity*.

The other factor is determining the *size and spread* of the cancer from its original site, which is called **staging.** A number of systems are used to describe staging. Some are specific to the type of cancer; others are general systems. If staging is determined by various diagnostic techniques, it is referred to as *clinical staging*. If it is determined by the pathologist's report, it is called *pathological staging*. An example is TNM staging. In this system, **T** stands for the **size** of the tumor, **N** stands for the number of lymph **nodes** positive for cancer, and **M** stands for the presence of distant **metastasis** (meh TAS tuh sis). Summary staging puts together the TNM to give one number as a stage. Again, this helps determine the type of treatment that is most effective. Fig. 7-6 illustrates a staging system. If the cancer cells appear only at the original site and have not invaded the organ of origin, it is called **carcinoma in situ (CIS).**

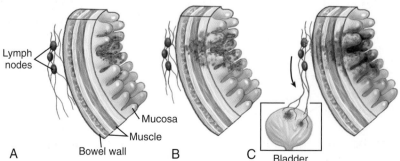

Fig. 7-6 Staging of colon cancer. **A,** stage I; **B,** stage II; **C,** stage III.

COMBINING FORMS FOR NEOPLASMS

MEANING	COMBINING FORM
connective tissue, flesh	sarc/o
cancer of epithelial origin	carcin/o
formation	plas/o
tumor	onc/o

⊠ BE CAREFUL!

Don't confuse *sarc/o*, meaning flesh, and *sacr/o*, meaning sacrum.

PREFIXES FOR NEOPLASMS

PREFIX	MEANING	PREFIX	MEANING
ana-	again, up, apart	hyper-	excessive
apo-	separate, away	meso-	middle
dys-	abnormal	meta-	beyond, change
ecto-	outer	neo-	new
endo-	inner		

SUFFIXES FOR NEOPLASMS

SUFFIX	MEANING
-oma	tumor, mass
-ptosis	falling
-sarcoma	cancer of connective tissue
-stasis	stopping, controlling

◈ Exercise 7-1: GENERAL ONCOLOGY TERMS

Match the word part with its correct meaning.

_____ 1. -stasis

_____ 2. -oma

_____ 3. plas/o

_____ 4. meta-

_____ 5. dys-

_____ 6. carcin/o

_____ 7. ana-

_____ 8. hyper-

_____ 9. neo-

_____ 10. sarc/o

A. again, up, apart
B. abnormal
C. connective tissue
D. new
E. cancer of epithelial tissue origin
F. stopping, controlling
G. beyond, change
H. tumor
I. excessive
J. formation

Circle the correct answer.

11. Tumors that are cancerous are considered to be *(benign, malignant)*.
12. The most common type of malignant cancer is *(carcinoma, sarcoma, leukemia, lymphoma, myeloma, mixed cell cancer)*.

13. Cancer composed of connective tissue is classified as (*carcinoma, sarcoma, leukemia, lymphoma, myeloma, mixed cell cancer*).
14. Cancer cells that derive from plasma cells in the bone marrow are classified as (*carcinoma, sarcoma, leukemia, lymphoma, myeloma, mixed cell tumors*).
15. Healthy cells are (*well, poorly*) differentiated.
16. A determination of the degree of dedifferentiation of cancer cells is called (*grading, staging*).
17. A system of determining how far a cancer has spread from its original site is called (*grading, staging*).
18. The site where the cancer originates is referred to as the (*primary, metastatic*) site.

PATHOLOGY

Signs and Symptoms

The signs and symptoms of cancer are manifestations of how cancer cells replace the functions of healthy tissue. Some examples include anorexia, bruising, leukocytosis, fatigue, cachexia (wasting), and thrombocytopenia.

Neoplasia by Body System

The following tables summarize characteristics of benign and malignant tumors by body system. Note that a particular system does not always have all one type of cancer because organs are composed of a variety of tissues with different embryonic origins. The integumentary system has both carcinomas and sarcomas.

Comparison of Benign and Malignant Neoplasms

CHARACTERISTICS	BENIGN	MALIGNANT
Mode of growth	Relatively slow growth by expansion; encapsulated; cells adhere to each other	Rapid growth; invades surrounding tissue by infiltration
Cells under microscopic examination	Resemble tissue of origin; well differentiated; appear normal	Do not resemble tissue of origin; vary in size and shape; abnormal appearance and function
Spread	Remains isolated	Metastasis; cancer cells carried by blood and lymphatics to one or more other locations; secondary tumors occur
Other properties	No tissue destruction; not prone to hemorrhage; may be smooth and freely movable	Ulceration and/or necrosis; prone to hemorrhage; irregular and less movable
Recurrence	Rare after excision	A common characteristic
Pathogenesis	Symptoms related to location with obstruction and/or compression of surrounding tissue or organs; usually not life threatening unless inaccessible	Cachexia; pain; fatal if not controlled

From Frazier MS, Drzymkowski JW: *Essentials of human diseases and conditions,* ed 2, Philadelphia, 2000, Saunders.

Neoplasms by Body System

BODY SYSTEM	ORGAN	BENIGN NEOPLASMS	MALIGNANT NEOPLASMS
Musculoskeletal	Bone	Osteoma	Ewing sarcoma, osteosarcoma
	Cartilage	Chondroma	Chondrosarcoma
	Muscle	Rhabdomyoma, leiomyoma	Rhabdomyosarcoma, leiomyosarcoma
Integumentary	Skin	Dermatofibroma	Basal cell carcinoma, squamous cell carcinoma, malignant melanoma, Kaposi sarcoma
Gastrointestinal	Esophagus	Leiomyoma	Adenocarcinoma of the esophagus, stomach, pancreas, colon, and/or rectum
	Stomach	Polyp	
	Pancreas	Gastric adenoma	
	Colon/rectum		
Urinary	Kidney	Nephroma	Hypernephroma/renal cell carcinoma, Wilms tumor/nephrosarcoma
	Bladder		Transitional cell carcinoma (bladder cancer)
Male Reproductive	Testis		Seminoma, teratoma
	Prostate	Benign prostatic hyperplasia	Adenocarcinoma of the prostate
Female Reproductive	Breast	Fibrocystic changes in the breast	Infiltrating ductal adenocarcinoma of the breast
	Uterus	Fibroids	Stromal endometrial carcinoma
	Ovaries	Ovarian cyst	Epithelial ovarian carcinoma
	Cervix	Cervical dysplasia	Squamous cell carcinoma of the cervix
Blood/Lymphatic/ Immune	Blood		Leukemia
	Lymph vessels		Non-Hodgkin lymphoma, Hodgkin lymphoma
	Thymus gland	Thymoma	Malignant thymoma
Cardiovascular	Blood vessels	Hemangioma	Hemangiosarcoma
	Heart	Myxoma	Myxosarcoma
Respiratory	Epithelial tissue of respiratory tract, lung, bronchus	Papilloma	Adenocarcinoma of the lung, small cell carcinoma, mesothelioma, bronchogenic carcinoma
Nervous	CNS (brain, spinal cord, meninges)	Neuroma, neurofibroma	Glioblastoma, meningioma, astrocytoma
	PNS		
Endocrine	Pituitary	Benign pituitary tumor	
	Thyroid		Thyroid carcinoma
	Adrenal medulla	Pheochromocytoma	
Eyes and Ears	Retina		Retinoblastoma
	Acoustic nerve	Acoustic neuroma	
	Middle ear	Cholesteatoma	

COMBINING FORMS RELATED TO ONCOLOGY

MEANING	COMBINING FORM	MEANING	COMBINING FORM
base	bas/o	kidney	nephr/o, ren/o
bone	oste/o	lymph	lymph/o
carcinoma, epithelial tissue cancer	carcin/o	connective tissue, flesh	sarc/o
			squam/o
cartilage	chondr/o	scale	semin/i
change	mut/a	semen	rhabdomy/o
embryonic	blast/o	skeletal muscle	dermat/o
fiber	fibr/o	skin	leiomy/o
gland	aden/o	smooth muscle	astr/o
glue	gli/o	star	

◈ Exercise 7-2: PATHOLOGY

Match the combining form with its correct meaning.

_____ 1. nephr/o	_____ 9. rhabdomy/o	A.	bone
		B.	semen
_____ 2. astr/o	_____ 10. chondr/o	C.	smooth muscle
		D.	embryonic
_____ 3. gli/o	_____ 11. blast/o	E.	cartilage
		F.	skeletal muscle
_____ 4. fibr/o	_____ 12. semin/i	G.	kidney
		H.	base
_____ 5. aden/o	_____ 13. oste/o	I.	scale
		J.	star
_____ 6. squam/o	_____ 14. leiomy/o	K.	epithelial tissue cancer
		L.	glue
_____ 7. carcin/o	_____ 15. bas/o	M.	fiber
		N.	connective tissue
_____ 8. sarc/o		O.	gland

Circle the correct answer.

16. An example of a benign muscle tumor is a *(rhabdomyoma, leiomyosarcoma)*.
17. Which of the following is a malignant tumor of the skin? *(dermatofibroma, basal cell carcinoma)*
18. A patient with fibroids has a *(benign, malignant)* growth.
19. Which of the following is NOT a malignancy? *(nephroma, lymphoma, seminoma, thymoma)*
20. An astrocytoma is a *(benign, malignant)* tumor of the nervous system.

Age Matters

Pediatrics

Childhood cancer is such a rarity that incidence rates are routinely expressed as the number of cases per million, instead of per 100,000 as with adult cancers. Still, certain cancers have a childhood form. Wilms tumor (children's kidney cancer), acute lymphocytic leukemia, retinoblastoma, and Ewing sarcoma are examples of cancers that seldom occur outside of childhood.

Geriatrics

The cumulative exposure to a lifetime of carcinogens reveals itself in cancer statistics that show cancer rates to increase as age increases. Lung, prostate, breast, colon, and skin cancers are common in elderly patients. Researchers estimate that 97% of men who have the prostate cancer gene will develop prostate cancer by the time they are 85.

DIAGNOSTIC PROCEDURES

Patient History

Along with the various clinical techniques described, the patient's history is especially important, including information regarding family history (for genetic information) and social history, such as tobacco and alcohol use, diet, and sexual history. A patient's smoking history is described in terms of "pack years." Pack years equals the average number of packs smoked per day multiplied by the number of years of smoking. For example: 1 pack/day × 25 years of smoking represents 25 pack years. A patient's current or former occupation may also shed light on the type of cancer. For example, exposure to asbestos, through an occupation of ship building or working with brake repair, may lead to a rare type of lung cancer, mesothelioma.

Tumor Markers

Tumor marker tests measure the levels of a variety of biochemical substances detected in the blood, urine, or body tissues that often appear in higher than normal amounts in individuals with certain neoplasms. Because other factors may influence the amount of the tumor marker present, they are not intended to be used as a sole means of diagnosis. Examples include the following:

AFP: Increased levels may indicate liver or germ cell cancer.
CA125: Used for ovarian cancer detection and management.
CA15-3: Levels are measured to determine the stage of breast cancer.
CA19-9: Levels are elevated in stomach, colorectal, and pancreatic cancers.
CA27-29: Used to monitor breast cancer; especially useful to test for recurrences.
CEA: Monitors colorectal cancer when the disease has spread or after treatment to measure the patient's response.
HCG: Used as a screen for choriocarcinoma.
LDH: Levels may be used to monitor Ewing sarcoma, non-Hodgkin lymphoma, testicular cancer, and some forms of leukemia.
NSE: Used to measure the stage and/or patient's response to treatment of small cell cancer and neuroblastoma.
PSA: Increased levels may be due to BPH or prostate cancer.

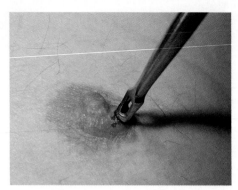

Fig. 7-7 Punch biopsy.

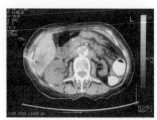

Fig. 7-8 CT scan of needle biopsy of the liver clearly shows the needle in the liver *on the left. (Courtesy Riverside Methodist Hospitals, Columbus, Ohio. From Mace JD, Kowalczy KN: Radiographic pathology for technologists, ed 4, St Louis, 2003, Mosby.)*

Biopsy (bx)

A **biopsy** is a viewing of a section of living tissue. **Excisional biopsies** are those in which the entire tumor may be removed with borders as a means of diagnosis and treatment. **Exfoliation** is a scraping or shaving off of samples of friable (easily crushed) lesions for a laboratory examination called an **exfoliative cytology.** An **incisional biopsy** is one in which larger tissue samples may be obtained by excising a wedge of tissue and suturing the incision. **Needle aspiration** is the removal of fluid from lesions to obtain samples for culture and examination. Finally, a **punch biopsy** is one in which a tubular punch is inserted through to the subcutaneous tissue, and the tissue is cut off at the base (Fig. 7-7).

Imaging

Computed tomography (CT) scans: CT scans provide information about a tumor's shape, size, and location, along with the source of its blood supply. They are useful in detecting, evaluating, and monitoring cancer, especially liver, pancreatic, bone, lung, and adrenal gland cancers. CT scans are also useful in staging cancer and guiding needles for aspiration biopsy (Fig. 7-8).

Magnetic resonance imaging (MRI): Areas of the body that are often difficult to image are possible to see with MRI because of its three-dimensional capabilities. MRI is useful in detecting cancer in the central nervous system (CNS) and musculoskeletal (MS) system. It is also used to stage breast and endometrial cancer before surgery and to detect metastatic spread of cancer to the liver.

Nuclear scans: Nuclear scans are useful in locating and staging cancer of the thyroid and the bone. A *positron emission tomography (PET) scan* provides information about the metabolism of an internal structure, along with its size and shape. It is used for images of the brain, colon, rectum, ovary, and lung. It may also help to identify more aggressive tumors. *Single-photon emission computed tomography (SPECT)* uses a rotating camera to create three-dimensional images with the use of radioactive substances. It is useful to determine metastases to the bone. *Monoclonal antibodies* are used to evaluate cancer of the prostate, colon, breast, and ovaries, and melanoma.

Radiography: Because tumors are usually more dense than the tissue surrounding them, they may appear as a lighter shade of gray (blocking more radiation). Abdominal x-rays may reveal tumors of the stomach, liver, kidneys, and so on, whereas chest x-rays are useful in detecting lung cancer. If a contrast medium is used, as in an upper or lower gastrointestinal (GI) series or intravenous urogram (IVU), tumors of the esophagus, rectum, colon, or kidneys may be detected. Another special type of x-ray is a **mammogram,** useful in the early detection of breast cancer.

Stereotactic (3-D) mammography may be used for an image-guided biopsy.

Self-Detection

Self-detection remains the most important method of discovering cancer. The American Cancer Society (ACS) has developed a series of reminders and rules to help individuals become aware of cancer signs and symptoms. For general detection of cancer, they have developed the following CAUTION criteria:

CAUTION CRITERIA

Change in bowel or bladder habits
A sore that does not heal
Unusual bleeding or discharge
Thickening or lump in the breast, testicles, or elsewhere
Indigestion or difficulty swallowing
Obvious change in the size, shape, color, or thickness of a wart, mole, or mouth sore
Nagging cough or hoarseness

For discovering skin cancer, the ACS has come up with the following ABCDE rule:

ABCDE RULE

A for **asymmetry:** A mole that, when divided in half, does not look the same on both sides.
B for **border:** A mole with edges that are blurry or jagged.
C for **color:** Changes in the color of a mole, including darkening, spread of color, loss of color, or the appearance of multiple colors, such as blue, red, white, pink, purple, or gray.
D for **diameter:** A mole larger than ¼ inch in diameter.
E for **elevation:** A mole that is raised above the skin and has an uneven surface.

The ACS also has criteria for breast and testicular self-examination.

 Exercise 7-3: DIAGNOSTIC PROCEDURES

Circle the correct answer.

1. A patient's history of smoking may be described as pack years, which is the number of *(cigarettes, packs)* smoked per day × the number of years smoking.
2. Information regarding previous diet, alcohol use, and family members with cancer may be found in the *(history, pathology)* section of a patient's medical record.
3. Levels of biochemical substances present in the blood that may indicate neoplastic activity are referred to as *(monoclonal antibodies, tumor markers)*.
4. Removal of a sample of tissue to be examined for signs of cancer is a *(tomography, biopsy)*.
5. Mammography may be done to test for cancer of the *(breast, colon)*.

Hamstead Memorial Hospital
532 13th St.
Hamstead, TX 75201

OPERATIVE REPORT

Preoperative diagnosis: History of colon cancer, multiple colon polyps

Postoperative diagnosis: Same

Surgery: Colonoscopy with polypectomy × 5

This 78-year-old female has colon polyps and a previous history of colon carcinoma. Patient was taken to the endoscopy suite and in the left lateral position, the long colonoscope was inserted without difficulty. The perirectal area was normal. Rectal ampulla was normal. The left colon showed a few diverticula. The right colon had multiple polyps, five of which were removed with hot forceps. The patient tolerated the procedure well and went to the recovery room in stable condition.

Raechel Perez, MD

◆ Exercise 7-4: OPERATIVE REPORT

Using the operative report above, fill in the blanks.

1. What are "polyps" and why do you think they were removed? _____

2. What is the medical term for "colon cancer"? _____

3. What type of procedures are done in an endoscopy suite? _____

4. What is a colonoscope? _____

5. Explain the meaning of the procedure "colonoscopy with polypectomy × 5." _____

≋ THERAPEUTIC INTERVENTIONS

Surgery

The primary treatment for cancer has always been and remains the removal of the tumor. When the tumor is relatively small and present only in the organ that is removed, surgery is most effective.

The amount of tissue removed varies with the stage and grade of the cancer. In breast cancer surgery, for example, the types of surgery are as follows:

En bloc resection: removal of the cancerous tumor and the lymph nodes.
Lumpectomy: removal of the tumor only.

Lymph node dissection: the removal of clinically involved lymph nodes. **Lymph node mapping** determines a pattern of spread from the primary tumor site through the lymph nodes. The **sentinel node** is the first node in which lymphatic drainage occurs in a particular area. If this node is negative for cancer upon dissection, then the lymph system is free of cancer.

Radical mastectomy: removal of the breast containing the cancer, along with the lymph nodes and the muscle under the breast. When the surgical report discusses **margins,** it refers to the borders of normal tissue surrounding the cancer. A **wide margin resection** means that the cancer is removed with a significant amount of tissue around the tumor to ensure that all the cancer cells are removed. If the margins are reported as negative, no cancer cells are seen. If positive, cancer cells have been detected by the pathologist.

Simple mastectomy: removal of the breast containing the cancer.

Radiotherapy

Approximately half of all cancer patients receive radiation. The goal of radiation therapy is to destroy the nucleus of the cancer cells, thereby destroying their ability to reproduce and spread.

Although radiation is usually started after removal of the tumor, sometimes it is done before removal to shrink the tumor. Some cancers may be treated solely with radiation.

Brachytherapy (brah kee THAYR uh pee): the use of radiation placed directly on or within the cancer through the use of needles or beads containing radioactive gold, cobalt, or radium (Fig. 7-9).

Gamma knife surgery: a noninvasive type of surgery that uses gamma radiation to destroy a brain tumor.

Systemic Therapy

Bone marrow transplant (BMT): Patients who are incapable of producing healthy blood cells are given bone marrow from a matching donor to stimulate normal blood cell growth. Patients with specific types of leukemia may receive bone marrow transplants after chemotherapy has effectively destroyed the functioning of their own bone marrow.

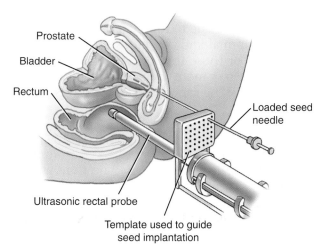

Fig. 7-9 Prostate brachytherapy. Radioactive seeds are implanted with a needle guided by ultrasound and a template grid.

Chemotherapy: Chemotherapy is the circulation of cancer-destroying medicine throughout the body. Chemotherapy may also be used as an adjuvant (aid) to other forms of treatment to relieve symptoms or slow down the spread of cancer. See the Pharmacology section for more details on chemotherapy drugs.

Complementary and alternative medicine (CAM) techniques: Prayer, massage, diet, exercise, and mind-body techniques encompass the majority of CAM methods used in cancer treatment. The U.S. government has established the National Center for Complementary and Alternative Medicine, which reports on results of research studies on the use of CAM techniques for various disorders (http://www.nccam.nih.gov).

Immunotherapy: Immunotherapy is the use of the body's own defense system to attack cancer cells. See the description of interleukins in the Pharmacology section.

 Exercise 7-5: THERAPEUTIC INTERVENTIONS

Circle the correct response.

1. Treatment with radioactive beads near or inside the cancer is called *(chemotherapy, brachytherapy)*.
2. A determination of the spread of the primary tumor through the lymph nodes is referred to as lymph node *(dissection, mapping)*.
3. The first node in which lymphatic drainage occurs is the *(sentinel, primary)* node.
4. Removal of the tumor and lymph nodes is *(lumpectomy, en bloc resection)*.
5. The borders of normal tissue surrounding the cancer are called *(stages, margins)*.
6. Use of the body's own defense system to attack cancer cells is called *(immunotherapy, BMT)*.
7. Prayer, massage, exercise, and mind-body techniques are examples of *(CAM, adjuvant therapy)*.

PHARMACOLOGY

Chemotherapy works by disrupting the cycle of cell replication. All cells go through a cycle of reproducing themselves, but, unlike cancer cells, they have a built-in mechanism that limits their growth. The side effects of cancer therapy, such as hair loss or nausea, are due to the inability of chemotherapeutic agents to differentiate between normal and cancerous cells. Thus cells that reproduce rapidly, such as hair cells or those that line the stomach, are also affected. It should also be noted that two or more chemotherapeutic agents are usually used together to effectively attack the cancer at various stages. This is referred to as a drug *protocol* or plan.

The majority of the pharmaceuticals prescribed to treat cancer are referred to as *antineoplastic agents*. They accomplish the goal of slowing or stopping the progression of cancer in different ways:

Alkylating agents: Interferes with DNA replication to lead to cancer cell death or dysfunction. Examples include cisplatin (Platinol AQ), nitrosoureas like carmustine (Gliadel), and nitrogen mustards like cyclophosphamide (Cytoxan).

Antimetabolites: Replace compounds that cancer cells need to grow and/or replicate. Examples are methotrexate and fluorouracil (5-FU).

Antineoplastic antibiotics: Prevent or delay cell replication. Examples include doxorubicin (Rubex, Adriamycin) and dactinomycin (Cosmegen).

Antineoplastic hormones: Interfere with receptors for growth-stimulating proteins. Examples include flutamide (Eulexin) and tamoxifen (Nolvadex).

Interleukins: Stimulate cells of the immune system to boost attack on cancer cells. An example is aldesleukin (Proleukin).

Mitotic inhibitors: Prevent cell division. An example is paclitaxel (Taxol).

Vinca alkaloids: Prevent formation of chromosome spindles necessary for cell duplication. Examples include vincristine (Oncovin) and vinblastine.

 Exercise 7-6: PHARMACOLOGY

Circle the correct answer.

1. Patients who are prescribed chemotherapy receive a drug *(protocol, adjuvant)*.
2. Side effects of chemotherapy frequently occur because the drugs used to kill cancer cells often *(stimulate, kill)* normal cells.
3. Most chemotherapeutic agents work by disrupting a phase of the cell *(cycle, movement)*.
4. Drugs that interfere with receptors for growth-stimulating proteins are *(antineoplastic hormones, antimetabolites)*.
5. Drugs that interfere with DNA replication are called *(antineoplastic antibiotics, alkylating agents)*.
6. Drugs that replace compounds that cancer cells need to grow or replicate are *(interleukins, antimetabolites)*.
7. Cell division is prevented by *(vinca alkaloids, mitotic inhibitors)*.

 Exercise 7-7: DISCHARGE SUMMARY

Using the discharge summary on p. 294, fill in the blanks.

1. This patient has "metastatic breast cancer." What does this mean? _____

2. Where has the cancer spread to? _____

3. What type of treatment has she received? _____

4. The patient is dehydrated and hyponatremia is noted. What is hyponatremia? _____

5. Explain what "her long-term prognosis is poor, probably in the range of months" means.

Hamstead Memorial Hospital
532 13th St.
Hamstead, TX 75201

DISCHARGE SUMMARY

DATE OF ADMISSION/DISCHARGE: 12/06/XX - 12/10/XX

Final Diagnosis: 1. Metastatic breast cancer

2. Dehydration with confusion

SUMMARY: This is a 65-year-old woman who developed breast cancer approximately 1 year ago. She had surgery, chemotherapy, seemed to be doing well, but this fall developed recurrence. This was present in the neck and liver. She underwent cycles of chemotherapy. Although the nodes in her neck subsided, she has had advancing cancer in the liver and does not seem to be responding to chemotherapy, and in fact, the chemotherapy is making her quite ill. This has been discussed with her family, and because this therapy is not going to cure her and is making her ill, she has decided to forego any more chemotherapy at this time, which seems appropriate.

She has had some right flank pain, I presume from the liver metastases. She has had a very poor appetite, poor oral intake, and has become quite dehydrated and confused. She came to the hospital in an extremely weak and confused condition. She was noted to have hyponatremia with sodium down to 125, extremely dry mucous membranes. White count was elevated to 16.5. Hemoglobin has been right around 10. Initial labs also suggested a urinary tract infection, although the culture did not grow anything.

She was admitted and treated with IV fluids, nausea medication, and started on Cipro for presumed UTI. Her condition improved so that she became mentally clear. She continues to have poor oral intake and needs a lot of encouragement, but is discharged home to be followed by hospice. Her long-term prognosis is poor, probably in the range of months.

Discharge medications include Cipro 500 mg for an additional 7 days. Compazine 10 mg po q 6 hr for nausea, Ultram 1 to 2 tablets tid for pain, and Senokot 1 to 2 tablets prn for constipation. Plan of care was discussed with her and her family, and hospice will be following her.

Melissa Landrey, MD

Abbreviations

Abbreviation	Meaning	Abbreviation	Meaning
AFP	Alpha-fetoprotein test	G	Grade
BSE	Breast self-examination	hCG	Human chorionic gonadotropin
bx	Biopsy	LDH	Lactate dehydrogenase (may be used to detect presence of cancer or to monitor certain cancers)
CA	Cancer		
CA125	Tumor marker primarily for ovarian cancer		
		mets	Metastases
CA15-3	Tumor marker to monitor breast cancer	NSE	Neuron-specific enolase (used to detect neuroblastoma, small cell cancer)
CA19-9	Tumor marker for pancreatic, stomach, and bile duct cancer		
		Pap	Papanicolaou test for cervical/vaginal cancer
CA27-29	Tumor marker to check for recurrence of breast cancer		
		PSA	Prostate-specific antigen
CEA	Carcinoembryonic antigen (used to monitor colorectal cancer)	SPECT	Single-photon emission computed tomography
CTR	Certified tumor registrar	TNM	Tumor-nodes-metastasis
FOBT	Fecal occult blood test	TSE	Testicular self-examination

◇ Exercise 7-8: ABBREVIATIONS

Write the meaning of the following abbreviations.

1. The patient appeared for a bx of a suspicious mole. _____

2. The prognosis was poor for the lung cancer patient with a G IV finding on his pathology report.

   _____

3. The 50-year-old woman made an appointment for a colonoscopy to check for CA after she had a

   positive finding on a home FOBT. _____

4. The CTR at Montgomery Memorial recorded the TNM stage for the patient's abstract.

   _____

5. SPECT was used to detect bone mets in the patient with advanced breast cancer.

   _____

Careers

Cancer Registrar

Cancer registrars (also called tumor registrars) are specialists in cancer data management. Their primary responsibility is to report and track patients with cancer who are diagnosed and/or treated at the registrar's health care facility. Registrars identify cancer patients, abstract demographic and medical information, and perform lifetime follow-up of these patients. Most registrars work in hospitals, but some work in regional or state registries. Patient contact is the exception, not the rule.

Cancer registrars are trained on the job through workshops or formal education programs. Several colleges along with the American Health Information Management Association (http://www.ahima.org) currently offer on-line courses. Students take courses in health care terminology, anatomy and physiology, cancer management, statistics, and cancer registry procedures. Individuals with the appropriate amount of education and/or experience may sit for a certification examination offered by the National Board for Certification of Registrars. A passing score earns a Certified Tumor Registrar (CTR) credential. These jobs are expected to grow faster than the average because of a new requirement for American College of Surgeons Approved Cancer Programs to hire CTRs in their registries.

Students interested in finding out more about the profession may check out the website for the National Cancer Registrars Association at http://www.ncra~usa.org.

Orthotist and Prosthetist

Closely related, yet performing different duties, orthotists and prosthetists help patients restore functioning and/or their appearance after injury or loss of a body part. Orthotists design, build, and fit external devices (termed *orthoses*) that help stabilize a body part, assist with functioning, prevent deformity, or prevent injury. Examples are leg braces, shoe inserts, and carpal tunnel support devices. Prosthetists design, build, and fit external devices (termed *prostheses*) that are substitutes for body parts that have been removed. A prosthesis could be an artificial arm, leg, breast, or testicle. Individuals may study for this profession through a baccalaureate, master's level, or post-baccalaureate certificate program. A 1-year residency is required to sit for the certification examination offered by the American Board for Certification in Orthotics and Prosthetics. For more information, visit the American Academy of Orthotics and Prosthetists at: www.opcareers.org.

Medical Illustrator

If you find that you are interested in medicine and art, a career as a medical illustrator may be for you. These individuals produce materials for medical, biological, and related fields including research groups. Most medical illustrators have undergraduate courses that concentrate on art and biology. A master's degree from an accredited graduate program in medical illustration is the next step in this field. Job settings include medical schools, medical centers, medical publishers, pharmaceutical companies, or freelance work. For more information, contact The Association of Medical Illustrators at http://www.ami.org.

Hamstead Memorial Hospital
532 13th St.
Hamstead, TX 75201

DISCHARGE SUMMARY

Patient Name: Clifford Walker   MR#: 163544
Physician: Albert Schwartz, MD   Adm: 12/01/02
                                        Disch: 12/04/02

Diagnosis: Sigmoid colon cancer by colonoscopy
Procedure: Sigmoid colectomy and appendectomy
History: This 45-year-old male with a significant family history of colon cancer came to my office after a colonoscopy demonstrated a carcinoma at 18 cm. He comes now after having an outpatient bowel preparation.
Hospital Course: The patient was admitted, and a sigmoid colectomy was performed. At that time, an appendectomy was also done. His postoperative course was unremarkable. His diet was slowly advanced, and by day 4, he was able to be discharged to home.

   His pathology report demonstrated a carcinoma through the wall with a microperforation. He had 12 nodes examined, all negative for carcinoma. His appendix was also positive for subacute appendicitis. He was scheduled for follow-up in my office in 10 days.
Discharge Medications: Percocet, Tylenol

                                        _____
                                        Albert Schwartz, MD

I. Health Care Report

52. What was the patient's diagnosis?

_____

53. How was his cancer diagnosed?

_____

54. What procedures were done?

_____

55. How do we know that there was no cancer in the lymph nodes?

_____

Reference

Mayo CH, Hendricks WA: Carcinomas of the right segment of the colon, *Ann Surg* 83: 357-363, 1926.

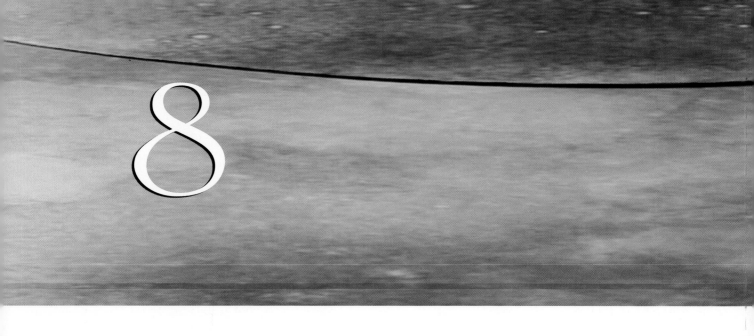

8

Objectives

You will be able to do the following after completing this chapter:

Key Terms
1. Define, appropriately use, and spell all the Key Terms for this chapter.

Film-Screen Radiography
2. Explain how electromagnetic energy is used to produce images on x-ray film.
3. List the four views that can be taken in a chest radiograph ("x-ray") and describe the patient positioning for each.
4. Explain the patient preparation necessary for accurate mammography.

Fluoroscopic Imaging
5. Explain the difference between film-screen radiographic imaging and fluoroscopic imaging.
6. Explain the purpose of contrast media, and state an important question to ask patients before contrast studies using iodine are performed.

Computer Imaging
7. Explain how ultrasonography uses sound waves to create images of soft tissue and internal organs.
8. Describe the patient preparation necessary for abdominal, gallbladder, kidney, and pelvic ultrasound tests.
9. Explain how magnetic resonance imaging (MRI) allows physicians to view detailed pictures from inside the body.
10. Describe the patient preparation necessary for MRI, and list three important questions to ask the patient before the procedure.
11. Explain how computed tomography (CT) scans create a cross-sectional image of a target organ or body area.
12. Describe the patient preparation necessary for a CT scan.
13. Explain how positron emission tomography (PET) scans pinpoint cancer sites or other abnormally functioning areas in the body.
14. Describe the patient preparation necessary for a PET scan.

Employee Safety
15. List two safety precautions for employees working in areas where they could be exposed to radiation.

Medical Assistant's Role
16. Identify two topics the medical assistant must address with the patient when scheduling x-ray examinations.
17. State the most important task for the medical assistant after patient testing.

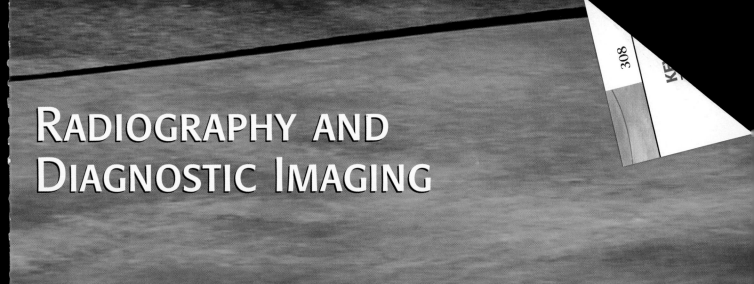

RADIOGRAPHY AND DIAGNOSTIC IMAGING

Patient-Centered Professionalism

18. Analyze a realistic medical office situation and apply your understanding of radiography and diagnostic imaging to determine the best course of action.
19. Describe the impact on patient care when medical assistants understand the concepts associated with radiography and diagnostic imaging and how patients are prepared for these procedures.

KEY TERMS

angiogram Diagnostic radiograph of the blood vessels using a contrast medium.

caliper Hinged instrument that measures thickness or diameter.

cholecystogram Radiograph of the gallbladder.

claustrophobia Fear of closed spaces.

computed tomography (CT) Computerized procedure that views the target organ or body area from different angles in a three-dimensional view.

computer imaging Techniques that display images with the use of contrast media.

contrast medium Radiopaque substance that enhances an image; plural *media.*

diagnostic imaging Techniques used to produce a picture image that does not involve the use of radiation.

digital radiographic imaging Radiography using computer imaging instead of conventional film or screen imaging.

dosimeter Device that monitors the quantity of x-ray exposure to health care workers.

film-screen radiography Radiography using special photographic film that blackens in response to the light from intensifying screens.

fluoroscopic imaging, fluoroscopy Radiographic imaging in which the view allows the radiologist to view images in motion.

intravenous pyelogram (IVP) Radiographic view of the kidneys using contrast dye injected intravenously.

lower gastrointestinal series (lower GI) Radiographic examination of the lower intestinal tract during and after

introduction of a contrast medium; also called *barium enema.*

magnetic resonance imaging (MRI) Procedure in which strong magnetic field and radio waves are used to produce images to view body structures.

mammogram X-ray record of breast tissue.

mammography X-ray technique used to detect abnormalities of the breast.

nuclear medicine Techniques that use radioactive material for patient diagnosis and treatment.

open MRI Imaging table with more space used for MRI imaging versus the enclosed narrow magnet tube.

positron emission tomography (PET) Procedure in which a sugar tracer is injected into the body and picked up by cancer cells that send out signals that can be picked up by a camera that forms pictures of various body parts. Also used with cerebral and arteriovascular diseases.

radiograph Picture or image created on film when exposed to x-rays; x-ray film.

radiography Process of producing an image using radiation (e.g., x-rays).

radiology Branch of medicine dealing with radioactive substances (e.g., x-rays, isotopes).

radiopaque Able to be seen using an x-ray technique.

tomography Radiography that views the body or organ as a whole in a cross-sectional view.

tracer Special radiographic medium that tags body cells, such as cancer cells.

CHAPTER 8

...Y TERMS—cont'd

transducer Device that is moved over the skin to record sound waves.

ultrasonography Use of high-frequency sound waves to produce images.

ultrasound Imaging of soft tissue and internal organs using high-frequency sound waves.

upper gastrointestinal series (upper GI) Radiographic examination of the esophagus, stomach, and upper small intestines during and after the introduction of a contrast medium; also called *barium swallow*.

x-ray film Special photographic film that blackens in response to light; also called a *radiograph*.

x-ray tube Vacuum tube that creates x-radiation.

What Would You Do?

Read the following scenario and keep it in mind as you learn about radiography and diagnostic imaging in this chapter.

Suzanne is a medical assistant who works for Dr. Sahara. Dr. Sahara has a medical office with the equipment for basic radiography. She sends her patients to specialized radiographic offices when more extensive testing is necessary. Dr. Sahara informs Suzanne that she has ordered these diagnostic imaging tests: (1) gallbladder ultrasound for middle-aged Mr. Donnolly, (2) baseline mammography for 40-year-old Mrs. Martens, (3) MRI for Mrs. Smith because of a possible brain lesion, and (4) chest radiograph for Mr. Charles, a patient with parkinsonism, because of possible pneumonia. Mr. Charles's chest x-ray film is inconclusive, so Dr. Sahara sends him back for a CT scan. When the CT scan arouses her suspicions, Dr. Sahara orders a PET scan for Mr. Charles 2 days later, and the results come back positive for cancer.

Would you be able to prepare patients for these procedures? Could you answer patient questions concerning the procedures?

Radiography is the diagnostic technique of producing an image with radiation, usually x-rays. Sound waves and other types of energy can also be used to produce images of specific body areas. In radiography, a radioactive substance sends out radiation, or rays of energy, in different directions. Typical x-ray films use the radiation to create a picture of a specific body area. Diagnostic radiographic imaging provides valuable information; the physician can use the images and pictures to diagnose fractures or other disorders and diseases of the body.

Some states require additional training to take x-ray films, whereas other states allow the medical assistant to perform these tasks in the medical office under the physician's guidance. In addition, the medical assistant may be required to (1) schedule various procedures with outside **radiology** offices or departments, (2) order supplies, (3) assist with positioning, and (4) provide patient instructions prior to imaging. Therefore understanding the basics of all forms of diagnostic radiographic imaging is essential.

There are three basic types of diagnostic imaging: film-screen radiography, fluoroscopic imaging, and computer imaging. (In specialty areas of radiology, radiation is also used to treat cancer.) Medical assistants need to understand safety precautions when performing radiography, as well as the need to properly prepare patients for these procedures.

FILM-SCREEN RADIOGRAPHY

In **film-screen radiography** the body part for which imaging is requested is placed between the **x-ray tube** and the **x-ray film.** These procedures can be performed on patients in a standing, sitting, or supine position (Fig. 8-1). Electromagnetic energy from the x-radiation is directed at the film. The film is sensitive to the energy and, when developed, the picture or image **(radiograph)** that appears is the result of the x-ray energy. The recorded image looks like a photo negative, as follows (Fig. 8-2):

- Maximum density areas are white because the x-ray beam could not penetrate them. Bone, a dense tissue, does not allow the radiation to pass through to the film, so bone appears on the film as a white or light-colored image.
- Minimal areas are gray because there was some penetration of energy or density. Muscle tissue

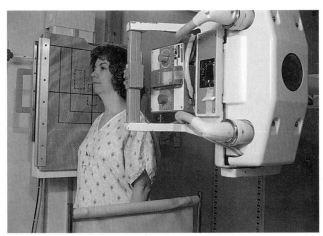

Fig. 8-1   Patient is positioned between the film and the x-ray tube. *(From Chester GA: Modern medical assisting, Philadelphia, 1998, Saunders.)*

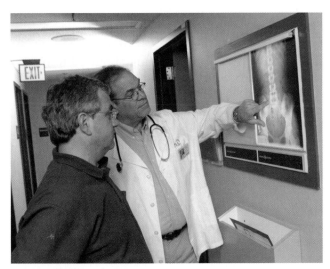

Fig. 8-2   Physician explains x-ray results to a patient.

does not absorb electromagnetic energy, so muscle tissue does not appear on the radiograph.

- Areas with no energy or little density are black because nothing stopped the radiation energy from reaching the film. Air, such as that within the lungs and intestines, does not absorb electromagnetic energy and appears black on the x-ray film.

The best images occur when the passage of energy is directed in a straight line through the desired area. Body structures do not lie at exact 90-degree angles to each other, so a body part may be rotated or positioned to allow for clear projection of the x-ray beam.

The x-ray machine is designed to prevent x-ray leakage and confines the area of the x-rays to a small, specific part of the body. A lead shield (to

---

BOX 8-1   Common Diagnostic Imaging Tests

- *Radiography (radiology) studies:* Radiation is used to show internal structures on x-ray films.
- *Ultrasonography:* High-frequency sound waves are used to create visual images of internal body structures.
- *Nuclear medicine:* Radionuclides are injected and travel throughout the body. Special equipment detects the material, and a computer creates an image.
- *Magnetic resonance imaging (MRI):* Specific parts of the body are exposed to an electromagnetic field. A scanner uses the information gathered to produce a three-dimensional image.
- *Computed tomography (CT scan):* Internal structures are examined using a selected body plane. Rotating x-ray beam scans a cross section, and a computer reconstructs the image.
- *Fluoroscopy:* Internal organs are viewed in motion. Procedure is used for viewing the function of the stomach and intestinal structures and for cardiac catheterization.

protect the gonads), collar (to protect the thyroid), and glasses (to protect eyes) are used to protect sensitive organs when they are not being studied. The high-speed film used means less radiation is required, but protection is still necessary.

Two types of film-screen radiography with which the medical assistant should be familiar are chest radiography (chest x-ray) and mammography (mammogram). If more diagnostic information is required, the physician may order tests from other departments, such as **nuclear medicine** or **diagnostic imaging.** Box 8-1 defines common diagnostic imaging tests. The type of medical imaging ordered by the physician depends on what part of the body is being examined and for what purpose.

Chest Radiography

The chest radiograph, or "chest x-ray," provides an image of the lungs, heart, and large blood vessels (Fig. 8-3). After the images are taken, a radiologist evaluates the results, and a report is sent to the primary physician. The following four views can be taken:

1. *Posteroanterior (PA) chest view* (posterior to anterior). The patient is facing the film holder,

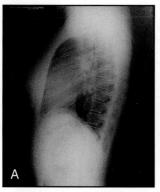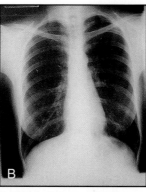

Fig. 8-3 Chest radiographs: **A,** lateral (side) view; **B,** AP (frontal) view (anterior to posterior). *(From Young AP, Kennedy DB: Kinn's the medical assistant, ed 9, Philadelphia, 2003, Saunders.)*

and the x-ray tube is to the back. The hands are placed low on the hips with the palms facing outward, the shoulders are rolled forward with the scapulae moved forward, and the chin is elevated. The x-ray beam passes through the patient from the back to the front. Note that there are several ways to obtain a PA view. Fig. 8-4, *A,* shows the patient with arms raised to obtain a PA view.

2. *Anteroposterior (AP) chest view* (anterior to posterior). The patient is facing the x-ray tube, and the film holder is to the back. The arms are at the patient's side, slightly abducted, with shoulders relaxed and slightly rotated forward (Fig. 8-4, *B*). The x-ray beam passes through the patient from front to back.
3. *Lateral chest view.* The patient's feet, hips, and shoulders are in lateral position to the film holder. The patient's arms are raised over the head with each hand grasping the opposite elbow and the chin elevated (Fig. 8-4, *C*).
4. *Oblique chest view.* The x-ray beam is directed at an angle through the body part (Fig. 8-4, *D*).

Patient Preparation

Before a chest x-ray film is taken, explain the procedure so that the patient knows what to expect (no advance preparation is necessary). Just before the procedure, remove all upper body jewelry. The patient is normally positioned in an upright position with the body weight equally distributed on both feet. The patient is asked to take a deep breath and hold it.

Mammography

Mammography is an x-ray examination of the breasts to detect abnormalities. It is considered to be one of the most effective methods for early detec-

tion of breast cancer. When scheduling a patient for a mammogram, keep in mind that the patient should make the appointment when her breasts are least tender (after her period). A **mammogram** is taken by positioning the patient's breast on a mammography machine and having a compression paddle apply pressure to the breast, flattening it (Fig. 8-5). Mammography is usually performed bilaterally (on both breasts). Mammography may also be performed on males who have possible abnormalities of breast tissue.

Patient Preparation

Patient preparation involves letting the patient know how to prepare for the mammography and what to expect during the procedure. The following areas should be addressed with the patient:

1. The patient should avoid caffeine for several days before the test.
2. No lotions, powders, or deodorant are to be used the morning of the examination.
3. The patient will be standing about 15 minutes for the procedures.
4. Explain that the x-ray machine will separately compress each breast both superior to inferior, and medial to lateral. There may be some discomfort, but full compression is necessary to achieve maximum results.
5. Advise patients to wear two-piece outfits, so only clothing from the waist up needs to be removed.

PATIENT-CENTERED PROFESSIONALISM

- How would the medical assistant explain the purpose of radiography to a patient?

FLUOROSCOPIC IMAGING

The film-screen radiographic imaging produces a view that is motionless, but in **fluoroscopic imaging,** or **fluoroscopy,** the image may include movement of contrast media through a body part. If you think of radiography as taking a snapshot or picture of a structure, think of fluoroscopic imaging as using a video camera.

Fluoroscopy is used when real-time visualization is necessary.

Contrast Media

Fluoroscopic imaging requires the use of a **contrast medium** (plural *media*). A contrast medium is a **radiopaque** substance that enhances the imaging characteristic of the x-ray film by providing

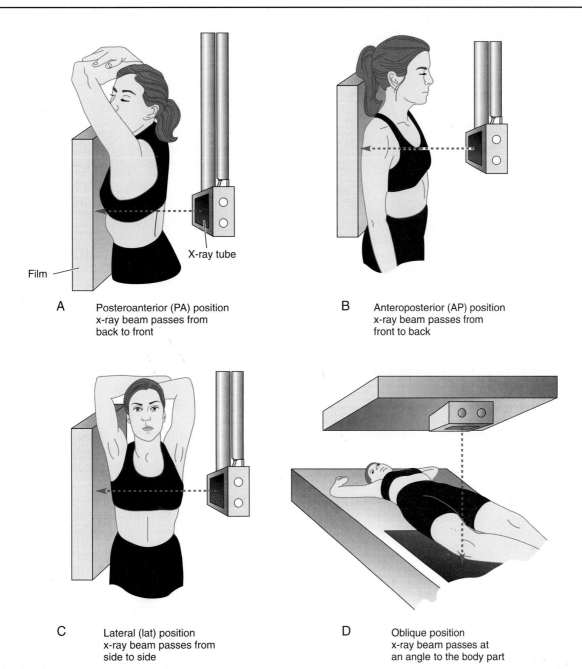

Film

X-ray tube

A   Posteroanterior (PA) position
x-ray beam passes from
back to front

B   Anteroposterior (AP) position
x-ray beam passes from
front to back

C   Lateral (lat) position
x-ray beam passes from
side to side

D   Oblique position
x-ray beam passes at
an angle to the body part

Fig. 8-4 Positions used for x-ray studies: **A,** posteroanterior; **B,** anteroposterior; **C,** lateral; **D,** oblique. *(From Hunt SA: Saunders fundamentals of medical assisting, Philadelphia, 2002, Saunders.)*

a difference in density. It provides for a better visual effect because it allows organs to be outlined and tissues to absorb radiation better, thus allowing them to stand out on radiographs. Contrast media can be introduced into the body by swallowing, through injection, or with an enema. Typical contrast media are barium and iodine. Table 8-1 lists major tests using contrast media.

Patient Preparation
A key question to ask patients for contrast studies using iodine concerns any possible allergy to any

iodine compound or to shellfish. As with other procedures, tell the patient what will be done during the procedure and what to expect. Advise the patient to call the physician if pain, swelling, or redness appears at the injection site.

PATIENT-CENTERED PROFESSIONALISM

- How would the medical assistant explain the purpose of fluoroscopy to a patient?

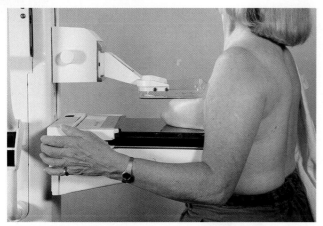

Fig. 8-5 Patient positioning for mammography. *(From Ballinger PW, Frank ED, editors: Merrill's atlas of radiographic positions and radiologic procedures, vol 2, ed 10, St Louis, 2003, Mosby.)*

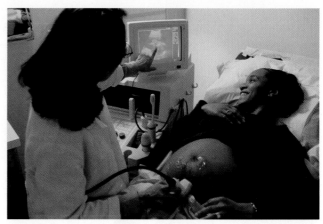

Fig. 8-6 Fetal ultrasound. Technician moves a transducer across the patient's abdomen, and image appears on a television monitor. *(From Hunt SA: Saunders fundamentals of medical assisting, Philadelphia, 2002, Saunders.)*

COMPUTER IMAGING

Computer imaging or **digital radiographic imaging** is used in ultrasound, magnetic resonance imaging, computed tomography, and nuclear medicine. Digital imaging reduces errors in processing because it does not rely on film, but rather computerized sensing and storage devices.

Ultrasonography

Instead of using ionizing radiation to diagnose, **ultrasonography** uses high-frequency sound waves to create an image **(ultrasound)** of soft tissue and internal organs. These sound waves are reflected by body tissues and recorded when a **transducer** (a computer mouse–like object) is moved over the skin, over the area to be examined.

Ultrasonography is a noninvasive and painless procedure that provides immediate feedback to the user. It can be used to visualize the abdominal area, the heart (echocardiogram), pelvic organs, and urinary organs. Table 8-2 lists patient preparations for various ultrasound studies. Newer uses include using a vaginal and rectal probe that can provide very clear images. A condom is typically used to cover the vaginal and rectal probe, making insertion easier.

Most people associate ultrasound examinations with pregnancy. It is frequently used in the first trimester to confirm pregnancy and to view the gestational sac, fetal heart, and body movements, as well as to detect any uterine abnormalities. As the pregnancy progresses, ultrasonography is used to determine fetal size, position, and head circum-

ference, as well as assess placental abnormalities and attachment (Fig. 8-6).

Patient Preparation

Depending on the type of ultrasound procedure, the specific body area to be examined, and the reason the patient is having the test, the patient may need to take specific steps to prepare for ultrasonography, such as fasting, or drinking to have a full bladder. Regardless of the nature of the ultrasound, the medical assistant needs to let the patient know what to expect during the procedure.

Magnetic Resonance Imaging

Magnetic resonance imaging (MRI) allows the physician to see detailed pictures inside the body without the use of x-rays. A strong magnetic field and radio waves are used to view anatomical structures. MRI is used to identify and evaluate blood clots, nerve damage, torn ligaments, and similar conditions. The MRI provides cross-sectional images of the body organs without the use of radiation.

MR images allow the physician to view anatomical structures more clearly than is possible with other forms of imaging. It basically creates a three-dimensional image of the body. MRI does not require the use of contrast media or radiation.

Patient Preparation

Patient preparation for MRI is simple. Patients can have a normal diet and continue to take their prescribed medications. Important questions to ask the patient include the following:

- Does the patient have any medical devices with metal (e.g., pacemaker, IUD [copper-7], surgical

TABLE 8-1	Common Diagnostic Tests Requiring Contrast Media		
Test	**Purpose**	**Patient Preparation**	**Procedure**
Upper gastrointestinal series (upper GI, barium swallow)	To examine esophagus, stomach, and small intestine for ulcers, obstructions, and inflammation	Light evening meal. NPO (nothing to eat or drink) after midnight.	Patient removes all clothing except shoes and socks; patient is gowned. Patient is positioned with the back against the film cassette. Patient drinks a barium solution through a straw while in front of a fluoroscope. Patient position is adjusted as needed for visualization. X-ray films are taken.
Lower gastrointestinal series (lower GI, barium enema)	To examine the colon for polyps, inflammation, diverticula, and other changes	Low-residue diet for 2 days before examination; no dairy products. Use of a special bowel preparation kit as ordered. Light meal and NPO after meal except water. Enema and rectal suppositories the morning of examination; NPO.	Patient removes all clothing except shoes and socks; patient is gowned. Patient is positioned in Sims' position. Barium sulfate is inserted as an enema. Frequent side-to-side turning movement is needed to allow barium to move through intestines. X-ray films are taken.
Intravenous pyelogram (IVP)	To examine the renal pelvis, ureters, and bladder for cysts, stones, and tumors	Light evening meal. Laxative taken the night before. NPO after midnight. Before the test, drink fluids. Empty bladder before procedure.	Dye is injected through intravenous (IV) catheter. As the kidneys excrete the dye, x-ray films are taken.
Cholecystogram	To study the gallbladder	Low-fat evening meal. Take oral medication the evening before. NPO after medication.	Series of x-ray films is taken. Fatty meal given to stimulate gallbladder after preliminary films. Additional x-ray films are taken.
Angiogram	To detect tumors and obstructions, as well as lung, heart, and other organ problems	NPO after midnight.	Sedative is given. Dye is injected into a vein using IV catheter. X-ray films are taken.

NPO, Latin *nil per os*, nothing by mouth.

TABLE 8-2   Patient Preparation for Ultrasound Test

Ultrasound	Preparation
Abdominal*	NPO after midnight.
Gallbladder	NPO after midnight.
Kidney	NPO after midnight.
Pelvic	No dietary restrictions.
	Patient must drink four to six 8-ounce glasses of fluid (water, juice, coffee, or tea) 1 hour before the examination.
	Patient must not empty the bladder until after the test is done.
	NOTE: A full bladder provides the physician with a point of reference when visualizing the urinary bladder full.

*Includes liver, gallbladder, kidneys, pancreas, spleen, and aorta.
NPO, Latin *nil per os*, nothing by mouth.

clips [e.g., aneurysm], metal prosthesis, hearing aids, dental bridges, glasses, wig with metal clips)? Metal disturbs the signals needed to produce the image, which can cause blurring. Also, because the magnetic pull is so strong, a loose metal fragment could be pulled away from the patient's body, causing injury to the patient. Because clothing harbors metal, a gown will be provided for the patient. Even eye shadow and transdermal patches must be removed because they may be composed of metallic compounds (e.g., some patches have an aluminum backing).

- Is there any chance of pregnancy? MR scans are not recommended for pregnant women because the effects of strong magnetic fields on a fetus are not well documented.
- Can the patient lie still for at least 30 minutes? Movement will blur the images.

The patient will be asked to lie flat (sometimes a small pillow is placed under the patient's knees for comfort), with arms at the side, on the scanning bed. Once the patient is comfortable, the bed is slid into the magnet tube (Fig. 8-7). Because motion will affect the image, the patient must be still. A covering may be given to the patient to provide warmth. Some patients may be anxious, and others may experience **claustrophobia** in enclosed areas. In these situations, a mild sedative may be prescribed before the examination. The patient will hear a humming or thumping sound, which can be lessened by wearing earplugs. After the examination, the patient can resume normal activities.

Technological advances have made **open MRI** a possibility for many patients. Instead of lying in the narrow magnet tube, the patient lies on an imaging table with more space around the body. Open MRI is often a good choice for children and for those who are claustrophobic or obese. Open MRI is now being used more frequently. The noise is less noticeable, and the feeling of being "closed in" is reduced.

Computed Tomography

Tomography is the use of radiography to see the body or an organ as a whole in a cross-sectional or "sliced" view. **Computed tomography (CT)** views the target organ or body area from different angles in a three-dimensional view; the CT scan is sometimes called a "CAT scan" (computerized axial tomography). Typical uses for CT scanning are the assessment of blood vessels (e.g., detecting aneurysms), the hepatic system, the kidney, and pulmonary systems. Box 8-2 lists other diagnostic uses of head, body, and cardiovascular CT scans.

The CT scanner x-ray tube focuses a narrow x-ray beam across a layer, or "slice," of the body. The x-ray energy is absorbed differently by the body structures. Receptors detect the amount of x-radiation passing through the body. This information is relayed and stored in the computer. The x-ray tube rotates around the body, constantly scanning. Numerous readings are stored in the computer. The computer analyzes the readings at the different angles and converts this information into a cross-sectional image. The radiologist interprets the resulting image and determines if further tests are needed.

Patient Preparation

If a contrast medium is used for a head and chest CT scan, the patient is advised to avoid food or fluids for 8 hours. The use of contrast media sharpens details better than the image produced by sound waves. It is important to ask the patient about any known allergies and to have the

Radiowave detector   Magnet   Radiowave pulses

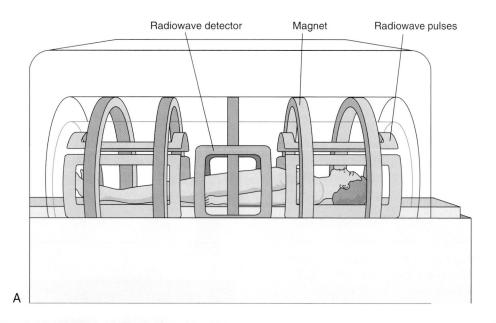

A

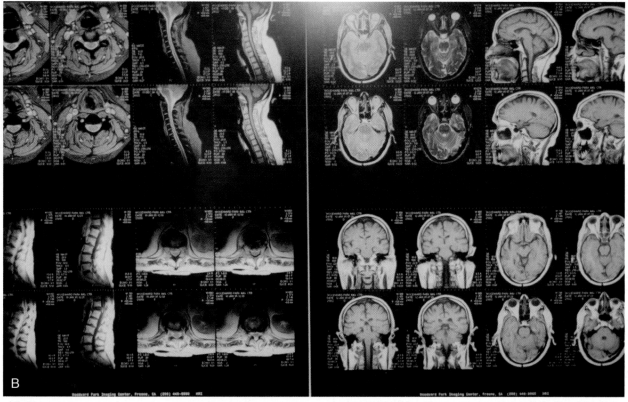

B

Fig. 8-7 **A,** Magnetic resonance imaging (MRI) unit. **B,** Magnetic resonance (MR) images. *(From Kinn ME, Woods MA: The medical assistant, ed 8, Philadelphia, 1999, Saunders.)*

patient remove any metal objects. The patient lies in a supine position in a cylinder, with the head secured in a cradle if a CT head scan is ordered (Fig. 8-8). Depending on what site is to be scanned, the average time needed for the scan is 1 hour.

An intravenous (IV) line is started to allow a site for the dye (contrast medium) to be injected, if needed. The patient must not move because blurs could result.

FOR YOUR INFORMATION

CT Scans
• Radiation exposure for CT scans is reported to be two to three times as much as for a typical x-ray film.
• CT scans often detect the smallest abnormalities, allowing treatment to begin early.

BOX 8-2   Purpose and Diagnostic Uses of CT Scans

Head Scans

To show brain structures and any abnormalities.

- Tumors growing in brain and spinal tissue.
- Blood clots forming because of a ruptured blood vessel in the brain.
- Enlarged ventricles resulting from cerebrospinal fluid not draining properly.
- Nerve and eye muscle abnormalities.
- Brain differences associated with mental illness, Alzheimer disease, and other disorders.

Body Scans

To distinguish among bone, tissue, fat, gas, fluid, and other body structures; can determine the size and shape of an organ and if a growth is solid or fluid filled.

- Lymph node enlargement caused by infection or other conditions.
- Pancreatic disease (can be diagnosed within 1 hour).
- Back problems, including ruptured vertebral discs.
- Lung cancer (growths can be viewed in areas not shown on regular x-ray films).

Cardiovascular Scans

To show heart structures and blood vessels and any abnormalities.

- Abnormal blood flow within blood vessels can be detected through the use of high-frequency sound waves (Doppler ultrasound).
- Structure and function of heart valves can be seen through the use of ultrasound (echocardiogram).

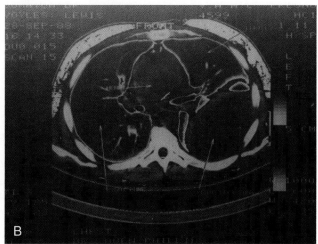

Fig. 8-8   **A,** Computed tomography (CT) total scanner. **B,** Example of CT scan. *(From Kinn ME, Woods MA: The medical assistant, ed 8, Philadelphia, 1999, Saunders.)*

Positron Emission Tomography

Positron emission tomography (PET) is an imaging method that can evaluate the entire body with a single procedure. A patient is injected with a sugar **tracer,** which is taken up and concentrated in cancer cells or other cells, such as the brain. These "sugar cells" (the cancer or other cells concentrated with sugar) send out signals that are picked up by a specialized camera. A computer in this camera converts these signals into pictures of the human body. Using this type of technology allows cancer and other sites to be pinpointed. CT scans and MRIs provide pictures of internal organs, but they do not identify abnormal functioning as the PET scan can.

In addition to oncological purposes, PET scanning is also used in cardiology and neurology. For example, PET is used to assess the potential benefits of coronary artery bypass surgery in high-risk patients and assists in the diagnosis of Alzheimer disease, Parkinson disease, and other neurological disorders.

Patient Preparation

The patient is asked to fast for at least 6 hours before the PET procedure. The patient is seated in a reclining chair and given an injection of the sugar tracer. After 45 minutes the patient is taken to an imaging table to lie down. The PET camera acquires information concerning the localization of the tracer in the body. These data are transmitted to a computer, and pictures of the body are formed. This part of the procedure takes another 45 minutes. A nuclear medicine physician reviews the PET scan in detail and sends a report to the primary physician.

EMPLOYEE SAFETY

The medical assistant working in a medical office with an x-ray machine, or any health care employee working in the radiology department, can be exposed to particles of radiation if safety procedures are not followed.

All employees working in an area where the possibility of exposure to radiation exists should wear a personal monitoring device called a **dosimeter** (Fig. 8-9). The dosimeter monitors the quantity of radiation exposure. It should be worn on the anterior surface, between chest and waist level. The device is usually referred to as a "film badge," and each employee is issued his or her own badge. To obtain an accurate exposure reading, the badge should not be shared among employees. It is usually worn clipped to the lab coat, uniform pocket, or collar.

The medical assistant should stand behind a lead barrier when performing radiography to ensure no exposure to radiation. Excessive exposure to radiation during pregnancy can result in birth defects and other problems in the child.

MEDICAL ASSISTANT'S ROLE

Depending on the policies of the medical facility and state and local regulations, medical assistants may or may not be allowed to perform radiography. However, all medical assistants need to understand their role in patient care associated with radiography and diagnostic imaging.

Questions to Ask Patients

Before making arrangements for a patient to have an x-ray examination or diagnostic imaging done, the medical assistant should routinely ask the patient the following:

1. Has the patient had other x-rays or diagnostic tests done, and for what?

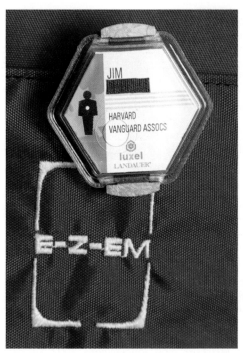

Fig. 8-9 Optically stimulated luminescence (OSL) dosimeter. *(From Young AP, Kennedy DP: Kinn's the medical assistant, ed 9, Philadelphia, 2003, Saunders.)*

2. If the patient is a female of childbearing age, is there a chance she could be pregnant? Asking the patient when her last menstrual period (LMP) occurred is a good indicator of pregnancy possibilities. Use the "10-day rule," which determines the patient is least susceptible to radiation to the gonads during the 10 days from the beginning of her menses, because it is unlikely the woman will become pregnant during this time.
3. If the patient will have a contrast medium injected, is he or she aware of any allergies to the dye? For example, patients who have an allergy to shellfish, which have naturally occurring iodine content, should avoid media that contain inorganic iodine compounds.

Scheduling and Patient Preparation

The medical office will routinely schedule patients for x-ray examinations. The medical assistant should review any special procedures that will be required of the patient and provide written instructions for the patient to take home. The patient needs to be informed of the following:

- Approximate length of time the examination will take.
- Special preparations required (e.g., fasting, bowel prep).

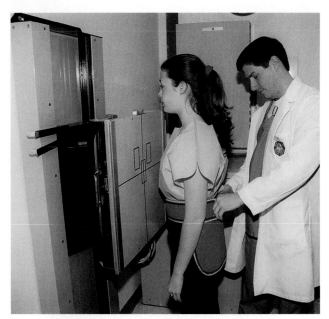

Fig. 8-10 Patient wears lead apron to protect reproductive organs. *(From Young AP, Kennedy DP: Kinn's the medical assistant, ed 9, Philadelphia, 2003, Saunders.)*

If the medical assistant helps in taking the x-ray film in the office, patient preparation includes the following:

1. Ensuring proper identification of the patient.
2. Measuring the body part with a **caliper** and properly marking the area to be surveyed.
3. Positioning the patient and the central x-ray correctly. Film accuracy requires that the patient be placed in the correct position and the position be held without moving.
4. Ensuring that children and adults of childbearing age have the reproductive organs covered with a gonad shield to prevent damage to these organs (Fig. 8-10). If the patient is pregnant, a release form must be signed stating that she understands the dangers from radiation to the fetus.
5. Providing reassurance as needed.
6. Developing the film properly, making certain the radiograph is free of artifacts. The film should be hung on the light box for the physician to view.

Postprocedural Duties

The medical assistant's most important task after patient testing is to be certain that a written report is received in the medical office for the physician to review. After review, the report must be filed in the patient's medical record. To make efficient use of the physician's and patient's time, the following can be done:

- Keep an x-ray log to monitor the return of diagnostic imaging reports.
- If a report is not received at the physician's office within a week, follow up with a call to the radiology department.
- The patient's medical record should be reviewed the day before the patient's visit to make certain all reports are available and signed off by the physician. Most physicians do not want to see patients without test results, and patients do not like to wait while results are being faxed.

PATIENT-CENTERED PROFESSIONALISM

- What is the medical assistant's role in preparing a patient for radiology studies?

CONCLUSION

Radiography has been a much-used diagnostic tool for nearly 100 years. In the last several decades, new technology has enabled digital computer imaging. These techniques enable physicians to diagnose illnesses and injuries quickly and efficiently. Diagnosing illness and injury in a timely manner allows the physician to determine the best course of treatment for patients and to implement the treatment plan more quickly.

Understanding the types of diagnostic imaging procedures, including film-screen radiography, fluoroscopy, and computer imaging, helps medical assistants provide better care to patients undergoing these tests, regardless of whether the assistant is directly involved in the procedure. Effectively preparing the patient allows the tests to run more smoothly and helps to produce better results.

SUMMARY

Reinforce your understanding of the material in this chapter by reviewing the curriculum objectives and key content points below.

1. Define, appropriately use, and spell all the Key Terms for this chapter.
   - Review the Key Terms if necessary.
2. Explain how electromagnetic energy is used to produce images on x-ray film.
   - Electromagnetic energy from the x-ray is directed at energy-sensitive film, with the

body part between the energy source and the film.

- White areas indicate no penetration of the energy (e.g., bones or total blockage) because of density, gray areas indicate some penetration of energy (some muscles and bones), and black areas indicate nothing blocking the penetration of radiation energy to the film (air) because of lack of density.

3. List the four views that can be taken in a chest radiograph ("x-ray") and describe the patient positioning for each.
   - The posteroanterior (PA) view is a frontal view (posterior to anterior). The patient stands facing the film holder, and the x-ray tube is to the back; hands are low on the hips, palms face outward, shoulders and scapulae are moved forward, and the chin is elevated.
   - The anteroposterior (AP) view is a back view (anterior to posterior). The patient stands facing the x-ray tube, and the film holder is to the back; arms are slightly abducted at the sides, with the shoulders relaxed and slightly rotated forward.
   - The lateral view is a side view. The patient stands sideways to the film holder; the arms are raised over the head, with each hand grasping the opposite elbow, and the chin is elevated.
   - The oblique view is accomplished when the x-ray beam is directed at an angle through the body part.

4. Explain the patient preparation necessary for accurate mammography.
   - Patients should be told to avoid caffeine for several days before the test.
   - Patients should be told not to use lotions, powders, or deodorant the morning of the examination.
   - Patients should be informed how long they will stand and what will happen during the procedure.
   - Tell patients to wear two-piece outfits so only clothing from the waist up needs to be removed.

5. Explain the difference between film-screen radiographic imaging and fluoroscopic imaging.
   - Film-screen imaging produces a still view; fluoroscopic imaging produces images in motion.

6. Explain the purpose of contrast media, and state an important question to ask patients before contrast studies using iodine are performed.
   - Contrast media are radiopaque substances that enhance the imaging characteristics of the radiograph.

- Before administering contrast media, always ask the patient if he or she is allergic to any iodine compound or shellfish.

7. Explain how an ultrasonography uses sound waves to create images of soft tissue and internal organs.
   - Sound waves are reflected by body tissues and organs and recorded when a transducer is moved over the skin outside the area to be examined.

8. Describe the patient preparation necessary for abdominal, gallbladder, kidney, and pelvic ultrasound tests.
   - Review Table 8-2.

9. Explain how magnetic resonance imaging (MRI) allows physicians to view detailed pictures from inside the body.
   - A three-dimensional image of the body area is generated by a strong magnetic field and radio waves. Images are more clearly delineated with MRI than with other forms of imaging.

10. Describe the patient preparation necessary for MRI, and list three important questions to ask the patient before the procedure.
    - Patients can have a normal diet and take their prescribed medications before MRI is performed.
    - The medical assistant should ask the patient questions about (a) medical devices with metal, (b) chance for pregnancy, and (c) whether the patient can lie still for 30 minutes.

11. Explain how computed tomography (CT) scans create a cross-sectional image of a target organ or body area.
    - CT scans view a target organ or body area from different angles in a three-dimensional view.
    - The body or organ as a whole is viewed in a cross-sectional, or "sliced," view.

12. Describe the patient preparation necessary for a CT scan.
    - If contrast medium is used for a head and chest CT scan, the patient should avoid fluid and foods for 8 hours, and the patient should be asked about allergies to iodine or shellfish. All metal objects should be removed from the patient.

13. Explain how positron emission tomography (PET) scans pinpoint cancer sites or other abnormally functioning areas in the body.
    - PET scans use tracers that are taken up by cancer or other cells. A specialized camera picks up the signals sent out by these cells, and a computer converts these signals into images.

14. Describe the patient preparation necessary for a PET scan.
    - Patients must fast for 6 hours before a PET scan.
15. List two safety precautions for employees working in areas where they could be exposed to radiation.
    - A dosimeter should be worn to monitor radiation exposure.
    - Employees should stand behind a lead barrier to block exposure to radiation.
16. Identify two topics the medical assistant must address with the patient when scheduling x-ray examinations.
    - Patients should be told (a) the approximate duration of the examination and (b) any special preparations required for the procedure.
17. State the most important task for the medical assistant after patient testing.
    - The medical assistant must be certain that a written report is received in the medical office for the physician to review.
18. Analyze a realistic medical office situation and apply your understanding of radiography and diagnostic imaging to determine the best course of action.

- Medical assistants need to know about the types of imaging procedures that are performed and why and how each is used.
19. Describe the impact on patient care when medical assistants understand the concepts associated with radiography and diagnostic imaging and how patients are prepared for these procedures.
    - Continuity of patient care is maintained when the medical assistant is aware of the functions of various forms of radiography and can answer patients' questions.
    - Proper patient preparation is necessary to provide the best results from diagnostic imaging procedures.

FOR FURTHER EXPLORATION

Research qualifications for becoming certified in your state to take x-ray films in the medical office.

Keywords: Use the following keywords in your search: office radiology, x-ray technician, radiologic technologist.

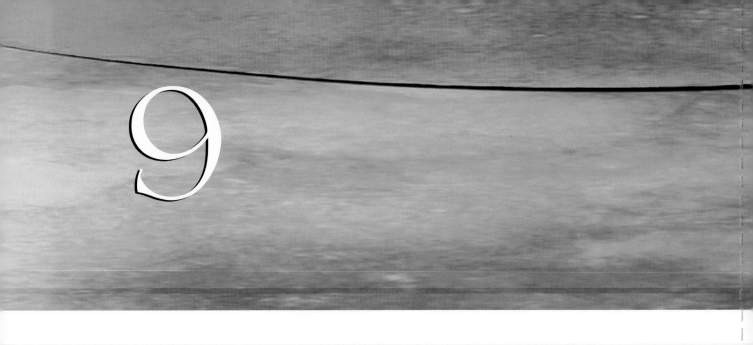

OBJECTIVES

After reading this chapter and working the exercises, you should be able to:

1. Identify the kind of information that appears in various medical reports.
2. Prepare a discharge summary, operative report, pathology report, radiology report, consultation report, autopsy protocol, and medicolegal report.
3. Know how to find acceptable formats for a variety of reports and medical documents.
4. Recognize the usefulness of a standard macro within a document.
5. Recognize the names of operative procedures, instruments, types of anesthesia, and suture materials and be familiar with how these terms should be transcribed.

PREPARATION OF MISCELLANEOUS MEDICAL REPORTS

This chapter continues the instruction for the preparation of "the basic four": the history and physical examination report, operative report, consultation report, and discharge summary. These and a variety of other medical reports concerning patients are transcribed by medical transcriptionists for the hospital or the facility or service contracted by the hospital. On a few occasions, a physician may want the medical transcriptionist who works for the office or clinic to transcribe some of these reports; in some medical facilities, the department medical transcriptionist transcribes the documents for that department only. For example, the pathology department may have laboratory reports and autopsy reports transcribed in the department. Consultation reports may be transcribed in the hospital or physician's office, and medicolegal reports are usually done by the private medical office medical transcriptionist or service employed. Some services hire medical transcriptionists with a legal background, as well as a medical background, and specialize in transcription of medicolegal reports. Private transcription agencies are prepared to perform a variety of medical transcribing. Because you do not know where you will seek employment, it is necessary for you to be prepared to transcribe the many different types of medical records.

Reports are sent to consultants who participated in the management of the patient, to insurance companies who want background information on patients, to third-party carriers to justify bills, to referring physicians, and to the Social Security Administration to assess a patient for total disability.

Accuracy and readability are the most important factors emphasized in reference to format. All headings and subheadings must follow the same format; therefore it is important to determine how you will set up the report before you begin. Topics of equal importance are given equal emphasis through the use of capital letters, lowercase letters, boldface, spacing, underlining, centering, and so on. The figures in this chapter give you a glimpse of possible headings; each physician/dictator/client chooses different words to emphasize. The sequence of the topic words may also be reversed in some dictations. The general guideline to follow is to transcribe exactly the sequence that is dictated and to determine the words requiring the most emphasis for major headings and those requiring less emphasis for subheadings. In some institutions, forms with preprinted headings necessitate that you reformat the dictation so that it is typed in the sequence given on the forms. There is an operational policy for individuals to consult when they select a format. Various professional groups have joined in an effort to standardize report formats.

DISCHARGE SUMMARIES

A discharge summary (clinical résumé or final progress note) is required for each patient who is discharged from a hospital. It contains the same information that is found in the patient's history and physical examination report with the addition of the admitting and discharge diagnoses, operations performed, laboratory and x-ray studies, consultations, hospital course, and the condition of the patient at the time of discharge, including medications on discharge, instructions for continuing care and therapy, and possibly a date for a follow-up postoperative office visit. The condition of the patient on discharge should be stated in terms that enable a specific measurable comparison with the condition on admission; the use of vague terminology such as "improved" should be avoided. Many medical transcriptionists have the documentation available and skill to assemble a discharge summary and are being asked to do so. If a resident or intern (house staff physician) dictates the discharge summary, it is usually approved by the attending physician (attending staff physician). If the patient or a legally qualified representative has provided written authorization, a copy of the discharge summary should be sent to any known medical practitioner or medical facility responsible for follow-up care of the patient. Often, discharge summaries for patients being transferred are transcribed on a stat basis. If stat material is processed at an offsite location, a facsimile is placed with the medical record and is replaced with the original report when the original is delivered to the facility.

In the case of a patient's death, a summary statement should be added to the record either as a final progress note or as a separate résumé. This final note should give the reason for admission, the findings and course in the hospital, and the events leading to death.

Figs. 9-1 and 9-2 are examples of complete discharge summaries, showing appearance, formats, and content.

OPERATIVE REPORTS

Whenever a surgical procedure is performed in the hospital, an outpatient surgical center, or a clinic, an operative report should be dictated or written in the medical record immediately after surgery. The report should contain a description of the findings, the technical procedures used, the specimens removed, the preoperative and postoperative diagnosis or diagnoses, the type of operation performed, and the name of the primary surgeon and any assistants. If the postoperative diagnosis is the same as the preoperative diagnosis, repeat the preoperative diagnosis exactly. The body of the report is a narrative of the procedure and findings and contains the type of anesthetic, incision, instruments used, drains, packs, closure, sponge count, tissue removed or altered, materials removed or inserted, blood loss and replacement, wound status, complications or unusual events, and condition of patient on leaving the surgical area. The completed operative report should be authenticated by the surgeon and filed in the medical record as soon as possible after surgery. When a delay in transcription or filing occurs, a comprehensive operative progress note should be entered in the medical record immediately after surgery to provide pertinent information

for other physicians who may be attending the patient. If a patient requires additional surgery after the initial surgery has been completed, the report may be transcribed on a stat basis.

See Fig. 9-3 for an example of an operative report. Notice that the first paragraph is one long paragraph. Although this format may seem awkward to you, this is how many surgeons dictate their operative records. However, some hospitals require that surgeons separate the report into subheadings, such as *Anesthesia, Incision, Findings, Procedure, Closure,* and so on. Fig. 9-4 illustrates another format for an operative report. Operative reports are more difficult to transcribe than other documents because of the thousands of procedures that are performed, the many instruments named during the procedure, the types and names of suture materials, placement (position) of the patient on the operating table, the type and substance used for anesthesia, and the types of incisions and closures made. The format itself is simple and straightforward.

PATHOLOGY REPORTS

As a medical transcriptionist, you can specialize by typing pathology or radiology reports. Pathology transcriptionists work in laboratories, hospital medical laboratories, and coroners' offices. A wide variety of job duties other than transcription exist, and these can consist of giving reports via the telephone; filing; retrieving diagnoses from *Systematized Nomenclature of Human and Veterinary Medicine (SNOMED International), Current Procedural Terminology* (CPT), and *International Classification of Diseases, Ninth Revision, Clinical Modification* (ICD-9-CM) coding; keeping tumor and autopsy logs; typing statistical reports; delivering reports; sorting and delivering mail; labeling and filing specimens; maintaining cross files; preparing procedure manuals throughout the laboratory; and performing other miscellaneous laboratory tasks, depending on the size of the workplace and the number of pathologists on the staff. Some of the departments in the laboratory include histology, chemistry, hematology, microbiology/bacteriology, immunology, and blood bank. Pathology consists of two divisions: anatomical (surgical and autopsy) and clinical (blood bank, microbiology, hematology, and chemistry).

When a surgical procedure is performed to remove tissue or fluid from the body, these specimens may be examined by the pathologist to determine the nature and extent of the disease. In some instances, a pathologist may render his or her opinion before the sutures are placed, as in the event of a malignant tumor, in which case more extensive surgery

Evans, Cornelia Elizabeth
97-32-11
July 16, 200X

DISCHARGE SUMMARY

ADMISSION DATE: June 14, 200X   DISCHARGE DATE: July 15, 200X

HISTORY OF PRESENT ILLNESS
This 19-year-old black female nulligravida was admitted to the hospital on June 14, 200X, with fever of 102°, left lower quadrant pain, vaginal discharge, constipation, and a tender left adnexal mass. Her past history and family history were unremarkable. Present pain had started 2 to 3 weeks prior to admission. Her periods were irregular, with the latest period starting on May 30, 200X, and lasting for 6 days. She had taken contraceptive pills in the past but had stopped because she was not sexually active.

PHYSICAL EXAMINATION
She appeared well developed and well nourished and in mild distress. The only positive physical findings were limited to the abdomen and pelvis. Her abdomen was mildly distended, and it was tender, especially in the left lower quadrant. At pelvic examination, the cervix was tender on motion, and the uterus was of normal size, retroverted, and somewhat fixed. There was a tender cystic mass, about 4 to 5 cm, in the left adnexa. Rectal examination was negative.

ADMITTING DIAGNOSES
1. Probable pelvic inflammatory disease (PID).
2. Rule out ectopic pregnancy.

LABORATORY DATA ON ADMISSION
Hemoglobin 8.8, hematocrit 26.5, WBC 8100 with 80 segs and 18 lymphs. Sedimentation rate 100 mm in 1 hour. Sickle cell prep+ (turned out to be a trait). Urinalysis normal. Electrolytes normal. SMA-12 normal. Chest x-ray negative. A 2-hour UCG negative.

HOSPITAL COURSE AND TREATMENT
Initially, she was given cephalothin 2 g IV q.6 h. and kanamycin 0.5 g IM b.i.d. Over the next 2 days, the patient's condition improved. Her pain decreased, and her temperature came down to normal in the morning and spiked to 101° in the evening. Repeat CBC showed hemoglobin 7.8, hematocrit 23.5. The pregnancy test was negative. On the 2nd night following admission, she spiked to 104°. The patient was started on antituberculosis treatment consisting of isoniazid 300 mg per day, ethambutol 600 mg b.i.d., and rifampin 600 mg daily. She became afebrile on the 6th postoperative day and was discharged on July 15, 200X, in good condition. She will be seen in the office in 1 week.

SURGICAL PROCEDURES
Biopsy of omentum for frozen section; culture specimens.

DISCHARGE DIAGNOSIS
Genital tuberculosis.

_____
Harold B. Cooper, MD

amd
D:7/15/200X
T:7/16/200X

Fig. 9-1 Discharge summary, full block format. (Under *ADMITTING DIAGNOSES,* "PID" was dictated, and the transcriptionist spelled out the diagnosis and put the abbreviation in parentheses.)

COLLEGE MEDICAL CENTER
1000 North Main Street • College Town, XY 12345-0001 • PHONE: (013) 123-4567 FAX; (013) 130-4599

DISCHARGE SUMMARY

DATE OF ADMISSION: July 9, 200X   DATE OF DISCHARGE: July 15, 200X

ADMITTING DIAGNOSES
1. Pneumonia.
2. Hypertension.
3. History of congestive heart failure.
4. Menopause.

BRIEF HISTORY
This is a 67-year-old woman with a complaint of chest tightness who was seen at Smith-Davis Urgent Care and was found to have bilateral pneumonia and hypoxemia. The patient was subsequently transferred to College Medical for admission.

HOSPITAL COURSE
The patient was admitted and placed on antibiotics and oxygen supplement. The patient improved, showing gradual resolution of hypoxemia. The patient was discharged in stable condition.

DISCHARGE DIAGNOSES
1. Pneumonia.
2. Hypertension.
3. History of congestive heart failure.
4. Menopause.

PROGNOSIS
Good. Discharged on medications. Ceftin 125 mg b.i.d. for 7 days. The patient is to follow up with Dr. Darnell in one week.

_____

Raul Garcia, MD

RG:mlt
D: 7/15/200X
T: 7/15/200X

_____

DISCHARGE SUMMARY

PT. NAME: MONTEZ, MARIA

IDNO: IT-890480
ROOM NO: 598
ATTENDING: RAUL GARCIA, MD

Fig. 9-2 Discharge summary, full block format. The bottom of the report illustrates the method used at some hospitals to insert the patient's identifying data.

Patient: Elaine J. Silverman
Hospital Number 84-32-11

Date: June 20, 200X
Room Number: 1308

OPERATIVE REPORT

PREOPERATIVE DIAGNOSES:
1. Menorrhagia.
2. Chronic pelvic inflammatory disease.
3. Perineal relaxation.

POSTOPERATIVE DIAGNOSES:
1. Menorrhagia.
2. Chronic pelvic inflammatory disease.
3. Perineal relaxation.

OPERATION:
1. Total abdominal hysterectomy.
2. Lysis of pelvic adhesions.
3. Bilateral salpingo-oophorectomy.
4. Appendectomy.
5. Posterior colpoplasty.

PROCEDURE: Under general anesthesia, the patient was prepared and draped for abdominal operation. The abdomen was opened through a Pfannenstiel incision, and examination of the upper abdomen was entirely normal. Examination of the pelvis revealed an enlarged uterus. The uterus was 3 degrees retroverted and adhered to the cul-de-sac. Both tubes and ovaries were involved in an inflammatory mass, with extensive adhesions to the lateral pelvic wall on both sides. The tubes revealed evidence of chronic pelvic inflammatory disease. The omentum was also attached to the fundus and to the left adnexa. The omentum was dissected by means of blunt and sharp dissection; the dissection was carried to each adnexa, freeing both tubes and ovaries by means of blunt and sharp dissection. The uterus was found to be approximately 2 times enlarged after freeing all the adhesions. The uterovesical fold of peritoneum was then incised in an elliptical manner, bladder was dissected off the lower uterine segment. The round ligament and the infundibulopelvic ligament on each side were identified, clamped, cut, and ligated. The uterine artery on each side was clamped, cut, and doubly ligated. Paracervical fascia was developed. Heaney clamps were placed on the cardinal ligaments, and the cardinal ligaments were cut, and the pedicles ligated. The vagina was circumscribed; the uterus, both tubes, and ovaries were removed from the operative field. The cardinal ligaments were then sutured into the lateral angles of the vagina by means of interrupted sutures; the vagina was then closed with continuous over-and-over stitch. The paracervical fascia was sutured into place with interrupted figure-of-eight suture; the lateral suture incorporated the stumps of the uterine arteries; the pelvis was then reperitonealized with a continuous length of GI 2-0 atraumatic suture. Appendix was identified, and appendectomy was done in the usual manner. The appendiceal stump was cauterized with phenol and neutralized with alcohol. Re-examination of the pelvis at this time revealed all bleeding well controlled. The abdominal wall was then closed in layers, and the skin was approximated with camelback clips. During the procedure, the patient received 1 unit of blood. Patient was then prepared for vaginal surgery.

Patient was placed in lithotomy position, prepared, and draped. Posterior colpoplasty was begun for repair of rectocele and perineal relaxation. The posterior vaginal mucosa was dissected from the perirectal fascia; the excess posterior vaginal mucosa was excised, and the perirectal fascia was brought together with continuous interlocking suture of 0 chromic. The posterior vaginal mucosa was closed with continuous interlocking suture of 0 chromic. Perineal body was closed with subcutaneous subcuticular stitch. There was a correct sponge count. The patient withstood the operation well. Patient left the operating room in good condition.

_____
Harold B. Cooper, MD

ftr
D: 6-20-0X
T: 6-22-0X

College Park Hospital
321 College Park Circle
Woods Creek, XX 98765

Fig. 9-3 Operative report, modified block format.

TUFTS MEDICAL CENTER OUTPATIENT CARE

PATIENT: Ouddy, Busaba
DATE: 11/15/0X
SURGEON: Henry D. Sousa, DPM
ANESTHESIOLOGIST: Jeffrey B. Morgan, MD
ANESTHESIA: 10 mL of equally mixed 2% Xylocaine plain and 0.5% Marcaine plain.
PROCEDURE TIME: The operation began at 0730 and ended at 0815.

OPERATIVE REPORT

PREOPERATIVE DIAGNOSIS: Hallux limitus, right foot.

POSTOPERATIVE DIAGNOSIS: Hallux limitus, right foot.

OPERATION PERFORMED: Cheilectomy, first metatarsophalangeal joint, right foot.

OPERATIVE TECHNIQUE IN DETAIL: The patient was brought to the operating room and placed in the supine position. Anesthesia was achieved with the use of the aforementioned anesthesia distributed in a Mayo block to the right foot. Following sterile preparation, application of Betadine solution, and sterile draping, with hemostasis obtained by the placement of a tourniquet to the level of the ankle and inflated to 250 mmHg, the following surgical procedures were performed:
        A linear incision was placed on the dorsal aspect of the right foot medial to the extensor hallucis longus tendon. This incision began proximally at the midshaft of the first metatarsal and extended distally to the midshaft of the first proximal phalanx. The wound edges were underscored, and all vital structures were retracted. Superficial bleeders were coagulated with the use of a Bovie unit. The incision was deepened via anatomical dissection to the level of the capsule and periosteal structures about the first metatarsophalangeal joint. Using an incision that paralleled the initial skin incision, the capsule and periosteal structures were dissected free, delivering the dorsal exostosis that was located on the first metatarsal and proximal phalanx into the surgical site. At this time, the first metatarsophalangeal joint was inspected, and there were free-floating ossicles that were excised from the wound sites. The cartilage was noted to have central erosions located on both the head of the first metatarsal and base of the proximal phalanx. The bony exostosis that was present on the medial dorsolateral aspect of the first metatarsal head and base of the proximal phalanx were resected entirely. The surgical site was then flushed with copious amounts of sterile saline, inspected, and found to be free of debris. The hypertropic synovium was then excised. The surgical site was then freed further with the use of a scoop. The surgical site was then flushed again with copious amounts of sterile saline, inspected, and found to be free of debris. The surgical site was then remodeled to make a more normal-appearing metatarsal head and base of the proximal phalanx. The surgical site was then again flushed with copious amounts of sterile saline, inspected, and found to be free of debris. The patient was then placed through a range of motion and was noted to have 70 degrees of motion at the time of the surgery procedure. This was in comparison to 40 degrees preoperatively, with the last 15 degrees of that 40 degrees being painful. The surgical site was then reapposed with the periosteum and capsular structures closed via 3-0 PDS. The subcutaneous tissues were closed in layers using simple interrupted sutures of 4-0 Vicryl. The skin edges were reapposed using subcutaneous stitching of 4-0 Prolene. The surgical site was then further maintained using tincture of benzoin and Steri-Strips. The surgical site was then covered with a dry, sterile dressing consisting of Adaptic, 3 x 3 Huffs, and a 3-inch roll of Kling. Tourniquet was released. Capillary filling time was noted to return to digits 1 through 5 on the right foot within normal limits. Prior to application of the dressing, 1 mL of Soluspan was injected into the surgical site. Dressing was further maintained using 3-inch Coban.

Patient tolerated surgical procedure well and left the operating room with vital signs stable.

_____
HENRY D. SOUSA, DPM
:reo
D: 11/15/0X
T: 11/15/0X

Fig. 9-4 Operative report, run-on format. Note that the dictator is a podiatrist.

may be required. This tissue examination, or biopsy report, is called a *pathology report* or *tissue report* (Fig. 9-5). It consists of a *gross description* of the specimen submitted, which means the way the specimen looks to the naked eye before the specimen is pre- pared for microscopic study. The *microscopic description* is the description of the tissue after it has been prepared and carefully examined under the microscope. The *diagnosis* is then given. Often, the gross descriptions (*grosses*) of all of the surgical specimens

College Hospital
2345 College Hospital Boulevard
Wood Creek, XX 98765

PATHOLOGY REPORT

Date:	June 20, 200X	Pathology No. 430211
Patient:	Elaine J. Silverman	Room No. 1308
Physician:	Harold B. Cooper, MD	

SPECIMEN SUBMITTED:

Tumor, right axilla.

GROSS DESCRIPTION

Specimen A consists of an oval mass of yellow fibroadipose tissue measuring 4 x 3 x 2 cm. On cut section, there are some small, soft, pliable areas of gray apparent lymph node alternating with adipose tissue. A frozen section consultation at time of surgery was delivered as NO EVIDENCE OF MALIGNANCY on frozen section, to await permanent section for final diagnosis. Majority of the specimen will be submitted for microscopic examination.

Specimen B consists of an oval mass of yellow soft tissue measuring 2.5 x 2.5 x 1.5 cm. On cut section, there is a thin rim of pink to tan-brown lymphatic tissue and the mid portion appears to be adipose tissue. A pathological consultation at time of surgery was delivered as no suspicious areas noted and to await permanent sections for final diagnosis. The entire specimen will be submitted for microscopic examination.

RTW:wfr

MICROSCOPIC DESCRIPTION

Specimen A sections show fibroadipose tissue and nine fragments of lymph nodes. The lymph nodes show areas with prominent germinal centers and moderate sinus histiocytosis. There appears to be some increased vascularity and reactive endothelial cells seen. There is no evidence of malignancy.

Specimen B sections show adipose tissue and 5 lymph node fragments. These 5 portions of lymph nodes show reactive changes including sinus histiocytosis. There is no evidence of malignancy.

DIAGNOSIS

A & B: TUMOR, RIGHT AXILLA: SHOWING 14 LYMPH NODE FRAGMENTS WITH REACTIVE CHANGES AND NO EVIDENCE OF MALIGNANCY.

_____
Stanley T. Nason, MD

STN:wfr
D: 6-18-0X
T: 6-18-0X

Fig. 9-5 Pathology report, full block format.

are dictated, transcribed, and given to the pathologist, who then dictates the microscopic descriptions *(micros)*. These are transcribed, and the completed pathology reports are given to the pathologist for signature. A copy of the report is given to each physician involved in the case, and a copy is retained in the laboratory. The original is placed in the patient's medical record. In addition to tissue and tumor reports, a pathology transcriptionist may

type second-opinion reports, fine-needle aspiration reports, muscle biopsy reports, renal biopsy reports, bone marrow examination reports, autopsy reports, forensic reports, and coroner reports. Pathology reports must be completed within 24 hours. Pathologists usually dictate in the present tense because they interpret the pathological findings as they look at the specimen. The history is in past tense, and the findings are in present tense. Each dictation may include certain headings, but the headings are not always used and are not always in the same sequence.

In dictation involving pathology, it is often the nonmedical term that puzzles the novice transcriptionist because it may be difficult to understand the mechanics behind the dictated words. A common phrase encountered and typed incorrectly is "The specimen is submitted in toto." This statement means that all of the specimen is submitted by the pathologist for further processing. Because many pathological terms cannot be found in standard references, always obtain a good word reference book or pathology/laboratory medicine dictionary if a great deal of your transcription deals with pathology. Macros of standard dictated material are very useful in this specialty.

RADIOLOGY AND IMAGING REPORTS

As mentioned previously, another way of specializing is to become a radiology transcriptionist for a group of radiologists or for the radiology department of a hospital.

An x-ray report (Fig. 9-6) is a description of the findings and interpretations of the radiologist who reviews the x-ray films taken of a patient. These can be bone and joint films, soft tissue films, or special studies of the internal organs that require the patient to take contrast medium (dye) orally or by injection. The contrast medium may be radiolucent (permitting the passage of some roentgen rays) or radiopaque (not permitting the passage of roentgen rays). For assistance in spelling the types of contrast media, refer to the back of the current *Physician's Desk Refer-*

```
                    College Hospital
                    4567 Broad Avenue
                  Woodland Hills, XY 12345



                    RADIOLOGY REPORT

Examination Date:  June 14, 200X        Patient:      Elaine J. Silverman
Date Reported:     June 14, 200X        X-ray No.:    43200
Physician:         Harold B. Cooper, MD  Age:          19
Examination:       PA Chest, Abdomen    Hospital No.: 80-32-11

Findings:

PA CHEST:          Upright PA view of chest shows the lung fields are clear,
                   without evidence of an active process.  Heart size is
                   normal.

                   There is no evidence of pneumoperitoneum.

IMPRESSION:        NEGATIVE CHEST.

ABDOMEN:           Flat and upright views of the abdomen show a normal gas
                   pattern without evidence of obstruction or ileus.  There
                   are no calcifications or abnormal masses noted.

IMPRESSION:        NEGATIVE STUDY.


                   Radiologist_____
                             Marian B. Skinner, MD

mtf
D:  6-14-200X
T:  6-14-200X
```

Fig. 9-6 Radiology report, modified block format.

ence (PDR), which has a comprehensive reference list. An examination of an organ with radioactive isotopes is called a *scan*. Radiologists' writing may change from present to past tense within the body of a report. As a rule, the procedure was performed (past tense), and the findings are given in the present tense. At some facilities, each physician has a set of normal phrases or paragraphs logged into computer memory in the form of macros. The physician may choose to dictate the radiological examination and say, "Add note N1," to access one of these phrases; if necessary, the phrase may be edited, depending on the case dictated.

Technology has produced methods to view structures in dimension (stereoscopy) or in layers (tomography). Through the use of x-rays with computers, a specific slice of the abdomen, chest, or head can be seen; this imaging technique is called *computed tomography* (CT) or *CT scanning*. A process for measuring temperature by photographically recording infrared radiations emanating from the surface of the body is called *thermography*. Use of high-frequency sound waves without the use of x-rays can give a composite picture of an area; the image is called a *sonogram* or an *echogram*. A system that produces sectional images of the body without the use of x-rays is *magnetic resonance imaging* (MRI), also called *nuclear magnetic resonance* (NMR) *imaging* (Fig. 9-7). In this method, a band of radio frequencies and a range of magnetic field strengths are used, so that information is obtained simultaneously from a large number of points in a volume. The information is processed by a computer with the use of mathematical techniques similar to those used to form CT images.

Some facilities provide radiotherapy for treatment or palliation of malignant tumors, and so radiotherapy summaries become part of the patient's medical record. Nuclear medicine diagnostic and therapeutic procedures require reports (Fig. 9-8) stating the interpretations, consultation, and therapy (e.g., specific preparation of the patient, identity, date, and amount of radiopharmaceutical used).

The radiology report provides preliminary information and the type of x-ray films taken or the x-ray examination performed: for example, "Chest x-ray, PA and lateral," at the top of the report. In order to avoid confusion, the date in the heading should reflect the date of service rather than the date of dictation. Dictation and transcription dates are best placed at the end of the report. The date in the heading is followed by the number and type of views taken and any special circumstances that may affect the examination: for example, whether the patient is fasting for a bowel study. Views obtained in addition to what is usual for a given study should

be noted. Documentation should also include the quality of the study (*clear* or *blurry*), positive findings (*abnormal*), negative findings (*normal*), incidental findings in other areas of the film, the radiologist's impression or interpretation and diagnosis, recommendations for additional studies or treatment, and the signature of the radiologist. Several x-ray examinations may be described in the same report. Radiology reports should be incorporated into the patient's medical record for use if the physician needs to prove that the study was medically necessary. Radiology examinations must be documented in sufficient detail to justify reimbursement.

Some of the types of radiology reports dictated are the following:

aortogram
arteriogram
arthrogram
barium enema
bronchogram
cardioangiogram
cholangiogram
cholecystogram
cineradiogram
computed tomogram (CT scan)
cystogram
echogram
encephalogram
esophagram
esophagogram
fluoroscopy (chest, colon, gallbladder, and stomach)
hysterosalpingogram (HSG)
intravenous cholangiogram (IVC)
intravenous pyelogram (IVP) a.k.a. intravenous urogram (IVU)
laminagram
lymphangiogram

magnetic resonance imaging (MRI)
myelogram, spinal
nephrotomogram
nuclear magnetic resonance (NMR) study
pneumoencephalogram
retrograde pyelogram (RP)
scan (blood and heart, bone, full body, brain, liver, lung, spleen, and thyroid)
sialogram
single-photon emission computed tomography (SPECT) (heart and brain)
sonogram
stereoscopy
thermogram
tomogram
ultrasonogram (bile ducts, gallbladder, kidneys, liver, ovaries, and uterus)
upper and lower gastrointestinal (GI) series
venogram
ventriculogram

CONSULTATION REPORTS

Often, an attending physician seeks the advice and opinions of a consulting physician. The consultant dictates a report (Fig. 9-9) that will be incorporated into the patient's hospital record. The physician may see the patient in consultation in the office, emergency room, or hospital; then a report is dictated and sent to the referring physician. Sometimes, a consultation associated with decisions relating to surgical intervention may be transcribed stat. The report may contain the present history, past history, x-ray and laboratory studies, physical examination, and impression and comments on findings, prognosis, and future course of treatment recommended. It

GrandView Magnetic Imaging Center
4500 River Road
Center City, XY 12345
(013) 647-0980

INTERPRETATION

PATIENT: Jeffrey Clauson   AGE: 27
NUMBER: 430-34-1276   DATE: August 30, 200X

MAGNETIC RESONANCE IMAGING, CERVICAL SPINE

HISTORY: Cervical radiculopathy

TECHNIQUE: Sag. GE 600/30/23. MR, 43 Nex, 5 mm, CC.
             Sag. SE 500/24. MR, 4 Nex, 5 mm, CC.
             Ax. SE 1000/30. HR, 2 Nex, 5 mm, CC.
FINDINGS

The sagittal sequences cover from the lower posterior fossa to approximately T4-5. The axial sequence covered from the upper odontoid process through mid T1.

There is mild reversal of the normal lordotic curve of the cervical spine.

The C2-3 and C3-4 interspaces are normal.

There is posterior osteophyte formation projecting broadly across the anterior aspect of the spinal canal at C4-5 level. On the sagittal sequences, this appears to contact the cord. There is no deformity identified with the cord to indicate compression. The foramina are patent.

The C5-6 level is unremarkable aside from some narrowing of the anterior subarachnoid space, probably a result of mild spurring and the effect of the reversal of the normal lordotic curve.

At C6-7 there are degenerative disk changes with disk space narrowing and osteophyte formation. There is no cord compression, although there is moderate left foraminal stenosis.

The C7-T1 level demonstrates moderate left foraminal stenosis.

There is either spur or disk bulge at the T1-2 level. This was only seen on the sagittal sequences. The abnormality appears to contact the cord but does not appear to cause any compression. There are no additional extradural abnormalities. There are no intradural extramedullary lesions. The cord is normal without abnormal intensity to indicate the presence of infarction or mass, and there is no evidence of a syrinx. This is mentioned in that the cerebellar tonsils project somewhat below the foramen magnum indicating the possibility of a Chiari II malformation.

IMPRESSION: CEREBRAL SPONDYLOSIS AS DESCRIBED ABOVE. PROBABLE CHIARI II
              MALFORMATION. NO CORD SYRINX.

rmt   Jason B. Iverson, MD

Fig. 9-7   Magnetic resonance imaging (MRI) report, full block format.

may be dictated in letter form or report form, with content and headings similar to a history and physical examination medical report.

AUTOPSY PROTOCOLS

When a patient dies while in the hospital or within 24 hours of discharge from the hospital, permission may be requested from the next of kin to perform an autopsy or postmortem examination of the body to determine the exact cause of death. The complete protocol should be made part of the record within 90 days after the death. Through autopsies, much knowledge has been gained that assists in the diagnosis and treatment of disease. Visual and microscopic examinations are done on every organ and related structure. When an organ is removed from

College Grove Hospital
4567 City College Avenue
Canyon Rim, XY 12345

RADIATION THERAPY CONSULTATION

Name: Theodore V. Valdez   Requested by: John L. Morris, MD
Room #499
MR #380780   Date: 6/15/200X

HISTORY OF PRESENT MEDICAL ILLNESS: This is a 72-year-old who underwent decompressive laminectomy and Harrington rod placement in 2004 for angiosarcoma. Postoperative radiation therapy at St. Mary's Hospital: 4025 cGy[1] in 23 fractions (175 cGy), 4 treatments per week, 2 to 1 PA to AP portals measuring 13 x 9 cm at 100 SSD on 8 Mv Linac, 5 HVL cord block at 3000 cGy. Dr. Davis estimates coverage T2 to T8. Myelogram and CT scan negative 2 years ago. However, developed cough and hemoptysis in past month. Chest x-ray and CT: Right perihilar mass extending into mediastinum with multiple central and 1 anterior mediastinal mass with postobstructive infiltrate, bilateral pleural effusion. Bronchoscopy: 75% narrowing right upper lobe orifice to subsegments, 50% narrowing right lower lobe orifice. Bleeding at right upper lobe orifice. Draining right pleural effusion and sclerodesis with negative cytology. Preliminary tissue diagnosis from right paratracheal area and mediastinoscopy: Probable angiosarcoma.

PAST MEDICAL HISTORY: Hypertension.

SOCIAL HISTORY: 50-year tobacco habit.

PHYSICAL EXAMINATION: General: Well-developed male in no acute distress. No palpable adenopathy. Lungs: Clear. Heart: Regular rate and rhythm. Abdomen: Unremarkable. Extremities: Without circulatory collapse or edema. Neurologic: Without focal deficit.

ASSESSMENT: Recurrent metastatic angiosarcoma with postobstructive pneumonitis and hemoptysis.

PLAN: 4000 cGy[1] to symptom-producing mediastinal disease. Initial 1000 cGy at 200 cGy fractions, then oblique off previously irradiated spinal cord and boost with 250 cGy fractions. No plans for chemotherapy. Discussed radiation therapy procedures, risks, and alternatives with patient, emphasizing possible long-term risks to spinal cord, lung, and heart as well as increased potential for morbidity resulting from prior irradiation. He agrees with treatment as outlined.

Sincerely

Barry T. Goldstein, MD
Radiology Medical Group, Inc.

trn
D: 06/15/200X
T: 06/16/200X

Fig. 9-8   Radiotherapy report, run-on format.

FAX
212.555.1247

TELEPHONE
212.555.0124

COLLEGE PARK HOSPITAL AND MEDICAL CENTER
555 LAKE VIEW DRIVE
BAY VILLAGE OH 44140

June 15, 200X

John F. Millstone, MD
5302 Main Street
Bay Village, OH 44151

Re: Waltrudis M. Tubbman

Dear Dr. Millstone:

This 91-year-old woman was seen at your request. The patient was admitted to the hospital yesterday because of chills, fever, and abdominal and back pain.

The history has been reviewed. A prominent feature of the history is the presence of intermittent, severe, shaking chills for 4 days with associated left lower back pain, left lower quadrant abdominal pain, and fever to as high as 103 or 104 degrees. The patient has had hypertension for a number of years and has been managed quite well with Aldomet 250 mg twice a day.

On examination, her temperature at this time is 100.6 degrees. The pulse is 110 and regular. Blood pressure is 190/100. The patient has partial bilateral iridectomies, the result of previous cataract surgery. Otherwise, the head and neck are not remarkable. Lung fields are clear throughout. The heart reveals a regular tachycardia; heart sounds are of good quality, no murmurs heard, and there is no gallop rhythm present. The abdomen is soft. There is no spasm or guarding. A well-healed surgical scar is present in the right flank area. There is considerable tenderness in the left lower quadrant of the left mid abdomen, but, as noted, there is no spasm or guarding present. Bowel sounds are present. Peristaltic rushes are noted, and the bowel sounds are slightly high-pitched in character. The extremities are unremarkable.

Diagnosis: I believe the patient has acute diverticulitis. She may have some irritation of the left ureter in view of the findings on the urinalyses. She appears to be responding to therapy at this time in that her temperature is coming down, and also there has been a slight reduction in the leukocytosis from yesterday. I agree with the present program of therapy, and the only suggestion would be to possibly increase the dose of ampicillin to 500 mg every 8 hours, rather than the 250 mg q.8 h. that she is now receiving.

Thank you for asking me to see this patient in consultation.

Sincerely,

Harold B. Cooper, MD

wpd

Fig. 9-9 Consultation report, letter form in modified block format with indented paragraphs and mixed punctuation.

a cadaver for the purpose of donation, there should be an autopsy report that includes a description of the technique used to remove and prepare or preserve the donated organ. All states have laws that govern autopsies. When someone dies unattended or there is suspicion of a crime (e.g., violent death, unusual death, child abuse, self-induced or criminal abortion, homicide, suicide, poisoning, drowning, fire, hanging, stabbing, exposure, starvation), an autopsy may be ordered by the court, or it may become the responsibility of the coroner's office to determine the cause of death. The professionals associated with the coroner's or medical examiner's office include the pathologist, forensic pathologist, forensic dentist, chemist, toxicologist, anesthesiologist, radiologist, odontologist, psychiatrist, and psychologist.

The written record of an autopsy is generally referred to as an *autopsy protocol*. In pathology, there are five forms: the narrative (in story form), the numerical form (by the numbers), the pictorial form (hand drawings or anatomical forms), protocols based on sentence completion and multiple-choice selection, and problem-oriented protocols (a supplement to the Problem-Oriented Medical Record System). A numerical format is an orderly description of all autopsy findings and tends to prevent omission of minor details that can be forgotten during narration. Numerical format is therefore usually a longer protocol and requires more time to complete.

Many hospital autopsy protocols (Fig. 9-10) contain the clinical history, which is a brief résumé of the patient's medical history and course in the hospital before death. It includes the pathological diagnosis made at autopsy, a report of the final summary, and the gross anatomy findings (visual examination of the organs of the body before any tissues are removed for preparation and examination). There is also a microscopic examination (an examination of the particular organs through the microscope). An epicrisis or final pathological

---

PITMAN COUNTY
OFFICE OF THE MEDICAL EXAMINER

AUTOPSY PROTOCOL

Bethany, Patricia M.   June 21, 200X

This is an autopsy on a prematurely born female infant weighing 1.25 kg. The body measures 39 cm in length. The body has not been embalmed prior to this examination.

<u>EXTERNAL EXAMINATION</u>:   The head, neck and chest are symmetrical. The abdomen is soft. The external genitalia are normal female. The extremities are symmetrical and show no evidence of developmental abnormality.

<u>INTERNAL EXAMINATION</u>

ABDOMINAL CAVITY: The abdominal cavity is opened, and the liver is enlarged, extending 4 cm below the costal margin in the right midclavicular line. The spleen appears enlarged. The intestinal coils are freely dispersed and contain gaseous fluid. All other organs are in normal position.

PLEURAL CAVITIES: The pleural cavities are opened, revealing the left lung to be collapsed and lying in the left pleural cavity. The right lung is partially expanded, and the pleura is smooth and glistening in both pleural cavities.

MEDIASTINUM: The mediastinum contains a moderate amount of thymic tissue.

PERICARDIAL SAC: The pericardial sac is opened and contains a few cubic centimeters of serous fluid. The heart is normal in position and appears to be average in size.

HEART: The heart weighs approximately 10 g. Thorough search of the heart fails to show any evidence of congenital abnormality. The foramen ovale has a thin membrane over the surface. The ductus arteriosus is noted and patent. There is no ventricular septal defect. All valves are competent. There is no rotation of the heart. The pulmonary artery is noted and appears normal. A few subendocardial and subepicardial petechiae and ecchymoses are noted.

LUNGS: The lungs weigh together 33 g. The left lung and the right lung sink in water, then slowly rise to the surface. The lungs are subcrepitant and atelectatic. (This is particularly noted in the left lung.) The bronchi contain a small amount of frothy mucus. The cut surfaces of the lungs are beefy and atelectatic. There are no cysts or tumors. The findings are consistent with hyaline membrane disease and pulmonary atelectasis.

LIVER: The liver weighs approximately 75 g. The liver appears enlarged and is reddish-brown and soft. The cut surface is reddish-brown and soft. There is no gross evidence of bile duct blockage. The gallbladder, cystic duct, and common bile duct are not remarkable.

(continued)

Fig. 9-10 Autopsy protocol, modified block format.

Continued

Bethany, Patricia M.
Autopsy Protocol, Page 2
June 21, 200X

INTERNAL EXAMINATION continued

PANCREAS: The pancreas appears average in size, weighing approximately 1.5 g. The pancreas is yellowish-white and soft on the cut surface. There is no gross evidence of cystic disease.

SPLEEN: The spleen weighs approximately 4 g and is bluish purple. The spleen on cut surface is reddish-brown and soft.

ADRENAL GLANDS: The adrenal glands weigh together approximately 4.5 g. The adrenal glands are soft and tan, and the cortical portion is distinct from the medullary portion. There is no gross evidence of hemorrhage, cysts, or tumors. Both adrenals are similar.

KIDNEYS: The kidneys weigh together approximately 13 g. The capsule strips with ease, leaving a faint fetal lobulation and a reddish-brown soft surface. The cut surface shows the cortex and medulla, both of which are distinct and in average proportions. The parenchyma is reddish-brown, moist and soft. Both kidneys are similar in appearance and consistency. The ureters are not remarkable.

URINARY BLADDER, UTERUS, TUBES, AND OVARIES: These organs are grossly not remarkable.

GASTROINTESTINAL TRACT: The esophagus is examined as well as the stomach. There is no evidence of reduplication, ulcer, or tumor. The small and large bowel are not remarkable.

BRAIN: The brain weighs approximately 230 g. The brain is slightly edematous. A few petechiae are observed. On sectioning, the brain anterior to posterior, the brain tissue is soft and somewhat edematous. The fluid in the ventricles is clear and watery. The cerebellum and cerebrum are symmetrical and grossly not remarkable. There is no gross evidence of hemorrhage or tumor.

SKELETAL SYSTEM: Not remarkable.

GROSS ANATOMICAL DIAGNOSES

1. Prematurity, 1.25 kg.
2. Pulmonary atelectasis.
3. Hyaline membrane disease.

STEPHEN M. CHOI, MD, CME

sw
D: June 21, 200X   0700
T: June 21, 200X   1350

Fig. 9-10, cont'd

diagnosis is given at the end of the protocol. The epicrisis is a critical analysis (actual finding) or discussion of the cause of disease after its termination.

In forensic pathology, an autopsy protocol may be organized under the following general guidelines:

1. External description
2. Evidence of injury
   a. External
   b. Internal
3. Systems and organs (cavities and organs)
4. Special dissections and examinations
5. Brain (and other organs) after fixation
6. Microscopic examination
7. Findings (diagnoses), factual and interpretative
8. Opinion or summary (conclusion), interpretative and opinion
9. Signature

Some autopsy procedures used for typing protocols are not necessarily seen in other types of medical dictation and transcription. Because autopsy records may be entered into a court of law to relate information about the cause of death, clarity is essential so that interpretation of the typed material is accurately understood. Because of this requirement, more words tend to be spelled out, and abbreviations are kept to a minimum. Many states require that military time be used when documenting the time a body is brought in for autopsy (e.g., "1400 hours"). Ciphers are used in stating the nonmilitary time (e.g., 9:00 a.m.). Units of measurement may be spelled out, such as pounds, inches, and grams. Quotation marks are never used to indicate inches but are used when indicating a marking on the body (e.g., tattoo device of the words "J.J. Tramp"). Temperature is typed "88 degrees Fahrenheit." Numbers may be typed as "2 fresh punctures" or "two (2) stab wounds."

Numbers may be typed numerically and then spelled out in parentheses when clarity is emphasized. Metric terms are given as abbreviations (e.g., 0.5 cm, 200 mL, 3 × 3 mm).

Forensic dentists work closely with forensic pathologists. They describe bite marks by size, shape, and location. They swab for saliva to determine blood type. They make impressions or molds of the mark and photograph and make impressions of the suspect's dentition. When two medical examiners are involved, the reference initials of both at the closing of the protocol must be shown (e.g., MB : DVW : mod). Only general guidelines for typing protocols are stated here. Each county has different practices and must meet various legal requirements.

MEDICOLEGAL REPORTS

Medicolegal reports originate from medical offices and hospitals. When they originate from the latter, they usually come from the medical records department, in which personnel make copies or abstracts of record entries rather than transcribing them (Fig. 9-11). The prudent physician responds to a request for medical information with a prompt and complete report and, in doing so, assists his or her patient in supporting claims for damages (probably including the physician's bill), facilitates the attorney's representation of a client, and can often spare himself or herself a trip to court. Usually, a report of this type involves an accident case or a workers' compensation case. The report is a legal document and is admissible as evidence in a court of law. Sometimes, the attorney abstracts data from the report and incorporates the information into a formal document presented to the physician for signature and subsequent notarization. Accuracy is essential.

The properly prepared medicolegal report follows a familiar format and is typed on the physician's letterhead stationery.

Patient Identification

The patient must be identified in the first paragraph. The patient's name; age, date of birth, or both; and address should be included. If the patient is a child, he or she should be identified as "the son or daughter of" his or her parents, whose names should also be included.

Date of Accident or Work-Related Injury

The date of the accident or injury must be noted, including the time of day, if known. (The physician should check the date of the accident given by the patient's attorney against that in the medical record. If the dates do not agree, telephone the patient to clarify the discrepancy.)

History

The history of the accident, injury, or work-related illness is described. Use the patient's own words, including quotation marks whenever possible. Be as detailed and complete as possible, listing all the facts.

Present Complaints

The patient's present complaints at the time of the first visit are recorded. (Sometimes these are referred to as *subjective complaints*.)

Past History

The past history should be described, along with any preexisting defects or injuries that might have a bearing on the present problem.

Physical Findings

The physical findings on examination are recorded in detail. (These are sometimes referred to as *objective findings*.)

Laboratory or X-Ray Findings

Laboratory or x-ray findings should be included in the report. In some instances, photocopies of x-ray, electrocardiograph, or operative reports should be made available. Consultation notes should also be photocopied and submitted with the medicolegal report.

CLARENCE F. STONES, MD
3700 LILAC LANE
GRANDVIEW, XX 00060

October 20, 200X

Aetna Casualty and Surety Company
3200 Roosevelt Boulevard
GrandView, XX 03030

Dear Madam or Sir:

RE: Injured: Howard P. Winston
     Date of Injury: July 27, 200X
     Employer: College Chemistry Company
     Case No.: 450-33-0821

EXAMINATION AND REPORT

HISTORY:
This 43-year-old white male was working with a chemical pump. It slipped and fell forward. He overcorrected and fell. The pump fell on the patient, striking him in the occiput area. The approximate weight of the pump was 325 pounds and was rolled off by a friend. The patient was knocked unconscious. He attended a meeting the following day in Round Valley. The pain occurred a day later in Round Valley. Then 3 days later, the pain was intense in the right shoulder and elbow. He went to Dr. John Garrett for physiotherapy. The left side then began to give him trouble also. He had a pressure type of pain in the left elbow, which was relieved by codeine. He entered College Hospital in GrandView under Dr. Garrett's service. The right leg, and later the right thigh, began getting numb. A myelogram was followed by fusion at C5-6 and C6-7. He wore a brace for 6 months. He still has right shoulder pain and neck pain with radiation into the right thumb and right mastoid. In June 200X, he was admitted to Community Hospital. The left eye began drooping, and there was no pupil dilation. He was improved 1 week later. A myelogram and brain scan were performed. There was pain on the left side, with pain into the rectum with spasms. He states that he fell several times. The surgery was postponed because of the eyes and the sudden loss of equilibrium.

FAMILY HISTORY:
The father died of burns in a fire in 1990. The mother died of kidney disease at age 82. He has two brothers and one sister, living and well. He is widowed. His wife had cancer of the uterus. He has four children, alive and well. There is no history of diabetes and no accidents.

ALLERGIES:
Penicillin and tetanus.

PHYSICAL EXAMINATION

GENERAL:
Blood pressure 122/78; pulse 84 and regular. The patient is cooperative and oriented to time and place.

(continued)

Fig. 9-11   Medicolegal report, modified block format with mixed punctuation.

Howard P. Winston
Page 2
October 20, 200X

PHYSICAL EXAMINATION   (continued)

HEENT: Head: Normal size and shape; no facial asymmetry. He
                                shows no evidence of elevated intracranial pressure.
Extraocular muscles intact. Pupils are equal and react briskly to light. At first, one gets the
impression that there might be a Horner syndrome on the left side because of inconstant ptosis
of the right eyelid, but this is not truly present.

NEUROLOGICAL EXAM: The patient walks with sparing of the left leg. There is no true
                                paralysis present.

REFLEXES: The right biceps and triceps are slightly reduced on the left
                                side but are present.

SENSORY: There is evidence of patchy hyperesthesia in the right upper
                                extremity but following no particular dermatomal pattern.

CEREBELLAR FUNCTION: Intact. Lower cranial nerves within normal limits. There were
                                no pathological reflexes elicited.

The remaining exam was deferred.

OPINION AND COMMENT: The patient continues to have slight dysfunction, principally in
                                left lower extremity and right upper extremity. It would seem to
me that the pupillary abnormality, which he experienced in June of 200X, merits some
investigation, including arteriography. For his cervical disc problems, I would think that
conservative treatment is warranted.

                                        Sincerely,

                                        Clarence F. Stones, MD

sw

Fig. 9-11, cont'd

Diagnosis

The diagnosis (or diagnoses in the case of multiple injuries) should be detailed.

Prescribed Therapy

The prescribed therapy must be described in detail. Each visit to the office should be listed, including any physical therapy treatments or medications prescribed.

Patient's Disability

The patient's disability should be outlined, describing work restrictions and including the dates of total or partial disability. The date on which the patient is permitted to return to work is given.

Prognosis

The prognosis is of paramount importance to the attorney and thus to the patient. The settlement may depend on the physician's estimate of continued pain and whether there will be future permanent disability.

Physician's Statement

The physician's statement of fees for services rendered is an integral part of the report to an attorney.

The statement should be itemized by date and service, making sure the statement correlates in detail with the dates of treatment mentioned in the report. The preparation of a report for an attorney is time consuming, and the physician is entitled to charge a fee. Documents requiring extensive research of hospital records and consultants' reports merit higher fees.

Although many cases are settled out of court, the few that go to trial justify painstaking care in preparation of the medical report. Remember that the value of a detailed document cannot be overemphasized when the physician is asked to testify in a trial 3 or 4 years after a patient's injury.

PSYCHIATRIC REPORTS

Psychiatry is one of the specialties of clinical medicine. It is a diverse field, and the language involves abnormal psychology, human behavior, and treatment terminology. Patients are referred to as *clients*. In a hospital setting, clients include mentally deficient and developmentally disabled persons, formerly referred to as *mentally retarded*.

For the mentally deficient client, an admission note might include a presentation of the problem stating the vital signs, current medications, allergies, medication taken in the previous 4 hours, present illness, psychological history, mental status examination, physical status examination, and a provisional diagnosis. Additional reports about the mentally disabled client might include a psychiatric evaluation, psychological evaluation, social history evaluation, rehabilitation therapy evaluation, discharge summary, and treatment planning conference. The conference is a program to establish the goals of treatment and track the progress that the client is making while under the treatment, with the ultimate goal of the client's being placed back into society as a fully functional person.

The reports for a developmentally disabled client might include a medical history, review of systems, release summary, and clinical record documentation system, which is equivalent to a treatment planning conference for a mentally deficient client. The reports are more detailed because these clients can be so low functioning that even the most basic self-care skills cannot be performed on admission. Members of the facility's staff attempt to teach these skills, with attainment of the highest potential of each client as a goal.

A report dictated by a clinical psychologist would not necessarily contain a physical examination of the body systems or a list of the medications, but it might describe motor skill problems. The main heading might be *Psychological Evaluation,* and subheadings might be given as follows: *Purpose of the Report, Psychosocial History, Results of the Psychological Assessment, Mental Status Examination, Test Results, Impressions, Diagnosis,* and *Recommendations.*

Because so many clients have legal problems (divorce, marriage, adoption procedures, negligence, physical abuse, disability, and so on), legal terminology is widely used. Some clients may be seen for chemical abuse, and drugs could be referred to by slang or street terms; often, these terms are unknown by the novice transcriptionist. These terms change from day to day, and the list is constantly enlarging. Most transcriptionists prepare lists of these slang terms for reference to assist in typing up the reports. An excellent reference for the names of street drugs is the *Pharmaceutical Xref* by Drake and Drake. Many of the words encountered in psychiatric reports do not appear in a standard English dictionary or a medical dictionary, and so the use of special reference books will assist you. The *Diagnostic and Statistical Manual of Mental Disorders, Fourth Edition, Revised* (DSM-IV-R) is used for psychiatric diagnoses for the mentally disabled. This is an excellent reference book for the transcriptionist because all mental diagnoses are given with their code numbers. However, for developmentally disabled clients, the *International Classification of Diseases, 9th Edition, Clinical Modification* (ICD-9-CM) code numbers and the etiology are used. If the psychiatrist wishes, the DSM-IV-R is also used for the diagnosis. Refer to Fig. 9-12 to see how the diagnoses and code numbers might be typed.

Reports that contain information about a person's mental stability are confidential. In fact, sometimes the information contained in the report is not divulged to the client. In order to obtain medical information, the signatures of the physician and the client are required on a special release-of-information form. If the client is developmentally disabled, the signatures of the physician and the guardian are needed. If authorized in writing by the client or his or her legally qualified representative and by the psychiatrist in charge of the case, a copy of the report is sent to the referring medical practitioner or medical facility responsible for follow-up care of the patient. Psychiatric information can be sent to a placement facility if a client is to live in the community in a residential facility. This information gives the receiving facility data regarding treatment and medication. At times, the court system may subpoena the medical records.

State of California—Health and Welfare Agency		Department of Mental Health

GUIDELINES	Date of Report: 11-09-0X Dictated: 11-09-0X Transcribed: 11-09-0X **PSYCHIATRIC EVALUATION**	Unit 99

A. PSYCHIATRIC HISTORY
  1. Identification data
  2. Source of information
  3. Chief complaint
  4. History of present illness (focus on recent illness, and include emotional behavior)
  5. History of past psychiatric episodes
  6. Relevant medical/ surgical/trauma/ medication history
  7. Developmental history (if applicable)
  8. Educational/Vocational
  9. Relevant family history
  10. Relevant social history
B. MENTAL STATUS EXAM
  11. Attitude/Cooperation
  12. General appearance (include speech)
  13. Motor activity
  14. Orientation
  15. Mood and affect
  16. Mental content
  17. Memory
  18. Fund of general knowledge
  19. Cognition and comprehension
  20. Abstraction ability
  21. Counting and calculating
  22. Judgement
  23. Insight regarding illness
  24. Patient strengths
  25. Suicide, homicide, dangerousness
C. SUMMARY OF PSYCHIATRIC ASSESSMENT
  26. Narrative summary (including Risk Potential)
  27. Diagnosis (DSM III R)
  28. Preliminary Treatment Plan
  29. Prognosis
  30. Signature and Title
	PSYCHIATRIC HISTORY
	1. This 17-year-old, single, Hispanic male patient was admitted to Greenvale Hospital on November 8, 20XX, on a temporary conservatorship 5353 from Pitman County. His birth date is September 24, 19XX. There is no religious reference. His mother is Mary Sanchez. Her address is 300 East Date Street, Woodland Hills, XY 12345. Telephone (555) 999-9999.
	
	2. Information obtained by interviewing the patient and reviewing the accompanying papers from Greenvale Center. The patient speaks only Spanish. The interview had to be done through an interpreter. His information is not very reliable.
	
	3. "I don't know why they sent me here."
	
	4. Pedro was admitted to Greenvale Medical Center on August 26, 200X, because of bizarre behavior for 5 days. According to the report, 5 days prior to admission, he smoked marijuana dipped in PCP. He also smoked cocaine. He demonstrated bizarre behavior such as running nude in the streets, sticking his fingers into light sockets and receiving electric shocks, crawling under a car and trying to set it on fire. He was not sleeping. He laughed and cried inappropriately. He broke a restraint in the hospital. The drug screening test 1 on August 26, 20XX, was positive for cocaine and negative for PCP and other drugs. Peabody test in Spanish revealed his IQ was about 76. Beery development test of visual motor integration did not suggest organicity. He was treated with Haldol and discharged to his mother on September 22, 20XX; however, he was readmitted to *Greenvale Medical Center Center on September 24, 20XX,* on a 5150. His mother stated that after discharge from the hospital, he was fearful and childish. He presented bizarre behavior such as collecting household articles, painting the walls, attempting to play with medicine bottles, refusing to eat or sleep, walking around the house nude, collecting piles of objects in his room, attempting suicide by jumping off an apartment building. He laughed and cried inappropriately. His mother stated that he did not take street drugs, and he took only Haldol and Cogentin. However, on one occasion, he went to the store without supervision. At the Greenvale Medical Center, he was confused, disorganized, and disoriented. It was difficult for him to attend to a conversation or to concentrate. He was not able to function in school. He needs close supervision and care. He had been in physical restraints many times because of assaultive behavior. He also banged the walls and screamed. He was treated with Haldol 10 mg t.i.d. A long-term hospitalization was...
	
	SANCHEZ, Pedro J. 999999-9 V.99 ☐ Continued

EVALUATION REPORT **PSYCHIATRIC** Confidential Client/Patient Information See W & I Code Section 5328	
MH 5702 (Revised 7/87) CRDM Reference 2410	

Fig. 9-12 Pages 1 and 4 of a psychiatric evaluation, full-block format. Note the diagnoses and code numbers at the end of the report: Axis I: substance abuse and other treatable conditions; Axis II: psychological disorders; Axis III: medical conditions; Axis IV: stressors; Axis V: global assessment of functioning (0-100). *GAF* means Global Assessment of Functioning Scale.

Continued

Date of Report: 11-09-0X
Dictated: 11-09-0X
Transcribed: 11-09-0X

Unit 99 -- PSYCHIATRIC EVALUATION

(Continued)

26.   Pedro's father deserted the family when Pedro was 11 years old. Around
        that time, he stopped going to school after finishing 6th grade. The reason
        for that was not clear. He lived with his grandmother after his mother left
        Honduras 4 years ago. About 8 months ago, he came to the United States
        to live with his mother because his grandmother was unable to handle him.
        He had been using cocaine and PCP for 6 or 7 months. It was felt that his
        first hospitalization at Greenvale Medical Center was due to PCP, Organic
        Mental Disorder. At this time, he appears retarded with residual
        symptoms of psychosis such as flat and inappropriate affect, loose associations,
        poverty of thoughts, no intention to go to school; and he needs constant
        supervision for daily living activities.

27.   Axis I: 298.9   Psychotic Disorder, NOS.
                           (Rule out 292.90 PCP, Organic Mental Disorder.)
                           306.90 Psychoactive Substance Abuse, NOS.
        Axis II: V71.09 No diagnosis.
                           (Rule out Mental Retardation.)
        Axis III: No somatic disorder.
        Axis IV: Discord with classmates.
        Axis V: GAF on admission 26; highest GAF last year unknown.

28.   Structured environment, special educational program, unit milieu, individual
        therapy, group therapy, and chemotherapy.

29.   Guarded.

30.

        _____
        Dan W. Stewart, MD

jrw

Page 4 SANCHEZ, Pedro J. 999999-9 U.99   ☐ Continued

CONTINUATION PAGE

☒ Assessment (Specify: __Psychiatric_____)
☐ Team Conference (Specify: _____)
☐ Consultation (Specify: _____)
☐ Other (Specify _____)

Confidential Client/Patient Information
See W & I Code Section 5378

MH 5705

Fig. 9-12, cont'd

Brief Review of Report Format Styles

FULL BLOCK FORMAT OR RUN-ON FORMAT		MODIFIED BLOCK FORMAT (CHANGES ONLY)
Statistical Data:	As determined by the facility. May be aligned on top or bottom of page.	
Margins and Spacing:	Half-inch margins. May double-space or single-space between topics. Single-spaced data.	Double space between topics.
Title:	Centered on the page or flush with left margin.	Centered on page.
Main Topic Titles:	Begun flush with left margin. Full caps. May be underlined. On a line alone or introducing data on same line.	
Subtopics:	Full caps or combination Begun flush with left margin.	Indented one tab stop under main topic for one or two lines.
Data:	Begun on same line as topic or subtopic. or Begun on left margin.	Always on the same line as topic or subtopic title with first and second line blocked under the first line.
Close:	As determined by facility. Dictator's name and signature area. Transcriptionist's initials. Date and time of dictation. Date and time of transcription.	

 Exercise 9-1: SELF-STUDY

Directions: *Retype the following data into discharge summary outline by using the full block format. Set margins at 0.5 and one tab stop at 4.5. Pay careful attention to punctuation and capitalization. The patient's name and other statistical data may be set up as you desire. Note topic changes and proper mechanics. The location of the headings for admitting diagnosis and discharge diagnosis may vary—occurring at the beginning of the report, in the natural order of dictation (as seen in Fig. 9-1), or at the end of the report—as specified by the individual facility.*

The patient is Marcia M. Bacon. The dictating physician is Henry R. Knowles, MD. The summary was dictated on May 10 and transcribed on May 11. The patient's hospital ID number is 52-01-96. The patient's room number is 248-C. The date of hospital admission is May 7, 200X, and she was discharged on May 9, 200X. Admission diagnosis: Torn medial meniscus, left knee. Discharge diagnosis: Torn medial meniscus, left knee; chondromalacia of the medial femoral condyle. History of present illness: The patient injured her left knee on April 11, 200X, while playing tennis. She subsequently had difficulty with persistent effusion and pain in the left knee. An arthrogram prior to admission revealed a tear of the medial meniscus. Physical examination: absence of tenderness to palpation of any of the joint structures. There was approximately 30-55 mL of fluid within the joint. Range of motion was full. Laboratory data: admission hemoglobin was 15.9, hematocrit 47%, with a white count of 7400 with normal differential. Urinalysis was within normal limits. Chem panel 19 showed an elevated cholesterol of 379 mg%. Chest x-ray was reported as negative. Treatment and hospital course: The patient was taken to the operating room on the same day as admission, at which time she underwent arthroscopy. This revealed that she had a tear of the medial meniscus. Arthrotomy was performed, with medial meniscectomy. A chondral fracture was noted in the medial femoral condyle, measuring approximately 5 mm in greatest diameter. The edges of this were sheathed. Postoperatively, the patient's course was benign. There was no significant temperature elevation. She became ambulatory with crutches on the first postoperative day with no difficulty with straight leg raising. Disposition: The patient is being discharged home ambulatory with crutches and an exercise program. She is to be seen in the office in 1 week for suture removal. Condition at the time of discharge: Improved. Complications: None. Medications: None.

 Exercise 9-2: PRACTICE TEST

Directions: *Retype the following data into an operative report by using the indented format and no variations. Set a 0.5 margin on right and left. Clear the tab stops and set a tab at 3.0 and 5.0. The patient's name and other statistical data may be set up as you desire. Pay attention to proper mechanics and capitalization. Date the report January 4, 200X.*

The patient's name is John P. Dwight, and his hospital ID number is 86-30-21. The surgeon is Felix A. Konig. The patient's room number is 582-B. The preoperative and postoperative diagnosis is: otosclerosis, left ear. The operation is a left stapedectomy. The findings, otosclerosis, footplate. Under local anesthesia, the ear was prepared and draped in the usual manner. The ear was injected with two percent Xylocaine and one to six thousand epinephrine. A stapes-type flap was elevated from the posterosuperior canal wall, and the bony overhang was removed with the stapes curet. The chorda tympani nerve was removed from the field. The incudostapedial joint was separated. The stapes tendon was cut. The superstructure was removed. The mucous membrane was reflected from the ear, stapes, and the facial nerve promontory. The footplate was then reamed with small picks and hooks. A flattened piece of Gelfoam was placed over the oval window, and a five millimeter wire loop prosthesis was inserted and crimped in the incus. The drum was reflected, and a small umbilical tape was placed in the ear canal. The patient tolerated the procedure well.

 Exercise 9-3: PRACTICE TEST

Directions: *Retype the following data into a pathology report by using run-on format and underline main topics. Date the report June 6, 200X. See pp. 338 and 343 for run-on format.*

The patient's name is Joan Alice Jayne, and her hospital ID number is 72-11-03. The referring physician is John A. Myhre, MD, and the pathologist is James T. Rodgers, MD. The date the specimen was removed was June 6, 200X. The patient's room number is 453-A. Pathology number is 532009. Specimen(s): The specimen consists of a four point five centimeter in diameter nodule of fibro-fatty tissue removed from the right breast at biopsy and enclosing a central, firm, sharply demarcated nodule one centimeter in diameter. Surrounding breast parenchyma reveals dilated ductiles (microcystic disease). Frozen section impression: Myxoid fibroadenoma of breast. Microscopic and diagnosis: Myxoid fibroadenoma occurring in right parenchyma, the site of microcystic disease of right breast.

 Exercise 9-4: SELF-STUDY

Directions: *Retype the following data into a radiology report by using the modified block format and no variations. Set margins at 0.5, clear tabs, and set new tabs at 2.0, 2.5, and 5.0. Remember to double-space between topics as done in full block format. Date the report June 8, current year. See p. 340 for modified block format.*

The patient's name is Donna Mae Weeser. Her x-ray number is 16-A2, and her hospital number is 52-80-44. This patient is age 46. The referring physician is George B. Bancroft, MD, and the radiologist is Clayton M. Markham, MD. The examination is mammography, right and left breasts. There are retromammary prosthetic devices in position. The anterior parenchyma is somewhat compressed. There is no evidence of neoplastic calcification or skin thickening demonstrated. No dominant masses are noted within the anteriorly displaced parenchyma. No increased vascularity is evident. Impression: mammography right and left breasts shows the presence of retromammary prosthetic devices in position. The demonstrated tissue appears within normal limits.

 Exercise 9-5: PRACTICE TEST

Directions: *Retype the following material into a consultation report. Use full block format, and the current date. Watch for proper topic changes, placement, and mechanics.*

The patient's name is Hazel R. Plunkett. This is for Glen M. Hiranuma, MD. The reason for the neurological consultation is for evaluation and treatment of chronic and recurrent headaches. In the past, the patient has had episodes of probably typical migraine occurring perhaps six or eight times in her life. She remembers that her mother had a similar complaint. This would begin with loss in the field of vision; and then, approximately fifteen minutes thereafter, she would have a relatively typical, unilateral throbbing pain of a significant degree which would often incapacitate her. These headaches disappeared many years ago and have never returned. However, for the last eight years approximately, the patient has had recurrent daily headaches, always right-sided, with associated pain beginning in the back of the neck with stiffness of the right side of the neck, radiating forward over the vertex to the right orbit, the nose, and the jaw. She also notes some pain in the right trapezius area. The pain tends to appear from 10 a.m. to noon, when she will take a Fiorinal, and often after she goes to sleep at night (at about 12:30 a.m.). She controls this pain by taking Fiorinal, one to four a day, and Elavil, 75 mg at bedtime. She estimates that the headaches occur approximately twice daily, are relatively short-lived but occasionally last a full day. The pain is dull and heavy, not throbbing, and worse at some times than at others. On examination she was a quiet woman, not in acute distress, and somewhat dour; but she gave a careful and concise history. Her gait and station were normal. The head functions were basically intact. The fundi showed only modest arteriosclerotic changes. The temporal arteries were normal. Facial motility and sensation was normal. There was a significant right carotid bruit present which was persistent and which could be heard all along the course of the right carotid artery. It was not transmitted from the neck. There were moderate pain and tenderness at the insertion of the great muscles of the neck and the occiput, and palpation over this area consistently reproduced the patient's symptoms. She also had a persistent area of tenderness in the right trapezius muscle. Otherwise, power, size, and symmetry of the arms and legs were essentially normal. The deep tendon reflexes were brisk. There were no long tract or focal signs, and sensation was intact.

Impression: 1. Muscle contraction headaches, chronic. 2. Localized myositis, right side of neck, right shoulder girdle. 3. Right carotid bruit, silent, asymptomatic. Comment: The findings were discussed in detail with the patient but no neurological studies were done. I suggested simple measures of physical therapy to the neck including the use of heat, hot packs, and massage and advised also that she purchase a cervical pillow on which to rest during the day. Motrin, 400 mg twice daily and Maolate, 400 mg at night were suggested in an attempt to provide antiinflammatory and muscle relaxant properties. It may also be necessary to inject these tender areas which are quite well localized. This can be determined after 30 to 60 days on the treatment regimen outlined above. The patient also has what seems to be a silent right carotid bruit. Certainly she is without symptoms. This should be brought to the attention of those who are caring for her, so that if transient ischemic attacks appear in the future, appropriate steps can be taken. I do not think that the right carotid bruit has anything to do with the patient's headaches, which are not vascular, and certainly there is no sign of cranial arteritis.

◇ Exercise 9-6: REVIEW TEST

Directions: *Retype the following material into a hospital autopsy protocol by using the full-block format with variation number one. The patient's name and other statistical data may be set up as you desire. Use a current date and correct punctuation. The dictator is Dr. Susan R. Foster, chief pathologist. See p. 339 for full-block format. Note that the main topic and subtopics vary from those shown in Fig. 9-10.*

I performed an autopsy on the body of Phyllis B. Dexter, Patient No. 65-43-90, at the College Hospital. Clinical Diagnosis: Congenital heart defect.

General Examination: The body is that of a well developed and well nourished newborn female infant, having been embalmed prior to examination through a thoracic incision and cannulization of the heart. The recorded birth weight is 7 pounds 2 ounces. Thorax opened: Considerable blood is present around the heart incident to the embalming procedure, and two incisions in the cardiac muscle are evident but the valves and great vessels do not appear to have been injured by the embalming procedure. Examination discloses a massive heart lying transversely in the midanterior thorax, the distended right ventricle exceeding in volume the ventricular mass. Examination discloses no enlargement of the ductus arteriosus or any significant deviation of the size of the great vessels. On exploration of the heart there is found to be a completely imperforate pulmonary artery at the level of the pulmonary valve, all 3 cusps of which appear to be adequately formed but fused by scar tissue slightly proximal to the free margins of the cusps. It is impossible to probe the existence of any opening in this area. The right heart is markedly hypertrophic, approximating three times the muscle mass of the normal infant heart. There is no evidence of an interventricular defect. There is a sacculation adjacent to the valve of the inferior vena cava as it enters the inferior right auricle and in the dome of this sacculated area the foramen ovale is demonstrated. The foramen is unusually small in diameter (estimated to be no more than 4 mm in diameter) and this is covered by a plica. It would appear that the pressure of the distended right auricle would further compromise the capacity of the foramen to transmit blood. In the absence of any interventricular defect, this would be the only way that blood could get from the right to the left side of the heart. The lungs are heavy and poorly serrated and the bronchial tree contains some yellowish fluid which, in the absence of feeding by mouth, must be assumed to be aspirated vernix. Abdomen Opened: The stomach contains some bloody mucus but no evidence of formula. The liver and abdominal viscera appear entirely negative throughout. Head: Not opened. Cause of Death on Gross Findings: Massive chylous pericardial effusion, etiology not established but presumptively related to defect in formation of thoracic duct tissue. Microscopic: Sections of the thymus gland revealed a generally normal histological architecture for the thymus of the newborn, epithelial elements still being distributed through the lymphoid tissues. Certainly no tumor is present in the thymic tissue. The pulmonary tissues are poorly expanded although the bronchi appear open. There are a general vascular congestion of pulmonary tissue and some apparent extravasation of blood into the poorly expanded alveoli. In addition, there are deposits of hyaline material on the surfaces of some of the air spaces that would indicate the existence of hyaline membrane disease. The liver shows marked congestion and a rather active hematopoiesis. The heart muscle is not remarkable and the epicardial surface does not appear thickened or unusual. The kidney tissue exhibits some punctate hemorrhages in the parenchyma consistent with anoxia. Microscopic Diagnosis: Renal hemorrhages incident to anoxia.

 Exercise 9-7: REVIEW TEST

Directions: *Retype the following data into an industrial accident report form and prepare an envelope. Use letterhead stationery. Use full block format, mixed punctuation, and the current date. Watch for proper paragraphing, placement, punctuation, and mechanics.*
   The letter concerns the patient George R. Champion and was dictated by Dr. James C. Taylor of 4532 Saint Charles Avenue, New Orleans, LA 70118. It is to be sent to an attorney, Ralph J. Claborne of 165 Colette, Suite A-1, New Orleans, LA 70120. Use a current date.

Dear Mr. Claborne. My patient Mr. George R. Champion was seen on September 14, 200X. History of injury: Mr. Champion was hit on the back of the head by a lettuce crate in April of 200X. He saw stars but was not knocked unconscious. Present complaints: The patient says he can see for an instant then the left eye blurs and also itches. He has had this problem since his accident in April 200X. When he is working and turns to the left he cannot see things out of that side since they are fuzzy. He can look at an object to the left and five seconds later it is gone. Physical examination: Visual acuity uncorrected: right eye, 20/80; left eye, 20/40. Manifest refraction: right eye, +1.75D = 20/30 Jaeger 1; left eye, +2.50 = 20/30 Jaeger 1–. Visual field: full centrally. Motility: Near point of convergence = 8 cm; Near point of accommodation = 3.5D. Prism cover test: Distance = no shift; Near = 8 prism diopters exophoria. Cycloplegic refraction: right eye = +2.50 + 0.50 × 30 = 20/25 – 2; left eye = +3.25 + 0.75 × 125 = 20/20 – 1. Slit-lamp examination revealed abnormal cornea, conjunctiva, iris and lens. Ocular tension was 11 mm Hg both eyes by applanation. Retinal examination revealed a normal optic disc, macula, vessels and periphery with direct and indirect ophthalmoscopy. Diagnosis: Compound hyperopic astigmatism with early presbyopia. Comments: I feel that this patient's focusing reserve was suddenly decreased by his accident when he was hit on the head. His basic problem of farsightedness coupled with a general weakness after the accident overcame his focusing reserve and caused his symptoms. I feel that glasses of the proper strength will enable him to see and focus. His problem of poor convergence and exophoria at near were also brought into prominence by the weakness he had after the accident. His age (38) means that he would have had symptoms within the next five or seven years due to his farsightedness. Recommended treatment: Glasses to be worn all the time. Eye exercises for convergence problem if the glasses do not relieve his symptoms. Disability: The condition is now stationary and permanent; and with the proper glasses, he should be able to resume his normal work load. Very truly yours.

 Exercise 9-8: REVIEW TEST

Directions: *Retype the following data into a psychiatric report form. Use letterhead stationery. Use full block format with variation number one, mixed punctuation, and the current date. Watch for proper paragraphing, punctuation, placement, and mechanics.*

The letter concerns the patient Tu Anh Dao and was dictated by Dr. Stephen B. Salazar of 5028 South Broadway, Exeter, NH 03833. It is to be sent to Department of Social Services Disability Evaluation Unit, 15 Kenneth Street, Exeter, NH 03833. Head this report Psychiatric Social Survey.

Presenting Problem: This 29 year old Vietnamese male was seen today at the request of the Department of Social Services Disability Evaluation Unit. Questions regarding mental status appearance simple repetitive tasks interests and daily activities and ability to relate and interact with public and coworkers were raised. The interview was conducted in the living room of the home in which he lives and has lived for the last three or four years. The claimant resides in this home with his mother and his 11 year old younger sister. His mother and an interpreter were present in the room during the interview. The interview lasted one hour. The claimant was very quiet and at some points hardly audible. He declined to answer questions quite often during the interview. Several times during the interview the mother interrupted and gave answers to him. He seemed to show some pressure of speech and memory difficulties during the interview. History: The history revealed that Mr. Dao was born in Hanoi Vietnam where he went to school up to the eighth grade. At the eighth grade he dropped out and began to farm doing rice farming. At age 26 he moved to Exeter. After arriving in Exeter he worked in a restaurant which he cannot name as a dishwasher for two or three months but he quit because the job in the first place was part time and temporary. He then worked for two years as a gardener and quit this job because of health problems he was always feeling sick. He also worked for one or two months as a carpenter but he quit because he did not have the money to buy the tools. In 1990 he was admitted to College Hospital where he had surgery and was in the hospital for one or two months during the winter of the year. He claims that the surgery was neurological although it could have been rather than on the brain an inner ear surgery due to vertigo and tinnitus problems. There is no history of any other hospitalizations. The claimant is the oldest son of five children he has two sisters and two brothers they are all living in the United States. Environment: The claimant has lived in his present house for one and a half years with his mother and his 11 year old sister. He states that he wakes at 8 or 9 am. He walks around in the yard for awhile and then he eats breakfast he does not eat lunch but does eat dinner. He said that during this time his appetite is good and he eats because he is hungry. Once a week he leaves the house to see a doctor who checks for the surgery and his neurological problems. He states that he had a ringing in the left ear which was partially a result of the surgery. He has not done any kind of work since the head surgery and he has not done anything around the house. He reports difficulty with memory. He rarely does anything with friends except when they come over to visit him and only leaves the house to walk around the yard or go to the doctor appointments. He is able to dress himself and bathe himself but does not do any chores of any kind around the house. He states that his mother cooks for him and he has never cooked for himself and he does not do anything around the yard either. His grooming showed him to be wearing a shirt slacks with no shoes or socks and he was clean shaven his hair styled and neatly brushed. He reports going to bed around 1 or 2 am. Most of his day is spent listening to the radio and watching television. While showing that he could ambulate he had significant difficulty walking on his toes; he was unable to do this but he was able to walk on his heels and his gait appeared to be normal. There was no significant psychomotor retardation noted. Mental status: The mental status reveals a 29 year old Vietnamese male who appears to be of average height and weight. He denied any paranoid ideations or auditory or visual hallucinations. He was oriented to time place and date and he was able to do 1 to 20 forward and backwards without any difficulty. He refused to do serial 7's although he was able to subtract 7 from 10 correctly. He showed difficulty with memory although he could remember that he had lived in the house that he lives in now for the last year and a half. He denied any headaches or visual difficulties or aura that might indicate seizure activity. He did have an affect of sadness and depression. When asked what he would change about himself he stated that he would change his bad health to good health. He has no goals at the present time. He is on no medication at the present time and he does not have a history of drug or alcohol use or abuse. He denied sleep or appetite problems or crying. There does appear to be some anhedonia. Medications: The claimant is taking no medications at the present time. Provisional Diagnosis: Axis I. Transient situational depression due to surgery mild to moderate. Axis II. Rule out organic brain syndrome. Observations and recommendations: Because there were no medical reports sent with this individual it would be recommended that there be a review to see if there actually was a surgery at College Hospital and what was the purpose of the surgery and what an update may be on his neurological function. In fact I would recommend a neurological evaluation to see if the depression emanates from the surgery itself or from some emotional disturbance. There is no indication that Mr. Dao could handle his own funds and it is recommended that a payee be appointed if he is approved for disability. Thank you for the consultation. Very truly yours

Exercise 9-9: FINAL REVIEW

Directions: *Examine the figures for operative reports in this chapter. Make a list of the following subjects on separate sheet of paper:*

Position of patient
Instruments and tools used
Type of anesthesia and material
Suture materials
Procedures performed

EXAMPLE

Position of patient
    Supine
    Prone jackknife
Instruments and tools used
    Scissors
    Bovie clamp
Type of anesthesia and material
    0.5% Marcaine
    Bupivacaine
Suture materials
    4-0 Prolene
    2-0 chromic
Procedures performed
    Excisional biopsy
    Hemorrhoidectomy

Appendix A Common Laboratory Test Values

NOTE: Common reference values may vary depending on the testing.

 NORMAL URINE REFERENCE VALUES

Urine Volume

Age	Normal Reference Range (mL/24 Hours)
Newborn	20-350
Child	300-1500
Adult	750-2000

Physical and Chemical Characteristics of Urine

Physical	Normal Reference Values	Average
Color	Straw (yellow) to amber, light to dark	Yellow
Turbidity	Clear to slightly hazy	Clear
Specific gravity	1.005-1.030	1.010-1.025
pH	5-8	6.5
Protein	Negative–trace	—
Glucose	Negative	—
Ketone	Negative	—
Bilirubin	Negative	—
Blood	Negative	—
Urobilinogen	0.1-1 EU/dL	0.1-1 EU/dL
Bacteria (nitrites)	Negative	—
Leukocyte esterase	Negative	—

Urine Sediment

Microscopic	Normal Reference Values
RBCs/HPF	Rare
WBCs/LPF	0-4
Epith/HPF	Occasional (may be higher in females)
Casts/LPF	Occasional hyaline
Bacteria	Negative
Mucus	Negative to 2+
Crystals	Only crystals such as cystine, leucine, and tyrosine are considered clinically significant.

Data from Pagana K, Pagana T: *Mosby's diagnostic and laboratory tests*, ed 2, St Louis, 2002, Mosby.
Epith, Epithelium; *HPF,* high-power field; *LPF,* lower power field; *RBCs,* red blood cells; *WBCs,* white blood cells.
NOTE: Results vary among laboratories.

NORMAL BLOOD CHEMISTRY REFERENCE VALUES

Test	Reference Range
Alanine transaminase (ALT) (SGPT)	4-36 U/L
Albumin	3.5-5 g/dL
Alkaline phosphatase (ALP)	30-120 U/L
Aspartate transaminase (AST) (SGOT)	0-35 U/L
Bicarbonate (HCO_3^-)	21-28 mEq/L
Bilirubin (total)	0.3-1 mg/dL
Blood urea nitrogen (BUN)	10-20 mg/dL
Calcium	9-10.5 mg/dL
Chloride	98-106 mEq/L
Cholesterol	<200 mg/dL
Creatinine	0.5-1.2 mg/dL
C-reactive protein	<1 mg/dL
Gamma glutamyl transferase (GGT)	8-38 U/L
Glucose	70-105 mg/dL
Iron	60-180 mcg/dL
Phosphorus	3-4.5 mg/dL
Potassium	3.5-5 mEq/L
Sodium	136-145 mEq/L
T_3 (triiodothyronine)	75-220 mcg/dL
T_4 (thyroxine)	4-12 mcg/dL
Total protein (albumin/globulin)	6.4-8.3 g/dL
Triglycerides (TGs)	40-160 mg/dL
Uric acid	2.7-8.5 mg/dL

NORMAL HEMATOLOGY REFERENCE VALUES

Test		Reference Range	
HEMOGLOBIN			
Newborns		16-23 g/dL	
1 year		9.5-14 g/dL	
6 years		10-15.5 g/dL	
Adult males		14-18 g/dL	
Adult females		12-16 g/dL	
MICROHEMATOCRIT			
Newborns		44%-64%	
1 year		30%-40%	
6 years		32%-44%	
Adult males		42%-52%	
Adult females		37%-47%	
LEUKOCYTE COUNTS			
Newborns	$9\text{-}30 \times 10^9$/L		9000-30,000/mm³
Children ≤2 years	$6.2\text{-}17 \times 10^9$/L		6200-17,000/mm³
Adults	$5\text{-}11 \times 10^9$/L		5000-11,000/mm³
ERYTHROCYTE COUNTS			
Newborn	$4.8 \times 7.1 \times 10^{12}$/L		4.8-7.1 million/mm³
1 year	$4 \times 5.5 \times 10^{12}$/L		4.0-5.5 million/mm³
6 years	$4 \times 5.5 \times 10^{12}$/L		4.0-5.5 million/mm³
Adult males	$4.5 \times 6 \times 10^{12}$/L		4.5-6 million/mm³
Adult females	$4.2 \times 5.4 \times 10^{12}$/L		4.2-5.4 million/mm³
ERYTHROCYTE INDICES			
Mean corpuscular volume (MCV)		80-95 mm³/cell	
Mean corpuscular hemoglobin (MCH)		27-31/pg	
Mean corpuscular hemoglobin concentration (MCHC)		32-36 g/dL	

PLATELET COUNT

Newborn	150,000-300,000/mm³
Children	150,000-400,000/mm³
Adult	150,000-400,000/mm³

ERYTHROCYTE SEDIMENTATION RATE (ESR)

Westergren method

Newborn	0-2 mm/hr
Children	0-10 mm/hr
Adult males	0-15 mm/hr
Adult females	0-20 mm/hr

ONE-HOUR SEDIPLAST ESR

Males	<50 years	0-15 mm
	>50 years	0-20 mm
Females	<50 years	0-20 mm
	>50 years	0-30 mm

PROTHROMBIN TIME

11-12.5 seconds

PARTIAL THROMBOPLASTIN TIME

60-70 seconds

Clotting times depend on the laboratory and the testing of that time for accurate clinical reference values for each test.

BLEEDING TIME

Ivy method   1-9 minutes

DIFFERENTIAL LEUKOCYTE COUNT

Leukocyte Type	**Adult Reference Range**
Neutrophil	55%-70%
Bands	3%-5%
Segs	54%-62%
Eosinophil	1%-4%
Basophil	0.5%-1%
Monocyte	2%-8%
Lymphocyte	25%-30%

Appendix B Core Skills Competency Checklists

_____   _____   _____
Student Name (print)   Instructor's Name (print)   Date

MEDICAL ASSISTANT
CORE SKILLS COMPETENCY GRADE SHEET

Core Skills	Points Earned	Points Possible	Instructor's Signature	Date
1. Perform Proper Handwashing for Medical Asepsis		100		
2. Apply and Remove Clean, Disposable (Nonsterile) Gloves		100		
3. Measure Oral Body Temperature Using a Mercury-Free Glass Thermometer (5)		100		
4. Measure Body Temperature Using a Disposable Oral Thermometer (5)		60		
5. Measure Body Temperature Using a Tympanic Thermometer		125		
6. Measure Radial Pulse (5)		75		
7. Measure Respiratory Rate (5)		50		
8. Measure Blood Pressure (5)		175		
9. Prepare a Parenteral Medication from a Vial		115		
10. Administer an Intradermal Injection (2)		245		
11. Administer a Subcutaneous Injection (2)		175		
12. Administer an Intramuscular Injection to an Adult (2 Deltoid, 2 Gluteal)*		210		
13. Administer an Intramuscular Injection Using the Z-Track Technique (2) **NOTE: 8th or 9th module students only**		215		
14. Perform Venipuncture Using the Evacuated-Tube Method (Collection of Multiple Tubes) (3)		250		
15. Perform Venipuncture Using the Syringe Method (1) **NOTE: 8th or 9th module students only**		255		
16. Perform Venipuncture Using the Butterfly Method (Collection of Multiple Evacuated Tubes) (1) **NOTE: 8th or 9th module students only**		250		

*Instructors will observe one intramuscular deltoid injection and one intramuscular gluteal injection for check off.

Core Skills	Points Earned	Points Possible	Instructor's Signature	Date
17. Charting		90		
18. Diagnostic Coding		100		
19. Procedural Coding		100		
20. Use *Physician's Desk Reference*		80		
21. Being a Professional		430		
	Total Points ÷ Earned	Total Points = Possible	Final Percentage	
	÷ 2580 (3300*) =			
	Instructor's Signature		Date	

Numbers in ( ) indicate minimum practice requirements

Student Name (print)   Instructor's Name (print)   Date

DOCUMENT EACH PATIENT IN PROPER CHARTING FORMAT.

VITAL SIGNS

	Date/Time	Patient	T	P	R	B/P	MA Signature
1.							
2.							
3.							
4.							
5.							

INJECTIONS

	Date/Time	Patient	Location	Reactions	MA Signature
INTRADERMAL					
1.					
2.					
SUBCUTANEOUS					
1.					
2.					
INTRAMUSCULAR (DELTOID)					
1.					
2.					
INTRAMUSCULAR (GLUTEAL-8th or 9th module students use Z-track technique)					
1.					
2.					

VENIPUNCTURE

	Date/Time	Patient	Location	Reactions	MA Signature
EVACUATED-TUBE METHOD					
1.					
2.					
3.					
SYRINGE METHOD [8th or 9th module students only]					
1.					
BUTTERFLY METHOD [8th or 9th module students only]					
1.					

Student Name _____   Date _____

CHECKLIST: PERFORM PROPER HANDWASHING FOR MEDICAL ASEPSIS

TASK: Prevent the spread of pathogens by aseptically washing hands, following Standard Precautions.

CONDITIONS: Given the proper equipment and supplies, the student will be required to demonstrate the proper method of performing handwashing for medical asepsis.

EQUIPMENT AND SUPPLIES
- Liquid antibacterial soap
- Nailbrush or orange stick
- Paper towels
- Warm running water
- Regular waste container

STANDARDS: Complete the procedure within _____ minutes and achieve a minimum score of _____%.

Time began _____   Time ended _____

Steps	Possible Points	First Attempt	Second Attempt
1. Assemble all supplies and equipment.	5		
2. Remove rings and watch or push the watch up on the forearm.	5		
3. Stand close to the sink, without allowing clothing to touch the sink.	5		
4. Turn on the faucets, using a paper towel.	5		
5. Adjust the water temperature to warm—not hot or cold. Explain why proper water temperature is important.	10		
6. Discard the paper towel in the proper waste container.	5		
7. Wet hands and wrists under running water, and apply liquid antibacterial soap. Hands must be held lower than the elbows at all times. Hands must not touch the inside of the sink.	10		
8. Work soap into a lather by rubbing the palms together using a circular motion.	10		
9. Clean the fingernails with a nailbrush or an orange stick.	5		
10. Rinse hands thoroughly under running water, holding them in a downward position and allowing soap and water to run off the fingertips.	10		
11. Repeat the procedure if hands are grossly contaminated.	10		
12. Dry the hands gently and thoroughly using a clean paper towel. Discard the paper towel in proper waste container.	10		
13. Using a dry paper towel, turn the faucets off, clean the area around the sink, and discard the towel in regular waste container.	10		
Total Points Possible	100		

Comments: Total Points Earned _____   Instructor's Signature _____

Student Name _____   Date _____

CHECKLIST: APPLY AND REMOVE CLEAN, DISPOSABLE (NONSTERILE) GLOVES

TASK: Apply and remove disposable (nonsterile) gloves properly.

CONDITIONS: Given the proper equipment and supplies, the student will be required to apply and remove nonsterile disposable gloves.

EQUIPMENT AND SUPPLIES
- Alcohol-based hand rub
- Nonsterile disposable gloves
- Biohazardous waste container

STANDARDS: Complete the procedure within _____ minutes and achieve a minimum score of _____%.

Time began _____   Time ended _____

Steps	Possible Points	First Attempt	Second Attempt
Applying Gloves			
1. Assemble all supplies and equipment.	5		
2. Select the correct size and style of gloves according to office policy.	5		
3. Sanitize hands.	10		
4. Apply gloves and adjust them to ensure a proper fit.	5		
5. Inspect the gloves carefully for tears, holes, or punctures before and after application.	5		
Removing Gloves			
1. Grasp the outside of one glove with the first three fingers of the other hand, approximately 1 to 2 inches below the cuff.	10		
2. Stretch the soiled glove by pulling it away from the hand, and slowly pull the glove downward off the hand. Usually the dominant hand is ungloved first.	10		
3. After the glove is pulled free from the hand, ball it in the palm of the gloved hand.	10		
4. Remove the other glove by placing the index and middle fingers of the ungloved hand inside the glove of the gloved hand; turn the cuff downward. Be careful not to touch the outside of the soiled glove.	10		
5. Stretch the glove away from the hand and pull the cuff downward over the hand and over the balled-up glove, turning it inside out with the balled glove inside.	10		
6. Carefully dispose of the gloves in a marked biohazardous waste container.	10		
7. Sanitize hands.	10		
Total Points Possible	100		

Comments: Total Points Earned _____   Instructor's Signature _____

Student Name _____   Date _____

CHECKLIST: MEASURE ORAL BODY TEMPERATURE USING A MERCURY-FREE GLASS THERMOMETER

TASK: Accurately measure and record a patient's oral temperature.

CONDITIONS: Given the proper equipment and supplies, the student will be required to role-play with another student or an instructor the proper method for measuring an oral body temperature using a mercury-free glass thermometer.

EQUIPMENT AND SUPPLIES
- Mercury-free glass oral thermometer
- Thermometer sheath
- Disposable gloves
- Biohazardous waste container
- Pen
- Patient's medical record

STANDARDS: Complete the procedure within _____ minutes and achieve a minimum score of _____%.

Time began _____   Time ended _____

Steps	Possible Points	First Attempt	Second Attempt
1. Assemble all supplies and equipment.	5		
2. Sanitize hands.	5		
3. Greet and identify the patient.	5		
4. Explain the procedure to the patient.	5		
5. Determine if the patient has recently had a hot or cold beverage to drink or has smoked.	5		
6. Put on gloves and remove the thermometer from its holder, without touching the bulb end with your fingers.	5		
7. Inspect the thermometer for chips or cracks.	5		
8. Read the thermometer to ensure that the temperature is well below 96.0° F. Shake down thermometer as necessary.	5		
9. Cover the thermometer with a protective thermometer sheath.	5		
10. Ask the patient to open his or her mouth and place the probe tip under the tongue.	5		
11. Ask the patient to hold, not clasp, the thermometer between the teeth and to close the lips snugly around it to form an airtight seal.	5		
12. Leave the thermometer in place for a minimum of 3 minutes.	5		
13. Remove the thermometer and read the results.	10		

Steps	Possible Points	First Attempt	Second Attempt
14. Holding the thermometer by the stem, remove the protective sheath and discard in a biohazardous waste container.	5		
15. Sanitize the thermometer following the manufacturer's recommendations.	5		
16. Remove gloves and discard in biohazardous waste container.	5		
17. Return the thermometer to its storage container.	5		
18. Sanitize hands.	5		
19. Document the results in the patient's medical record.	5		
Total Points Possible	100		

Comments: Total Points Earned _____   Instructor's Signature _____

Student Name _____   Date _____

CHECKLIST: **MEASURE BODY TEMPERATURE USING A DISPOSABLE ORAL THERMOMETER**

TASK: Accurately measure and record a patient's oral temperature using a disposable thermometer.

CONDITIONS: Given the proper equipment and supplies, the student will be required to perform the proper method for measuring an oral temperature using a disposable oral thermometer.

EQUIPMENT AND SUPPLIES
- Disposable thermometer
- Disposable gloves
- Biohazardous waste container
- Pen
- Patient's medical record

STANDARDS: Complete the procedure within _____ minutes and achieve a minimum score of _____%.

Time began _____   Time ended _____

Steps	Possible Points	First Attempt	Second Attempt
1. Assemble all supplies and equipment.	5		
2. Sanitize hands.	5		
3. Greet and identify the patient.	5		
4. Explain the procedure to the patient.	5		
5. Determine if the patient has recently had a hot or cold beverage to drink or has smoked.	5		
6. Put on disposable gloves.	5		
7. Open the thermometer packaging.	5		
8. Place the thermometer under the patient's tongue and wait 60 seconds.	5		
9. Remove the thermometer and read the results by looking at the colored dots.	5		
10. Discard the thermometer and gloves in a biohazardous waste container.	5		
11. Sanitize hands.	5		
12. Document results in the patient's medical record.	10		
Total Points Possible	65		

Comments: Total Points Earned _____   Instructor's Signature _____

Student Name _____   Date _____

CHECKLIST: MEASURE BODY TEMPERATURE USING A TYMPANIC THERMOMETER

TASK: Accurately measure and record a patient's temperature using a tympanic thermometer.

CONDITIONS: Given the proper equipment and supplies, the student will be required to role-play with another student the proper method for measuring the tympanic temperature using a tympanic thermometer.

EQUIPMENT AND SUPPLIES
- Tympanic thermometer
- Disposable probe cover
- Pen
- Patient's medical record
- Biohazardous waste container

STANDARDS: Complete the procedure within _____ minutes and achieve a minimum score of _____%.

Time began _____   Time ended _____

Steps	Possible Points	First Attempt	Second Attempt
1. Assemble all supplies and equipment.	5		
2. Sanitize hands.	5		
3. Greet and identify the patient.	5		
4. Explain the procedure to the patient.	5		
5. Remove the thermometer from the charger.	5		
6. Check to be sure the mode for interpretation of temperature is set to "oral" mode.	10		
7. Check the lens probe to be sure it is clean and not scratched.	5		
8. Turn on the thermometer.	5		
9. Insert the probe firmly into a disposable plastic probe cover.	5		
10. Wait for a digital "READY" display.	5		
11. With the hand that is not holding the probe, pull adult patient's ear up and back to straighten the ear canal. For a small child, pull the patient's ear down and back to straighten the ear canal.	10		
12. Insert the probe into the patient's ear and tightly seal the ear canal opening.	10		
13. Position the probe.	5		
14. Depress the activation button.	5		
15. Release the activation button and wait 2 seconds.	5		
16. Remove the probe from the ear and read the temperature.	5		

Steps	Possible Points	First Attempt	Second Attempt
17. Note the reading, making sure that the screen displays "oral" as the mode of interpretation.	5		
18. Discard the probe cover in a biohazardous waste container.	5		
19. Replace the thermometer on the charger base.	5		
20. Sanitize hands.	5		
21. Document results in the patient's medical record using ① to indicate a tympanic temperature was obtained.	10		
Total Points Possible	125		

Comments: Total Points Earned _____   Instructor's Signature _____

Student Name _____   Date _____

CHECKLIST: MEASURE RADIAL PULSE

TASK: Accurately measure and record the rate, rhythm, and quality of a patient's pulse.

CONDITIONS: Given the proper equipment and supplies, the student will be required to role-play with another student or an instructor the proper method for measuring a patient's radial pulse.

EQUIPMENT AND SUPPLIES
- Watch with a second hand
- Patient's medical record
- Pen

STANDARDS: Complete the procedure within _____ minutes and achieve a minimum score of _____%.

Time began _____   Time ended _____

Steps	Possible Points	First Attempt	Second Attempt
1. Assemble all supplies and equipment.	5		
2. Sanitize hands.	5		
3. Greet and identify the patient.	5		
4. Explain the procedure to the patient.	5		
5. Observe the patient for any signs that may indicate an increase or a decrease in the pulse rate due to external conditions.	5		
6. Position the patient.	5		
7. Place the index and middle fingertips over the radial artery while resting the thumb on the back of the patient's wrist.	10		
8. Apply moderate, gentle pressure directly over the site until the pulse can be felt.	10		
9. Count the pulse for 60 seconds.	10		
10. Sanitize hands.	5		
11. Document the results in the patient's chart; include the pulse rate, rhythm, and volume.	10		
Total Points Possible	75		

Comments: Total Points Earned _____   Instructor's Signature _____

Student Name _____   Date _____

CHECKLIST: MEASURE RESPIRATORY RATE

TASK: Accurately measure and record a patient's respiratory rate.

CONDITIONS: Given the proper equipment and supplies, the student will be required to role-play with another student the proper method for measuring a patient's respiratory rate.

EQUIPMENT AND SUPPLIES
- Watch with a second hand
- Patient's medical record
- Pen

STANDARDS: Complete the procedure within _____ minutes and achieve a minimum score of _____%.

Time began _____   Time ended _____

Steps	Possible Points	First Attempt	Second Attempt
1. Assemble all supplies and equipment.	5		
2. Sanitize hands.	5		
3. Greet and identify the patient.	5		
4. Explain the procedure to the patient.	5		
5. Count each respiration for 30 seconds and multiply by 2. (If breathing pattern is irregular, count for 1 full minute.)	15		
6. Sanitize hands.	5		
7. Document the results in the patient's chart; include the respiratory rate, rhythm, and depth. Document any irregularities found.	10		
Total Points Possible	50		

Comments: Total Points Earned _____   Instructor's Signature _____

Student Name _____   Date _____

CHECKLIST: MEASURE BLOOD PRESSURE

TASK: Accurately measure and record a patient's blood pressure by palpation and auscultation.

CONDITIONS: Given the proper equipment and supplies, the student will be required to role-play with another student the proper method for measuring a patient's blood pressure.

EQUIPMENT AND SUPPLIES
- Stethoscope
- Aneroid sphygmomanometer in proper size for patient
- Alcohol wipe
- Patient's medical record
- Pen

STANDARDS: Complete the procedure within _____ minutes and achieve a minimum score of _____%.

Time began _____   Time ended _____

Steps	Possible Points	First Attempt	Second Attempt
1. Assemble all supplies and equipment.	5		
2. Sanitize hands.	5		
3. Greet and identify the patient.	5		
4. Explain the procedure to the patient.	5		
5. Position the patient comfortably in a sitting or supine position.	5		
6. Palpate the brachial artery.	10		
7. Position the blood pressure cuff; wrap the cuff snugly and evenly around the patient's arm and secure the end.	10		
8. Position the aneroid gauge for direct viewing at a distance of no more than 3 feet.	10		
9. Measure the systolic pressure by palpation.	15		
10. Deflate the cuff completely and wait at least 60 seconds before re-inflating.	10		
11. Clean the stethoscope.	5		
12. Place the earpieces of the stethoscope in your ears, with the earpieces directed slightly forward.	5		
13. Position the head of the stethoscope over the brachial artery of the arm.	5		
14. Close the valve to the manometer.	5		
15. Pump the cuff at a smooth rate to approximately 20 to 30 mm Hg above the palpated systolic pressure.	10		

Steps	Possible Points	First Attempt	Second Attempt
16. Loosen the thumbscrew slightly to open the valve and release the pressure on the cuff, slowly and steadily.	10		
17. Obtain the systolic reading.	10		
18. Continue to release the air from the cuff at a moderately slow rate.	5		
19. Listen for the disappearance of the Korotkoff sounds; obtain diastolic pressure.	10		
20. Release the air remaining in the cuff quickly by loosening the thumbscrew to open the valve completely.	5		
21. Remove the earpieces of the stethoscope from your ears, and remove the cuff from the patient's arm.	5		
22. Sanitize hands.	5		
23. Document the results in the patient's chart.	10		
24. Clean the earpieces and diaphragm with an alcohol wipe, and properly store the equipment.	5		
Total Points Possible	175		

Comments: Total Points Earned _____   Instructor's Signature _____

Student Name _____   Date _____

CHECKLIST: PREPARE A PARENTERAL MEDICATION FROM A VIAL

TASK: From a vial, measure the ordered medication dosage into a 3-mL hypodermic syringe for injection.

CONDITIONS: Given the proper equipment and supplies, the student will prepare a parenteral medication from a vial in a 3-mL syringe.

EQUIPMENT AND SUPPLIES
- Vial of medication as ordered by physician
- 70% isopropyl alcohol wipes
- 3-mL syringe for ordered dose
- Needle with safety device appropriate for site of injection
- 2 × 2-inch gauze squares
- Biohazardous waste container
- Patient's medical record

STANDARDS: Complete the procedure within _____ minutes and achieve a minimum score of _____%.

Time began _____   Time ended _____

Steps	Possible Points	First Attempt	Second Attempt
1. Sanitize hands.	5		
2. Verify the order, and assemble equipment and supplies.	5		
3. Check expiration date of the medication.	10		
4. Follow the "seven rights" of medication administration.	10		
5. Check the medication against the physician's order three times before administration.	10		
6. Check the patient's medical record for drug allergies or conditions that may contraindicate the injection.	10		
7. Calculate the correct dose to be given, as necessary.	10		
8. Prepare the vial, needle, and syringe.	5		
9. Draw the amount of air into the syringe for the amount of medication to be administered.	5		
10. Remove the cover from the needle and insert the needle into the vial.	10		
11. Inject the air into vial and fill the syringe with the medication.	10		
12. Remove any air bubbles and recap the needle as necessary.	10		
13. Compare the medication to the vial label, and return the medication to its proper storage.	5		
14. Sanitize hands.	10		
Total Points Possible	115		

Comments: Total Points Earned _____   Instructor's Signature _____

Student Name _____   Date _____

CHECKLIST: ADMINISTER AN INTRADERMAL INJECTION

TASK
- Identify the correct syringe, needle gauge, and length for an intradermal injection.
- Select and prepare an appropriate site for an intradermal injection.
- Demonstrate the correct technique to administer an intradermal injection.
- Document an intradermal injection correctly in the medical record.

CONDITIONS: Given the proper equipment and supplies, the student will prepare and administer an intradermal injection.

EQUIPMENT AND SUPPLIES
- Nonsterile disposable gloves
- Medication as ordered by physician
- Tuberculin syringe for ordered dose
- Needle with safety device (26 or 27 gauge, ⅜ inch to ½ inch)
- 2 × 2-inch sterile gauze
- 70% isopropyl alcohol wipes
- Written patient instructions for post testing as appropriate
- Sharps container
- Biohazardous waste container
- Patient's medical record

STANDARDS: Complete the procedure within _____ minutes and achieve a minimum score of _____%.

Time began _____   Time ended _____

Steps	Possible Points	First Attempt	Second Attempt
1. Sanitize hands.	5		
2. Verify the order, and assemble equipment and supplies.	5		
3. Check expiration date of the medication.	10		
4. Follow the "seven rights" of medication administration.	10		
5. Check the medication against the physician's order three times before administration.	10		
6. Check the patient's medical record for drug allergies or conditions that may contraindicate the injection.	10		
7. Calculate the dose to be given, if necessary.	15		
8. Follow the correct procedure for drawing the medication into syringe.	10		
9. Greet and identify the patient, and explain the procedure to the patient.	10		
10. Select an appropriate injection site and properly position the patient as necessary to expose the site adequately.	10		
11. Apply gloves.	5		

Steps	Possible Points	First Attempt	Second Attempt
12. Prepare the injection site.	10		
13. While the prepared site is drying, remove the cover from the needle.	10		
14. Pull the skin taut at the injection site.	10		
15. Inject the medication between the dermis and epidermis. Create a wheal.	10		
16. Withdraw the needle from the injection site at the same angle as it was inserted, and activate the safety device immediately.	10		
17. Dab the area with the gauze. Do not rub.	5		
18. Discard in the syringe sharps container. Remove gloves and discard in a biohazardous container.	5		
19. Sanitize the hands.	5		
20. Check the patient.	5		
21. Read or discuss with the patient the test results.	10		
22. Sanitize hands.	5		
23. Document the procedure.	10		
Mantoux Test			
24. Check to be sure test was given 48 to 72 hours earlier.	10		
25. After sanitizing the hands and applying nonsterile gloves, gently rub the test site with a finger and lightly palpate for induration.	10		
26. Using the tape that comes with the medication, measure the diameter of the area of induration from edge to edge.	10		
27. Record the area of induration and notify the health care provider of the measurement if not within the negative range.	10		
28. Record the reading in the medical record.	10		
Total Points Possible	245		

Comments: Total Points Earned _____   Instructor's Signature _____

Student Name _____   Date _____

CHECKLIST: ADMINISTER A SUBCUTANEOUS INJECTION

TASK
- Identify the correct syringe, needle gauge, and length for a subcutaneous injection.
- Select and prepare an appropriate site for a subcutaneous injection.
- Demonstrate the correct technique to administer a subcutaneous injection.
- Document a subcutaneous injection correctly in the medical record.

CONDITIONS: Given the proper equipment and supplies, the student will prepare and administer a subcutaneous injection.

EQUIPMENT AND SUPPLIES
- Nonsterile disposable gloves
- Medication as ordered by physician
- Appropriate syringe for ordered dose of medication
- Appropriate needle with safety device
- 2 × 2-inch sterile gauze
- 70% Isopropyl alcohol wipes
- Sharps container
- Biohazardous waste container
- Patient's medical record

STANDARDS: Complete the procedure within _____ minutes and achieve a minimum score of _____%.

Time began _____   Time ended _____

Steps	Possible Points	First Attempt	Second Attempt
1. Sanitize hands.	5		
2. Verify the order, and assemble equipment and supplies.	5		
3. Check expiration date of the medication.	10		
4. Follow the "seven rights" of medication administration.	10		
5. Check the medication against the physician's order three times before administration.	10		
6. Check the patient's medical record for drug allergies or conditions that may contraindicate the injection.	10		
7. Calculate the correct dose to be given, if necessary.	15		
8. Follow the procedure for drawing the medication into the syringe.	5		
9. Greet and identify the patient, and explain the procedure.	10		
10. Select an appropriate injection site and properly position the patient as necessary to expose the site.	10		
11. Apply gloves.	5		
12. Prepare the injection site.	10		

Steps	Possible Points	First Attempt	Second Attempt
13. While the prepared site is drying, remove the cover from the needle.	5		
14. Pinch the skin at the injection site and puncture the skin quickly and smoothly, making sure the needle is kept at a 45-degree angle.	10		
15. Aspirate the syringe to check for blood. If no blood is present, inject the medication.	10		
16. Place a gauze pad over the injection site and quickly withdraw the needle from the injection site at the same angle at which it was inserted.	10		
17. Massage the injection site, if appropriate.	5		
18. Discard the syringe and needle into a rigid biohazardous container.	5		
19. Remove gloves and discard in a biohazardous waste container.	5		
20. Sanitize the hands.	5		
21. Check on the patient.	5		
22. Document procedure.	10		
Total Points Possible	175		

Comments: Total Points Earned _____   Instructor's Signature _____

Student Name _____   Date _____

CHECKLIST: **ADMINISTER AN INTRAMUSCULAR INJECTION TO AN ADULT**

TASK
- Identify the correct syringe, needle gauge, and length for an adult intramuscular injection.
- Select and prepare an appropriate site for a pediatric intramuscular injection.
- Demonstrate the correct technique to administer an intramuscular injection.
- Document an intramuscular injection correctly in the medical record.

CONDITIONS: Given the proper equipment and supplies, the student will prepare and administer an intramuscular injection to an adult patient.

EQUIPMENT AND SUPPLIES
- Nonsterile disposable gloves
- Medication as ordered by physician
- Appropriate syringe for ordered medication dose
- Appropriate needle with safety device (21 or 25 gauge, 1 inch to 1½ inch)
- 2 × 2-inch sterile gauze
- 70% isopropyl alcohol wipes
- Sharps container
- Biohazardous waste container
- Patient's medical record

STANDARDS: Complete the procedure within _____ minutes and achieve a minimum score of _____%.

Time began _____   Time ended _____

Steps	Possible Points	First Attempt	Second Attempt
1. Sanitize hands.	5		
2. Verify the order, and assemble equipment and supplies.	5		
3. Follow the "seven rights" of medication administration.	10		
4. Check the medication against the physician's order three times before administration.	10		
5. Check the patient's medical record for drug allergies or conditions that may contraindicate the injection.	10		
6. Check expiration date of the medication.	10		
7. Calculate the correct dose to be given.	20		
8. Greet and identify the patient, and explain the procedure.	10		
9. Select an appropriate injection site by amount and density of medication. Properly position the patient as necessary to expose the site adequately.	10		
10. Apply gloves.	5		
11. Prepare the injection site.	10		
12. While the prepared site is drying, remove the cover from the needle.	10		

Steps	Possible Points	First Attempt	Second Attempt
13. Secure the skin at the injection site.	10		
14. Puncture the skin quickly and smoothly, making sure the needle is kept at a 90-degree angle.	10		
15. Aspirate the syringe.	10		
16. Inject medication using proper technique for density of medication.	10		
17. Place a gauze pad over the injection site and quickly withdraw the needle from the injection site at the same angle at which it was inserted. Activate the safety shield over the needle.	10		
18. Massage the injection site if appropriate for medication.	10		
19. Discard the syringe and needle into a sharps container.	5		
20. Remove gloves and discard in a biohazardous waste container.	5		
21. Sanitize the hands.	5		
22. Check on the patient.	10		
23. Document procedure.	10		
Total Points Possible	210		

Comments: Total Points Earned _____   Instructor's Signature _____

Student Name _____   Date _____

CHECKLIST: ADMINISTER AN INTRAMUSCULAR INJECTION USING THE Z-TRACK TECHNIQUE

TASK: Demonstrate the correct technique to administer an intramuscular injection using the Z-track technique.

CONDITIONS: Given the proper equipment and supplies, the student will prepare and administer an intramuscular injection using the Z-track technique.

EQUIPMENT AND SUPPLIES
- Nonsterile disposable gloves
- Medication order by physician
- Appropriate syringe for ordered dose
- Appropriate needle with safety device
- 2 × 2-inch sterile gauze
- 70% isopropyl alcohol wipes
- Biohazardous waste container
- Patient's medical record

STANDARDS: Complete the procedure within _____ minutes and achieve a minimum score of _____%.

Time began _____   Time ended _____

Steps	Possible Points	First Attempt	Second Attempt
1. Sanitize hands.	5		
2. Verify the order, and assemble equipment and supplies.	5		
3. Follow the "seven rights" of medication administration.	10		
4. Check the medication against the physician's order three times before administration.	10		
5. Check the patient's medical record for drug allergies or conditions that may contraindicate the injection.	10		
6. Check expiration date of the medication.	10		
7. Calculate the correct dose to be given.	20		
8. Follow the correct procedure for drawing the medication into syringe.	10		
9. Greet and identify the patient, and explain the procedure to the patient.	15		
10. Select an appropriate injection site and properly position the patient.	5		
11. Apply disposable gloves.	5		
12. Prepare the injection site.	5		
13. While the prepared site is drying, remove the cover from the needle.	5		

Steps	Possible Points	First Attempt	Second Attempt
14. Secure the skin at the injection site by pushing the skin away from the injection site.	10		
15. Puncture the skin quickly and smoothly, making sure the needle is kept at a 90-degree angle.	10		
16. Continue to hold the tissue in place while aspirating and injecting the medication.	15		
17. Inject the medication.	10		
18. Withdraw the needle.	10		
19. Release the traction on the skin to seal the track as the needle is being removed. Activate safety shield over needle.	10		
20. Discard the syringe and needle into a rigid biohazardous container.	5		
21. Remove gloves and discard in a biohazardous waste container.	5		
22. Sanitize the hands.	5		
23. Check on the patient.	5		
24. Document the procedure.	5		
25. Clean the equipment and examination room.	10		
Total Points Possible	215		

Comments: Total Points Earned _____   Instructor's Signature _____

Student Name _____   Date _____

CHECKLIST: PERFORM VENIPUNCTURE USING THE EVACUATED-TUBE METHOD (COLLECTION OF MULTIPLE TUBES)

TASK: Obtain a venous blood specimen acceptable for testing using the evacuated-tube system.

CONDITIONS: Given the proper equipment and supplies, the student will be required to perform a venipuncture using the evacuated-tube system method of collection.

EQUIPMENT AND SUPPLIES
- Nonsterile disposable gloves
- Personal protective equipment (PPE) as required
- Tourniquet (latex-free)
- Evacuated tube holder
- Evacuated tube multidraw needle (21 or 22 gauge, 1 or 1½ inch) with safety guards
- Evacuated blood tubes for requested tests with labels (correct nonadditive or additive required for ordered test)
- Alcohol wipe
- Sterile 2 × 2-inch gauze pads
- Bandage (latex-free) or nonallergenic tape
- Sharps container
- Biohazardous waste container
- Laboratory requisition form
- Patient's medical record

STANDARDS: Complete the procedure within _____ minutes and achieve a minimum score of _____%.

Time began _____   Time ended _____

Steps	Possible Points	First Attempt	Second Attempt
1. Sanitize hands.	5		
2. Verify the order, and assemble equipment and supplies.	5		
3. Greet the patient, identify yourself, and confirm the patient's identity. Escort the patient to the proper room. Ask the patient to sit in phlebotomy chair.	5		
4. Confirm that the patient has followed the needed preparation (e.g., fasting).	10		
5. Explain the procedure to the patient.	5		
6. Prepare the evacuated tube system.	5		
7. Open the sterile gauze packet and place the gauze pad on the inside of its wrapper, or obtain sterile gauze pads from a bulk package.	10		
8. Position the remaining needed supplies for ease of reaching with nondominant hand. Place tube loosely in holder with label facing downward.	10		
9. Position and examine the arm to be used in the venipuncture.	10		
10. Apply the tourniquet.	10		
11. Apply gloves and PPE.	5		

Steps	Possible Points	First Attempt	Second Attempt
12. Thoroughly palpate the selected vein.	5		
13. Release the tourniquet.	5		
14. Prepare the puncture site using alcohol swabs.	10		
15. Reapply the tourniquet.	10		
16. Position the holder while keeping the needle covered, being certain to have control of holder. Uncover the needle.	10		
17. Position the needle so that it follows the line of the vein.	5		
18. Perform the venipuncture.	5		
19. Secure the holder. Push the bottom of the tube with the thumb of your nondominant hand so that the needle inside the holder pierces the rubber stopper of the tube. Follow the direction of the vein.	10		
20. Change tubes (minimum of two tubes) as required by test orders.	10		
21. Gently invert tubes that contain additives to be mixed with the specimen.	10		
22. While the blood is filling the last tube, release the tourniquet and withdraw the needle. Cover the needle with the safety shield.	10		
23. Apply direct pressure on the venipuncture site, and instruct the patient to raise the arm straight above the head and maintain pressure on the site for 1 to 2 minutes.	10		
24. Discard the contaminated needle and holder into the sharps container.	10		
25. Label the tubes as appropriate for lab.	10		
26. Place the tube into the biohazard transport bag.	5		
27. Check for bleeding at puncture site and apply a pressure dressing.	5		
28. Remove and discard the alcohol wipe and gloves.	5		
29. Sanitize the hands.	5		
30. Record the collection date and time on the laboratory requisition form, and place the requisition in the proper place in the biohazard transport bag.	10		
31. Ask and observe how the patient feels.	5		
32. Clean the work area using Standard Precautions.	5		
33. Document the procedure, indicating tests for which blood was drawn and the labs to which blood will be sent.	10		
Total Points Possible	250		

Comments: Total Points Earned _____   Instructor's Signature _____

Student Name _____   Date _____

CHECKLIST: PERFORM VENIPUNCTURE USING THE SYRINGE METHOD

TASK: Obtain a venous blood specimen acceptable for testing using the syringe method.

CONDITIONS: Given the proper equipment and supplies, the student will be required to perform a venipuncture using the syringe method of collection.

EQUIPMENT AND SUPPLIES
- Nonsterile disposable gloves
- Personal protective equipment (PPE) as required
- Tourniquet (latex-free)
- Test tube rack
- 10-cc (10-mL) syringe with 21- or 22-gauge needle and safety guards
- Proper evacuated blood tubes for tests ordered
- Alcohol wipe
- Sterile 2 × 2-inch gauze pads
- Bandage (latex-free) or nonallergenic tape
- Sharps container
- Biohazardous waste container
- Laboratory requisition form
- Patient's medical record

STANDARDS: Complete the procedure within _____ minutes and achieve a minimum score of _____%.

Time began _____   Time ended _____

Steps	Possible Points	First Attempt	Second Attempt
1. Sanitize hands.	5		
2. Verify the order. Assemble equipment and supplies.	5		
3. Greet the patient, identify yourself, and confirm the patient's identity. Escort the patient to the room for the blood draw. Position the patient in phlebotomy chair or on examination table.	5		
4. Confirm any necessary preparation has been accomplished (e.g., fasting). Explain the procedure to the patient.	5		
5. Prepare the needle and syringe, maintaining syringe sterility. Break the seal on the syringe by moving the plunger back and forth several times. Loosen the cap on the needle and check to make sure that the hub is screwed tightly onto the syringe.	15		
6. Place the evacuated tubes to be filled in a test tube rack on a work surface in order of fill.	15		
7. Open the sterile gauze packet and place the gauze pad on the inside of its wrapper, or obtain sterile gauze pads from a bulk package.	5		
8. Position and examine the arm to be used in the venipuncture.	10		
9. Apply gloves and PPE.	5		

Steps	Possible Points	First Attempt	Second Attempt
10. Thoroughly palpate the selected vein.	10		
11. Release the tourniquet.	10		
12. Prepare the puncture site and reapply tourniquet.	10		
13. If drawing from the hand, ask the patient to make a fist or bend the fingers downward. Pull the skin taut with your thumb over the top of the patient's knuckles.	15		
14. Position the syringe and grasp the syringe firmly between the thumb and the underlying fingers.	10		
15. Follow the direction of the vein and insert the needle in one quick motion at about a 45-degree angle.	10		
16. If drawing from AC vein, with your nondominant hand pull the skin taut beneath the intended puncture site to anchor the vein. Thumb should be 1 to 2 inches below and to the side of the vein.	15		
17. Position the syringe and grasp the syringe firmly between the thumb and the underlying fingers.	10		
18. Follow the direction of the vein and insert the needle in one quick motion at about a 15-degree angle.	10		
19. Perform the venipuncture. If flash does not occur, gently pull back on the plunger. Do not move the needle. If blood still does not enter the syringe, slowly withdraw the needle, secure new supplies, and retry the draw.	10		
20. Anchor the syringe, and gently continue pulling back on the plunger until the required amount of blood is in the syringe.	10		
21. Release the tourniquet.	5		
22. Remove the needle and cover the needle with safety shield without locking.	10		
23. Apply direct pressure on the venipuncture site, and instruct the patient to raise the arm straight above the head. Instruct the patient to maintain pressure on the site for 1 to 2 minutes.	5		
24. Transfer the blood to the evacuated tubes as soon as possible.	10		
25. Properly dispose of the syringe and needle.	10		
26. Label the tubes and place into biohazard transport bag.	10		
27. Check for bleeding at venipuncture site and place a pressure dressing.	10		
28. Remove and discard the alcohol wipe and gloves.	5		
29. Sanitize the hands.	5		
30. Record the collection date and time on the laboratory requisition form, and place the requisition in the biohazard transport bag.	10		

Steps	Possible Points	First Attempt	Second Attempt
31. Ask and observe how the patient feels.	5		
32. Clean the work area using Standard Precautions.	5		
33. Document the procedure.	10		
Total Points Possible NOTE: Awards points for Steps 13-14-15 OR 16-17-18, not both	255		

Comments: Total Points Earned _____   Instructor's Signature _____

Student Name _____   Date _____

CHECKLIST: PERFORM VENIPUNCTURE USING THE BUTTERFLY METHOD (COLLECTION OF MULTIPLE EVACUATED TUBES)

TASK: Obtain a venous blood specimen acceptable for testing using the butterfly method.

CONDITIONS: Given the proper equipment and supplies, the student will perform a venipuncture using the butterfly method of collection.

EQUIPMENT AND SUPPLIES
- Nonsterile disposable gloves
- Personal protective equipment (PPE) as required
- Tourniquet (latex-free)
- Test tube rack
- Winged-infusion set with Luer adapter and safety guard
- Multidraw needle (22 to 25 gauge) and tube holder, or 10-cc (10-mL) syringe
- Evacuated blood tubes for requested tests with labels (correct nonadditive or additive required for ordered tests)
- Alcohol wipe
- Sterile 2 × 2-inch gauze pads
- Bandage (latex-free) or nonallergenic tape
- Sharps container
- Biohazardous waste container
- Laboratory requisition form
- Patient's medical record

STANDARDS: Complete the procedure within _____ minutes and achieve a minimum score of _____%.

Time began _____   Time ended _____

Steps	Possible Points	First Attempt	Second Attempt
1. Sanitize hands.	5		
2. Verify the order. Assemble equipment and supplies.	5		
3. Greet the patient, identify yourself, and confirm the patient's identity. Escort the patient to the proper room for venipuncture.	5		
4. Ask the patient to have a seat in the phlebotomy chair or on the examination table.	5		
5. Confirm any necessary preparation has been followed (e.g., fasting). Explain the procedure to the patient.	10		
6. Prepare the winged infusion set. Attach the winged infusion set to either a syringe or an evacuated tube holder.	15		
7. Open the sterile gauze packet and place the gauze pad on the inside of its wrapper, or obtain sterile gauze pads from a bulk package.	5		
8. Position and examine the arm to be used in the venipuncture.	10		
9. Apply the tourniquet.	10		
10. Apply gloves and PPE.	5		
11. Thoroughly palpate the selected vein.	10		

Steps	Possible Points	First Attempt	Second Attempt
12. Release the tourniquet.	10		
13. Prepare the puncture site and reapply the tourniquet.	5		
14. If drawing from the hand, ask the patient to make a fist or bend the fingers downward. Pull the skin taut with your thumb over the top of the patient's knuckles.	10		
15. Remove the protective shield from the needle of the infusion set, being sure the bevel is facing up. Position needle over vein to be punctured.	10		
16. Perform the venipuncture. With your nondominant hand, pull the skin taut beneath the intended puncture site to anchor the vein. Thumb should be 1 to 2 inches below and to the side of the vein. Follow the direction of the vein and insert the needle in one quick motion at about a 15-degree angle.	20		
17. After penetrating the vein, decrease the angle of the needle to 5 degrees until a "flash" of blood appears in the tubing.	5		
18. Secure the needle for blood collection.	10		
19. Insert the evacuated tube into the tube holder or gently pull back on the plunger of the syringe. Change tubes as required by the test ordered.	10		
20. Release the tourniquet and remove the needle.	10		
21. Apply direct pressure on the venipuncture site, and instruct the patient to raise the arm straight above the head. Maintain pressure on the site for 1 to 2 minutes, with the arm raised straight above the head.	10		
22. If a syringe was used, transfer the blood to the evacuated tubes as soon as possible.	10		
23. Dispose of the winged infusion set.	5		
24. Label the tubes and place the tube into the biohazard transport bag.	5		
25. Check for bleeding and place a bandage over the gauze to create a pressure dressing.	5		
26. Remove and discard the alcohol wipe and gloves.	5		
27. Sanitize the hands.	5		
28. Record the collection date and time on the laboratory requisition form, and place the requisition in the biohazard transport bag.	10		
29. Ask and observe how the patient feels.	5		
30. Clean the work area using Standard Precautions.	5		
31. Document the procedure.	10		
Total Points Possible	250		

Comments: Total Points Earned _____   Instructor's Signature _____

Student Name _____   Date _____

CHECKLIST: CHARTING

TASK: Create new medical records, organize contents, interview patients, and document subjective and objective data.

CONDITIONS: Given the proper equipment and supplies, the students will be required to create new medical records by labeling them correctly and organizing sample forms and/or reports within each appropriately. The student will then role-play with another student or an instructor to demonstrate how to interview a patient. Finally, using the list of common charting abbreviations (as directed) from the student handbook, the student will record the "patient's" chief complaint (subjective data) as well as every procedure in this module using the sample documentation provided on the procedure competency checklists (objective data).

EQUIPMENT AND SUPPLIES
- File folders
- Blank file labels
- Color-coded year labels
- Alphabetical labels
- Medical alert labels
- Other labels as appropriate
- Sample forms and/or reports
- Sample documentation (on procedure competency checklists)

STANDARDS: Complete the procedure within _____ minutes and achieve a minimum score of _____%.

Time began _____   Time ended _____

Steps	Possible Points	First Attempt	Second Attempt
1. Assemble all equipment and supplies.	5		
2. Create a file label (patient name).	5		
3. Attach other labels as appropriate (year, initials, medical alert).	5		
4. Organize preprinted forms appropriately within the folder.	10		
5. Review medical history form with the patient (subjective data).	10		
6. Record chief complaint (in patient's own words/subjective data).	10		
7. Document all procedures on appropriate forms using correct terminology and abbreviations (objective data).	10		
8. Record all information legibly.	10		
9. Maintain HIPAA privacy guidelines.	10		
10. Maintain professional qualities as defined.	10		
11. Clean area when finished.	5		
Total Points Possible	90		

Comments: Total Points Earned _____   Instructor's Signature _____

Student Name _____   Date _____

CHECKLIST: **DIAGNOSTIC CODING**

TASK: Assign the proper *International Classification of Diseases (ICD-9-CM)* code based on medical documentation to the highest degree of specificity.

CONDITIONS: Given the proper equipment and supplies, the student will assign the proper *ICD-9-CM* code based on medical documentation to the highest degree of specificity.

EQUIPMENT AND SUPPLIES
- Current *ICD-9-CM* codebook
- Medical dictionary
- Patient's medical records
- Pen or pencil
- Work product (see next pages)

STANDARDS: Complete the procedure within _____ minutes and achieve a minimum score of _____%.

Time began _____   Time ended _____

Steps	Possible Points	First Attempt	Second Attempt
1. Assemble all supplies and equipment.	5		
2. Identify the key term in the diagnostic statement.	10		
3. Locate the diagnosis in the Alphabetic Index (Volume 2, Section 1) of the *ICD-9-CM* codebook.	20		
4. Read and use footnotes, symbols, or instructions.	15		
5. Locate the diagnosis in the Tabular List (Volume 1).	10		
6. Read and use the inclusions and exclusions noted in the Tabular List.	10		
7. Assign the code to the highest degree of specificity appropriate.	20		
8. Document in the medical record.	10		
9. Ask yourself these final questions (NO points awarded for this section).	0		
a. Have you coded to the highest degree of specificity?			
b. Are there any secondary diagnoses or conditions addressed during the encounter that need to be coded?			
Total Points Possible	100		

Comments: Total Points Earned _____   Instructor's Signature _____

≋ WORK PRODUCT FOR DIAGNOSTIC CODING

Diagnosis Codes

For the following diagnosis codes, use Volume 1 and 2 of the *ICD-9-CM*. Remember, look in the alphabetical listing of Volume 2 first. Then locate the exact entry in Volume 1. Write the correct code in the space provided:

1. Hematuria — *791.2*

2. Urinary obstruction, unspecified — *599.60*

3. Urethral stricture — *598.9*

4. Acute cystitis — *595.0*

5. Hypertrophy of kidney — *593.1*

6. Hypoglycemia, unspecified — *251.2*

7. Iron deficiency anemia — *280.9*

8. Hemophilia — ~~280.9~~ *286.0*

9. Vitamin K deficiency — ~~286.0~~ *269.0*

10. Thrombocytopathy — *287.1*

11. Kidney stone — *592.0*

12. UTI — *599.0*

13. Phimosis — *605*

14. Urinary retention — *788.20*

15. Cystitis, unspecified — *585.9*

16. Chronic renal failure — *582.1*

17. Chronic glomerulonephritis — *582.9*

18. Screening for sickle-cell disorder — *282.6*

19. Leukemia — *208.9*

20. Bladder cancer — *596.9*

239.4

Student Name _____   Date _____

CHECKLIST: PROCEDURAL CODING

TASK: Assign the proper *Current Procedural Terminology* (CPT) code to the highest degree of specificity based on medical documentation for auditing and billing purposes.

CONDITIONS: Given the proper equipment and supplies, the student will assign the proper (CPT) code to the highest degree of specificity based on medical documentation for auditing and billing purposes.

EQUIPMENT AND SUPPLIES
- Current *CPT* codebook
- Medical dictionary
- Patient's medical records
- Pen or pencil
- Work product (see next pages)

STANDARDS: Complete the procedure within _____ minutes and achieve a minimum score of _____%.

Time began _____   Time ended _____

Steps	Possible Points	First Attempt	Second Attempt
1. Assemble all supplies and equipment.	5		
2. Read the introduction, guidelines, and notes of a current *CPT* codebook.	10		
3. Review all service and procedures performed on the day of the encounter; include all medications administered and trays and equipment used.	20		
4. Identify the main term in the procedure.	15		
5. Locate the main term in the alphabetical index. Review any subterms listed alphabetically under the main term.	10		
6. Verify the code sets in the tabular (numerical) list. Select the code with the greatest specificity.	10		
7. Determine if a modifier is required.	20		
8. Assign the code using all necessary steps for proper code determination.	10		
9. Ask yourself these final questions (NO points awarded for this section).	0		
a. Have you coded to the highest degree of specificity?			
b. Are there any secondary diagnoses or conditions addressed during the encounter that need to be coded?			
Total Points Possible	100		

Comments: Total Points Earned _____   Instructor's Signature _____

≋ WORK PRODUCT FOR PROCEDURAL CODING

Procedure Codes

Find the following CPT codes in the *CPT* book. The codes are listed under the section in the *CPT* where they appear. Remember to use the index in the back to help locate a code. Write the correct code in the space provided:

1. MRI, neck without contrast materials   _____

2. CAT SCAN, abdomen with contrast materials   _____

3. Barium enema, with or without KUB   _____

4. Endoscopic catheterization of the pancreatic ductal system, with S&I   _____

5. Cystography, minimum of three views, S&I   _____

6. Perineogram   _____

7. Orthoroentgenogram   _____

8. Bone density study, one or more sites   _____

9. Radiological examination, surgical specimen   _____

10. Mammography, unilateral   _____

11. Angiography, extremity, unilateral S&I   _____

12. Thyroid uptake, single determination   _____

13. Chlamydia culture   _____

14. Pregnancy test, urine   _____

15. Hepatitis C antibody   _____

16. Total serum cholesterol   _____

17. KOH slide prep   _____

18. CAT SCAN, head or brain, without contrast material   _____

19. Transurethral resection of prostate   _____

20. Bone marrow transplant   _____

Student Name _____   Date _____

CHECKLIST: USE *PHYSICIAN'S DESK REFERENCE*

TASK: Demonstrate understanding of *Physician's Desk Reference's* organization by creating a fact sheet for each drug listed on a prepared document.

CONDITIONS: Given proper equipment and supplies, the student will be required to identify the trade and generic names for each listed drug, its classification, one indication for its use, one contraindication for its use, its usual dosage and administration, and any possible side effects.

EQUIPMENT AND SUPPLIES
- *Physician's Desk Reference*
- List of drugs (on following pages)
- Pen or pencil

STANDARDS: Complete the procedure within _____ minutes and achieve a minimum score of _____%.

Time began _____   Time ended _____

Steps	Possible Points	First Attempt	Second Attempt
1. Assemble all equipment and supplies.	5		
2. Create a fact sheet for each medication listed on the prepared drug list (see next page) to include the following:			
• Trade name, generic name, and drug classification	10		
• Identify indications for assigned medications	10		
• Identify contraindications for assigned medications	10		
• Identify dosage and administration of assigned medications	10		
• Identify side effects of assigned medications	10		
3. Display professional abilities through penmanship.	10		
4. Clean area.	5		
5. Proofread and correct your work and submit to your instructor. Demonstrate professionalism throughout procedure and accept constructive feedback with a problem-solving attitude.	10		
Total Points Possible	80		

Comments: Total Points Earned _____   Instructor's Signature _____

WORK PRODUCT FOR USE *PHYSICIAN'S DESK REFERENCE*

Drug	Generic Name	Classification	Indication(s)	Contraindication(s)	Dosage and Administration	Side Effects
Agenerase	amprenavir					
Trisenox	arsenic trioxide					
Suprax	cefixime					
Aranesp	darbepoetin					

Continued

Drug	Generic Name	Classification	Indication(s)	Contraindication(s)	Dosage and Administration	Side Effects
Ferrlecit	ferric gluconate					
Urispas	flavoxate					
Dalmane	flurazepam					
Heparin Leo	heparin					

Continued

Crixivan	Venofer	Glucophage	Novantrone
indinavir	iron sucrose	metformin	mitoxantrone

Drug	Generic Name	Classification	Indication(s)	Contraindication(s)	Dosage and Administration	Side Effects
Ditropan	oxybutynin					
Trental	pentoxifylline					
Pyridium	phenazopyridine					

smz-tmp	tinzaparin	tolterodine
Zotrim	Innohep	Detrol

Student Name _____   Date _____

CHECKLIST: BEING A PROFESSIONAL

TASK: Complete a self-survey checklist to increase your awareness of areas needing improvement before entering the job market.

CONDITIONS: Using the checklist as a tool, assess your professional characteristics, abilities and image. Discuss expectations with your instructor.

EQUIPMENT AND SUPPLIES
- Checklist and pen/pencil

STANDARDS: Complete the procedure within _____ minutes and achieve a minimum score of _____%.

Time began _____   Time ended _____

Steps	Possible Points	Student	Instructor
PROFESSIONAL CHARACTERISTICS			
1. Dependability			
a. I am punctual.	10		
b. I am efficient.	5		
c. I am reliable.	10		
2. Loyalty			
a. I turn in quality work.	10		
b. I manage my time wisely.	10		
c. I display consistent work habits.	10		
d. I accept decisions.	5		
e. I display ethical behavior.	15		
3. Positive attitude			
a. I am enthusiastic.	10		
b. I set goals.	10		
c. I seek out learning opportunities.	10		
d. I am a team player.	10		
e. I accept constructive criticism.	5		
f. I adapt to change.	5		
g. I am a good non-verbal communicator.	10		

Steps	Possible Points	Student	Instructor
4. Integrity			
a. I am trustworthy.	15		
b. I keep information confidential.	10		
c. I make ethical decisions.	15		
5. Diplomacy			
a. I use tact when dealing with classmates.	10		
b. I display courtesy and empathy when appropriate.	10		
6. Confidence			
a. I display leadership.	10		
b. I make decisions based on consensus.	5		
c. I prioritize assignments.	5		
PROFESSIONAL ABILITIES			
7. Competence			
a. I complete assignments on time.	10		
b. I request assistance when unfamiliar with assignment and/or instructions.	15		
8. Dexterity			
a. I display quality manual skills.	10		
b. I am able to assist with lifting or positioning.	10		
9. Effective communication			
a. I use correct grammar.	10		
b. I spell correctly.	10		
c. I have good penmanship.	5		
10. Nonverbal communication			
a. I smile when communicating with others.	10		
PROFESSIONAL IMAGE			
11. Personal hygiene			
a. I bathe or shower, use deodorant, and brush my teeth every morning.	20		

Steps	Possible Points	Student	Instructor
12. Grooming			
a. My hair is neat and off my face and collar. I don't use extreme hair colors or highlights or any ornaments or decorations in my hair.	10		
b. My fingernails are clean and short. I don't use colored nail polish or artificial nails.	10		
c. If I use makeup and/or wear perfume/after shave, it is minimal.	10		
d. I wear minimal jewelry, no more than a wedding ring, a wristwatch, and/or a single pair of nondangling earrings. I do not have any visible body piercings except perhaps for earrings.	10		
13. Dress			
a. I wear a uniform that is clean, pressed, in good condition, and that fits properly over appropriate undergarments.	20		
b. I wear clean stockings without holes or tears.	10		
c. I wear clean and polished closed-toe shoes (not Crocs) with clean laces.	10		
14. Professional appearance			
a. I don't chew gum.	10		
b. I don't smell like cigarette smoke.	10		
c. I don't slouch.	5		
d. If I have tattoos, they are hidden from view.	10		
Total Points Possible	430		

Comments: Total Points Earned _____   Instructor's Signature _____

Appendix C Module E
Procedure Competency Checklists

Student Name (print)   Instructor's Name (print)   Date

MEDICAL ASSISTANT
MODULE E
PROCEDURE COMPETENCY GRADE SHEET

Module E Skills	Points Earned	Points Possible	Instructor's Signature	Date
1. Use Methods of Quality Control		100		
2. Focus the Microscope		150		
3. Complete a Laboratory Requisition Form		100		
4. Collect a Specimen for Transport to an Outside Laboratory (2)		100		
5. Screen and Follow up on Patient Test Results		30		
6. Collect a Specimen for CLIA-Waived Throat Culture and Rapid Strep Test (2)		250		
7. Mono Test (2)		90		
8. Instruct a Patient in Collection of Midstream Clean-Catch Urine Specimen		50		
9. Use a Sterile Disposable Microlancet for Skin Puncture (3)		150		
10. Separate Serum from Whole Blood (3)		100		
11. Urinalysis Using Reagent Strips (3)		175		
12. Prepare a Urine Specimen for Microscopic Examination (3)		100		
13. Perform a Urine Pregnancy Test (1)		100		
14. Perform a Microhematocrit Test (3)		200		
15. Determine a Hemoglobin Measurement Using a HemoCue (3)		150		
16. Perform Glucose Testing (3)		100		
17. Obtain a Bacterial Smear from a Wound Specimen (2)		150		
	Total Points ÷ Points = Earned Possible	Total	Final Percentage	
	÷ 2095 =			
	Instructor's Signature	Date		

Numbers in ( ) indicate minimum practice requirements

Student Name (print)   Instructor's Name (print)   Date

DOCUMENT EACH PATIENT IN PROPER CHARTING FORMAT.

COLLECT A SPECIMEN FOR TRANSPORT TO AN OUTSIDE LABORATORY

	Date/Time	Patient	MA Signature
1.			
2.			

COLLECT A SPECIMEN FOR CLIA-WAIVED THROAT CULTURE AND RAPID STREP TEST

	Date/Time	Patient	MA Signature
1.			
2.			

MONO TEST

	Date/Time	Patient	MA Signature
1.			
2.			

USE A STERILE DISPOSABLE MICROLANCET FOR SKIN PUNCTURE

	Date/Time	Patient	MA Signature
1.			
2.			
3.			

SEPARATE SERUM FROM WHOLE BLOOD

	Date/Time	Patient	MA Signature
1.			
2.			
3.			

URINALYSIS USING REAGENT STRIPS

	Date/Time	Patient	MA Signature
1.			
2.			
3.			

PREPARE A URINE SPECIMEN FOR MICROSCOPIC EXAMINATION

	Date/Time	Patient	MA Signature
1.			
2.			
3.			

PERFORM A URINE PREGNANCY TEST

	Date/Time	Patient	MA Signature
1.			

PERFORM A MICROHEMATOCRIT TEST

	Date/Time	Patient	MA Signature
1.			
2.			
3.			

DETERMINE A HEMOGLOBIN MEASUREMENT USING A HEMOCUE

	Date/Time	Patient	MA Signature
1.			
2.			
3.			

PERFORM GLUCOSE TESTING

	Date/Time	Patient	MA Signature
1.			
2.			
3.			

OBTAIN A BACTERIAL SMEAR FROM A WOUND SPECIMEN

	Date/Time	Patient	MA Signature
1.			
2.			

Student Name _____   Date _____

CHECKLIST: USE METHODS OF QUALITY CONTROL

TASK: Practice quality control procedures in the medical laboratory to ensure accuracy of test results through detection and elimination of errors.

CONDITIONS: Given the proper equipment and supplies, the student will demonstrate the proper methods of quality control.

EQUIPMENT AND SUPPLIES
- Quality control logbook
- Quality control samples (as provided in CLIA-waived prepackaged test kits)
- Patient sample
- Copy of CLIA 88 guidelines
- Copy of state regulation and guidelines
- Patient's medical record

STANDARDS: Complete the procedure within _____ minutes and achieve a minimum score of _____%.

Time began _____   Time ended _____

Steps	Possible Points	First Attempt	Second Attempt
1. Sanitize hands.	5		
2. Assemble equipment and supplies.	5		
3. Obtain the quality control (QC) sample provided in a CLIA-waived prepackaged kit.	5		
4. Check the expiration date on the prepackaged test kit and on each QC specimen.	10		
5. Perform QC using the test kit supplied.	5		
6. Obtain the specimen from the patient, and identify the specimen as belonging to the patient.	15		
7. Perform testing of the specimen following the specific protocols outlined for the sample by the manufacturer.	20		
8. Perform QC testing as outlined by the manufacturer's protocols for the specimen being tested.	10		
9. Determine the results for both the patient's specimen and the QC sample.	10		
10. Sanitize the hands.	5		
11. Document the results in the QC logbook and the patient's medical record.	10		
Total Points Possible	100		

Comments: Total Points Earned _____   Instructor's Signature _____

Student Name _____   Date _____

CHECKLIST: FOCUS THE MICROSCOPE

TASK: Focus the microscope on a prepared slide from low power to high power and oil immersion.

CONDITIONS: Given the proper equipment and supplies, the student will be required to demonstrate the proper method for focusing a microscope.

EQUIPMENT AND SUPPLIES
- Microscope with cover
- Lens paper
- Lens cleaner
- Specimen slide
- Soft cloth
- Tissue or gauze

STANDARDS: Complete the procedure within _____ minutes and achieve a minimum score of _____%.

Time began _____   Time ended _____

Steps	Possible Points	First Attempt	Second Attempt
1. Sanitize hands.	5		
2. Assemble equipment and supplies.	5		
3. Clean the ocular and objective lenses of the microscope with lens paper and lens cleaner.	10		
4. Turn on the light source, and adjust the ocular lenses to fit your eye span.	5		
5. Place the slide on the stage and secure it in the slide clip.	10		
6. Rotate the nosepiece to the scanning objective (×4) or to the low-power objective (×10) if the scanning objective is not attached to your microscope.	10		
7. Adjust the coarse focus adjustment knob.	5		
8. Open the diaphragm to allow in the maximum amount of light.	10		
9. Focus the specimen.	5		
10. Further focus the specimen into finest detail by using the fine focus adjustment knob.	10		
11. Adjust the diaphragm and condenser to regulate and adjust the amount of light focused on the specimen to obtain the sharpest image.	10		
12. Rotate the nosepiece to high power and use fine adjustment as needed to bring specimen in focus.	10		

Steps	Possible Points	First Attempt	Second Attempt
13. Examine the specimen by scanning the slide using the stage movement knob to move it in four directions.	10		
14. Examine the specimen as required for the procedure or test, and report the results.	10		
15. Upon completion of the examination of the specimen, lower the stage or raise the objective, turn off the light, and remove the slide from the stage.	10		
16. Return objectives to highest placement and turn objective to lowest power.	10		
17. Clean the stage with lens paper or gauze.	5		
18. Once clean, cover the microscope with a dust cloth and return it to storage.	5		
19. Sanitize the hands.	5		
Total Points Possible	150		

Comments: Total Points Earned _____   Instructor's Signature _____

CHECKLIST: COMPLETE A LABORATORY REQUISITION FORM

TASK: Accurately complete a laboratory requisition form for specimen testing.

CONDITIONS: Given the proper equipment and supplies, the student will be required to complete a laboratory requisition form.

EQUIPMENT AND SUPPLIES
- Physician's written order for laboratory tests
- Laboratory requisition form
- Patient's medical record
- Pen

STANDARDS: Complete the procedure within _____ minutes and achieve a minimum score of _____%.

Time began _____   Time ended _____

Steps	Possible Points	First Attempt	Second Attempt
1. Obtain the patient's medical record, and confirm the physician's orders for laboratory test(s).	5		
2. Obtain the laboratory requisition form for the laboratory where the test will be performed; be sure the lab is acceptable for patient's insurance policy.	10		
3. Complete the section of the requisition requiring the physician's name and address.	5		
4. Complete the patient's demographic information.	5		
5. Complete the section of the requisition requiring the patient's insurance and billing information.	10		
6. Complete the desired laboratory test(s) information.	10		
7. Complete the section of the requisition requiring date and time of specimen collection.	10		
8. Enter the patient's diagnosis code on the requisition as required.	10		
9. Enter the type and amount of medication the patient is taking if appropriate for test to be performed.	10		
10. Complete the patient authorization to release and assign the benefits portion as applicable.	10		
11. Attach copy of insurance identification cards if required by lab.	5		
12. Attach the laboratory requisition securely to the specimen before sending it to the laboratory.	5		
13. Document in the patient's medical record and in the laboratory logbook showing the lab where specimen was sent for testing.	5		
Total Points Possible	100		

Comments: Total Points Earned _____   Instructor's Signature _____

Student Name _____   Date _____

CHECKLIST: COLLECT A SPECIMEN FOR TRANSPORT TO AN OUTSIDE LABORATORY

TASK: Collect a specimen to be sent to an outside laboratory.

CONDITIONS: Given the proper equipment and supplies, the student will be required to demonstrate the proper method of collecting a specimen for transport to an outside laboratory.

EQUIPMENT AND SUPPLIES
- Specimen and container
- Laboratory request form
- Patient's medical record
- Laboratory logbook
- Pen

STANDARDS: Complete the procedure within _____ minutes and achieve a minimum score of _____%.

Time began _____   Time ended _____

Steps	Possible Points	First Attempt	Second Attempt
1. Be sure the patient has followed any advance preparation or special instructions necessary for test accuracy.	5		
2. Review the requirements in the laboratory directory for collection and handling of the specimen ordered by the physician.	5		
3. Complete the laboratory requisition form.	10		
4. Sanitize hands.	5		
5. Assemble equipment and supplies.	5		
6. Greet and identify the patient, and escort the patient to the examination room.	5		
7. Collect the specimen using OSHA standards. Be sure specimen has been collected according to laboratory specifications.	10		
8. Process the specimen further as required by the outside laboratory.	5		
9. Clearly label the tubes and specimen containers and prepare for transport to outside lab.	10		
10. Record information about the collection in the patient's medical record and the laboratory logbook.	10		
11. Properly handle and store the specimen, according to the laboratory's specifications.	10		
12. Remove gloves and sanitize the hands.	5		

Steps	Possible Points	First Attempt	Second Attempt
13. When the laboratory report is returned to the physician's office, screen the test results and place in location for review. Indicate abnormal results.	10		
14. File report after evaluation by proper personnel.	5		
Total Points Possible	100		

Comments: Total Points Earned _____   Instructor's Signature _____

Student Name _____   Date _____

CHECKLIST: SCREEN AND FOLLOW UP ON PATIENT TEST RESULTS

TASK: Follow up with a patient who has abnormal test results.

CONDITIONS: Given the proper equipment and supplies, the student will screen and follow up with a patient's test results.

EQUIPMENT AND SUPPLIES
- Laboratory test results
- Tickler file (3 × 5-inch cards or computer software program) or laboratory log of patient results
- Follow-up reminder cards
- Pen
- Patient's medical record

STANDARDS: Complete the procedure within _____ minutes and achieve a minimum score of _____%.

Time began _____   Time ended _____

Steps	Possible Points	First Attempt	Second Attempt
1. Review the test results as returned from the laboratory.	5		
2. Attach the laboratory report to the patient's medical record, and submit it to the physician for review.	5		
3. If the physician requests that you schedule the patient for a follow-up appointment, determine the most appropriate method of contact, using HIPAA guidelines.	10		
4. Contact the patient and schedule an appointment.	10		
Total Points Possible	30		

Comments: Total Points Earned _____   Instructor's Signature _____

Student Name _____   Date _____

CHECKLIST: COLLECT A SPECIMEN FOR CLIA-WAIVED THROAT CULTURE AND RAPID STREP TEST

TASK: Collect an uncontaminated throat specimen to test for group A beta-hemolytic streptococci, and perform a rapid strep test.

CONDITIONS: Given the proper equipment and supplies, the student will collect a specimen to perform a CLIA-waived throat culture and rapid strep.

EQUIPMENT AND SUPPLIES
- Nonsterile disposable gloves
- Sterile polyester (Dacron) swab
- Face mask
- Culture transport system
- Test tube rack
- Tongue depressor
- Gooseneck lamp
- Timer
- Biohazardous waste container
- Patient's medical record

STANDARDS: Complete the procedure within _____ minutes and achieve a minimum score of _____%.

Time began _____   Time ended _____

Steps	Possible Points	First Attempt	Second Attempt
Specimen Collection for Throat Culture			
1. Sanitize hands.	5		
2. Assemble equipment and supplies.	5		
3. Obtain the patient's medical record.	5		
4. Greet and identify the patient, and escort the patient to the examination room.	5		
5. Instruct the patient to have a seat on the end of the examination table, and explain the procedure to the patient.	5		
6. Put on gloves and face mask.	5		
7. Prepare the culture transport system.	5		
8. Prepare the polyester (Dacron) swab.	5		
9. Visually inspect the patient's throat.	5		
10. Remove the culture transport system from the peel-apart package, being careful to prevent contamination caused by touching tip to any extraneous objects.	5		

Steps	Possible Points	First Attempt	Second Attempt
11. Remove the Dacron swab from the paper wrapper, again being careful not to contaminate it by touching the tip.	5		
12. Place both swabs in your right hand with the tips close together, almost like one swab.	5		
13. Ask the patient to tilt the head back and open the mouth.	5		
14. Use a tongue depressor to hold the tongue away from testing materials.	5		
15. Carefully insert the swabs into the patient's mouth without touching the inside of the mouth, tongue, or teeth.	10		
16. Ask the patient to say "Ahh. . . ."	5		
17. Firmly swab the back of the throat (posterior pharynx) with a figure-eight motion between the tonsillar areas.	10		
18. Continue to hold down the tongue with the depressor, and carefully remove the swabs from the patient's mouth without touching the tongue, teeth, or inside of the cheeks.	10		
19. Discard the tongue depressor in a biohazardous waste container.	5		
20. Remove and discard the cap from the tube, and place the swab from the transport system firmly into the bottom of the tube so that it is dampened with the transport medium and secure tightly. Return the Dacron swab to the original wrapper.	10		
21. Label the transport tube and swab, with the patient's name.	10		
22. Once the specimens have been returned to their individual packaging, remove personal protective equipment (PPE) and sanitize the hands.	5		
Rapid Strep Test (QuickVue)			
23. Sanitize the hands.	5		
24. Put on PPE (if not already applied).	5		
25. Assemble equipment and supplies, being sure to have sufficient supplies for quality control.	5		
26. Unwrap each of the three cassettes that are wrapped in foil pouches.	5		
27. Record the lot number and expiration date of the kit on the logsheets.	10		
28. Label each cassette for the controls and the patient.	10		
29. Insert the swab into the swab chamber of the cassette.	5		
30. Make sure a glass ampule is inside. Break ampule.	5		
31. Shake the bottle vigorously five times to mix the solution.	5		

Steps	Possible Points	First Attempt	Second Attempt
32. Fill the swab chamber to the rim with the extraction solution and remove the required amount.	10		
33. Set the timer for the required time, and do not move the cassette during that time.	5		
34. Examine the results window at the end of minutes. Check for positive or negative test results.	10		
35. Sanitize hands.	5		
36. Record the known controls on the quality control logsheet.	10		
37. Record the results from the patient's cassette, including the internal quality assurance.	10		
38. Document the test results.	10		
Total Points Possible	250		

Comments: Total Points Earned _____   Instructor's Signature _____

Student Name _____   Date _____

CHECKLIST: MONO TESTING (IMMUNOLOGY TESTING)

TASK: To correctly perform immunological testing.

CONDITIONS: Given procedure, proper equipment, and supplies, the student will be required to accurately perform a Mono test using a commercial kit.

EQUIPMENT AND SUPPLIES
- Mono test kit
- Nonsterile disposable gloves
- Alcohol wipes
- Sterile disposable lancet
- Sterile 2 × 2-inch gauze square
- 10% bleach solution
- Sharps container
- Biohazardous waste container
- Patient's medical record
- Laboratory quality control logsheet
- Timer

STANDARDS: Complete the procedure within _____ minutes and achieve a minimum score of _____%.

Time began _____   Time ended _____

Steps	Possible Points	First Attempt	Second Attempt
1. Verify the order and assemble all supplies and equipment.	5		
2. Sanitize hands and apply gloves.	5		
3. Perform the quality test as recommended by the manufacturer and document in the laboratory quality control logsheet if first test from a new box.	10		
4. Greet, identify the patient, and introduce self.	5		
5. Explain the procedure to the patient.	5		
6. Perform capillary puncture and dispose of the lancet in the sharps container. Wipe away the first drop of blood with a gauze pad.	20		
7. Properly collect the specimen by filling the capillary tube to the line.	10		
8. Follow manufacturer's direction by adding the specimen to the well and adding developer as directed. Wait the required time, and read and record the results.	10		
9. Report the results to the physician and provide patient with any follow-up action needed.	5		
10. Disinfect work area with bleach solution and return supplies to appropriate area.	5		

Steps	Possible Points	First Attempt	Second Attempt
11. Remove gloves and sanitize hands.	5		
12. Document the results in the patient's medical record and the laboratory logbook.	5		
Total Points Possible	90		

Comments: Total Points Earned _____   Instructor's Signature _____

Student Name _____   Date _____

CHECKLIST: INSTRUCT A PATIENT IN COLLECTION OF MIDSTREAM CLEAN-CATCH URINE SPECIMEN

TASK: Instruct a patient in the correct method for obtaining a midstream clean-catch urine specimen.

CONDITIONS: Given the proper equipment and supplies, the student will be required to demonstrate the proper method for instructing a patient in the collection of a midstream clean-catch urine specimen.

EQUIPMENT AND SUPPLIES
- Midstream urine collection kit OR
- Sterile specimen container with lid and three antiseptic towelettes

STANDARDS: Complete the procedure within _____ minutes and achieve a minimum score of _____%.

Time began _____   Time ended _____

Steps	Possible Points	First Attempt	Second Attempt
1. Sanitize hands.	5		
2. Assemble equipment and supplies and verify the order.	5		
3. Greet and identify the patient, and escort the patient to the examination room.	5		
4. Label the container with the patient's name and clinic identification number.	10		
5. Instruct the patient to wash and dry his or her hands.	10		
6. Instruct the patient to loosen the top of the collection container and to not touch the inside of the container.	10		
7. Provide the patient with instructions for collecting the specimen.	5		
Total Points Possible	50		

Comments: Total Points Earned _____   Instructor's Signature _____

Student Name _____   Date _____

CHECKLIST: USE A STERILE DISPOSABLE MICROLANCET FOR SKIN PUNCTURE

TASK: Obtain a capillary blood specimen acceptable for testing using the index or middle finger.

CONDITIONS: Given the proper equipment and supplies, the student will be required to use a sterile disposable microlancet for puncturing the skin to obtain a capillary sample.

EQUIPMENT AND SUPPLIES
- Nonsterile disposable gloves
- Alcohol wipes
- Sterile disposable microlancet with semiautomated lancet device or semiautomatic, one-use lancet system
- Sterile 2 × 2-inch gauze pads
- Sharps container
- Bandage and adhesive
- Patient's medical record

SUPPLIES FOR ORDERED TEST
Depending on the test ordered, the following supplies must be available
- Unopette
- Microhematocrit capillary tubes
- Microcontainers
- Glass slides
- Glucometer or cholesterol device
- Clay sealant tray

STANDARDS: Complete the procedure within _____ minutes and achieve a minimum score of _____%.

Time began _____   Time ended _____

Steps	Possible Points	First Attempt	Second Attempt
1. Sanitize hands.	5		
2. Assemble equipment and supplies, and verify order.	5		
3. Greet and identify the patient, and escort the patient to the examination room.	5		
4. Explain the procedure to the patient.	5		
5. Open the sterile gauze packet and place the gauze pad on the inside of its wrapper.	5		
6. Open the sterile lancet system.	5		
7. Position the patient comfortably either sitting or lying down with the palmer surface of the hand facing up and the arm supported.	10		
8. Select the appropriate puncture site.	10		
9. Warm the site to increase blood flow.	10		
10. Don gloves.	5		

Steps	Possible Points	First Attempt	Second Attempt
11. Cleanse the puncture site with an alcohol wipe, and allow to air-dry.	10		
12. Prepare the lancet as appropriate to perform the puncture.	5		
13. Dispose of the lancet in biohazardous sharps container.	5		
14. Wipe away the first drop of blood with dry gauze.	10		
15. If necessary, massage the finger by applying gentle, continuous pressure from the knuckles to the puncture site to increase the blood flow.	15		
16. Allow a second well-rounded drop of blood to form, and collect the specimen in the correct manner for the test ordered.	10		
17. Provide the patient with a clean gauze square and instruct to apply pressure directly over the site upon completion of collection.	10		
18. Bandage the puncture site as appropriate.	10		
19. Remove the gloves and sanitize the hands before transporting the specimen to the laboratory for processing.	10		
Total Points Possible	150		

Comments: Total Points Earned _____   Instructor's Signature _____

Student Name _____   Date _____

CHECKLIST: SEPARATE SERUM FROM A BLOOD SAMPLE

TASK: Transfer serum separated from whole blood through the process of centrifugation into a transfer tube.

CONDITIONS: Given the proper equipment and supplies, the student will transfer serum separated from whole blood through the process of centrifugation into a transfer tube.

EQUIPMENT AND SUPPLIES
- Nonsterile disposable gloves
- Personal protective equipment (PPE)
- Clotted blood specimen
- Laboratory requisition form

STANDARDS: Complete the procedure within _____ minutes and achieve a minimum score of _____%.

Time began _____   Time ended _____

Steps	Possible Points	First Attempt	Second Attempt
1. Sanitize hands.	5		
2. Assemble equipment and supplies, and verify order.	5		
3. Put on gloves and other appropriate PPE.	5		
4. Verify orders against the laboratory requisition form and the specimen tube.	5		
5. Place two-stoppered red-top tubes in the centrifuge to balance the centrifuge, and close and latch the centrifuge lid securely.	10		
6. Set timer for 15 minutes.	10		
7. When the time has elapsed, allow the centrifuge to come to a complete stop before opening the lid and removing the tube.	10		
8. Properly remove the stopper or apply a transfer device.	10		
9. Separate the serum from the top of the tube into a transfer tube using the transfer device or a disposable pipette. If a red/gray (marbled), speckled, or Hemogard gold tube is used, the serum may be poured into a transfer tube.	10		
10. Label the tubes and attach the laboratory requisition form.	10		
11. Properly dispose of all waste material in the appropriate waste receptacle.	5		
12. Package the specimen for transport to the laboratory.	10		
13. Remove gloves and sanitize the hands.	5		
Total Points Possible	100		

Comments: Total Points Earned _____   Instructor's Signature _____

Student Name _____   Date _____

CHECKLIST: URINALYSIS USING REAGENT STRIPS

TASK: Observe, record, and report the physical and chemical properties of a urine sample using Multistix 10-SG.

CONDITIONS: Given the proper equipment and supplies, the student will perform a urinalysis using reagent strips.

EQUIPMENT AND SUPPLIES
- Nonsterile disposable gloves
- Personal protective equipment (PPE)
- Multistix 10-SG reagent strips
- Normal and abnormal quality control reagent strips
- Laboratory report form
- Quality control logsheet
- Urine specimen container
- Conical urine centrifuge tubes
- Digital timer or watch with second hand
- Paper towel
- 10% bleach solution
- Biohazardous waste container
- Patient's medical record
- Laboratory log

STANDARDS: Complete the procedure within _____ minutes and achieve a minimum score of _____%.

Time began _____   Time ended _____

Steps	Possible Points	First Attempt	Second Attempt
1. Sanitize hands.	5		
2. Verify the order. Assemble equipment and supplies.	5		
3. Greet and identify the patient, and escort the patient to the examination room or laboratory area. Explain the procedure to the patient.	5		
4. Ask the patient to collect a midstream clean-catch urine specimen.	10		
5. Apply gloves and other PPE as indicated.	5		
6. While waiting for the patient to collect the specimen, record the lot number and expiration date of Multistix 10-SG on the laboratory quality control logsheet.	5		
7. Place controls from the manufacturer's container into the urine centrifuge tubes and record the lot number and expiration date on the tubes if the first samples of the day.	10		
8. Observe and record the physical properties of the control samples as appropriate.	10		
9. Remove one strip from container. Recap the bottle immediately.	5		

Steps	Possible Points	First Attempt	Second Attempt
10. Dip the strip in the abnormal control specimen and draw it out, pulling along the edge of the tube top to remove excess urine.	5		
11. Read each test on the strip after the manufacturer's recommended time has elapsed.	5		
12. Check the second hand on a watch to read the results after the recommended time has elapsed.	5		
13. Once the reagent strip has been interpreted and documented on the logsheet, discard the reagent strip in the biohazardous waste container.	5		
14. Repeat the process for the normal control specimen.	10		
15. Check controls to be sure recommended ranges have been achieved.	10		
16. After the reagent strip has been read, interpreted, and documented on the logsheet, discard the reagent strip in the biohazardous waste container.	10		
17. Prepare the patient specimen for testing.	5		
18. Perform steps 9 through 16 on the patient sample and record the result on the laboratory report form.	10		
19. Clean and disinfect the work area with a 10% bleach solution.	5		
20. Remove gloves and dispose of in a biohazardous waste container.	10		
21. Sanitize the hands.	10		
22. Document the results and provide to the physician.	10		
23. Document the procedure.	10		
24. After the physician has reviewed the results, place the laboratory report form if applicable in the patient's medical record.	5		
Total Points Possible	175		

Comments: Total Points Earned _____   Instructor's Signature _____

Student Name _____   Date _____

CHECKLIST: PREPARE A URINE SPECIMEN FOR MICROSCOPIC EXAMINATION

TASK: Prepare a urine sample for examination using a microscope.

CONDITIONS: Given the proper equipment and supplies, the student will prepare a urine specimen for microscopic examination.

EQUIPMENT AND SUPPLIES
- Nonsterile disposable gloves
- Personal protective equipment (PPE)
- Urine specimen container
- Comical urine centrifuge tubes with caps
- Disposable pipette
- Microscope slide and coverslip
- Centrifuge
- Paper towel
- Biohazardous waste container
- Laboratory logbook

NOTE: Perform Procedure 1-8 and then Procedure 2-1 in preparation for a microscopic urinalysis.

STANDARDS: Complete the procedure within _____ minutes and achieve a minimum score of _____%.

Time began _____   Time ended _____

Steps	Possible Points	First Attempt	Second Attempt
1. Sanitize the hands.	5		
2. Assemble equipment and supplies, and verify the order.	5		
3. Put on gloves and other PPE as indicated.	5		
4. Prepare a urine sediment sample by centrifuging. Properly fill tube and centrifuge before starting centrifuge.	10		
5. When the centrifuge stops, remove the cap from the specimen and discard it in the biohazardous waste container. Decant the supernatant fluid.	10		
6. Mix sediment with remaining urine in the bottom of the tube.	10		
7. Place a microscope slide on a paper towel, and pipette a drop of the mixed urine sediment in the center of the slide. Place coverslip on slide.	10		
8. Mount the slide on the microscope stage and adjust the coarse focus.	10		
9. Remove gloves and dispose of in a biohazardous waste container.	5		
10. Sanitize the hands.	5		

Steps	Possible Points	First Attempt	Second Attempt
11. Inform the physician that the slide is ready for viewing.	10		
12. Record the results in the laboratory logbook and medical record as reported by the physician and as office policy.	15		
Total Points Possible	100		

Comments: Total Points Earned _____   Instructor's Signature _____

Student Name _____   Date _____

CHECKLIST: PERFORM A URINE PREGNANCY TEST

TASK: Perform a urine pregnancy test using a commercially prepared CLIA-waived test (QuickVue).

CONDITIONS: Given the proper equipment and supplies, the student will be required to correctly perform a urine pregnancy test.

EQUIPMENT AND SUPPLIES
- Nonsterile disposable gloves
- Personal protective equipment (PPE)
- Urine specimen (preferably first morning specimen)
- Urine pregnancy testing kit (QuickVue)
- Biohazardous waste container
- Laboratory logbook
- Patient's medical record

STANDARDS: Complete the procedure within _____ minutes and achieve a minimum score of _____%.

Time began _____   Time ended _____

Steps	Possible Points	First Attempt	Second Attempt
1. Sanitize hands.	5		
2. Verify the order. Assemble equipment and supplies.	5		
3. Perform the quality control test as recommended by the manufacturer and document results in the laboratory logbook.	10		
4. Greet and identify the patient, and escort the patient to the examination room.	5		
5. If a urine specimen is to be collected in the office, explain the procedure to the patient.	10		
6. Provide the patient with the collection container and instructions as needed.	5		
7. Put on gloves and other PPE as indicated.	5		
8. Obtain a pregnancy test and prepare for testing according to manufacturer's directions.	5		
9. Time the test according to manufacturer's direction.	15		
10. Interpret the test results, and dispose of the test cassette in a biohazardous waste container.	10		
11. Remove gloves and dispose of in a biohazardous waste container.	10		
12. Sanitize the hands.	5		
13. Document the results in the patient's medical record and the laboratory logbook.	10		
Total Points Possible	100		

Comments: Total Points Earned _____   Instructor's Signature _____

Student Name _____   Date _____

CHECKLIST: PERFORM A MICROHEMATOCRIT TEST

TASK: Collect a capillary blood sample for performing a microhematocrit.

CONDITIONS: Given the proper equipment and supplies, the student will perform a microhematocrit.

EQUIPMENT AND SUPPLIES
- Nonsterile disposable gloves
- Personal protective equipment (PPE), as indicated
- Microhematocrit capillary tubes (heparinized)
- Sealing compound
- Alcohol wipe
- Sterile disposable microlancet
- Sterile 2 × 2-inch gauze squares
- 10% bleach solution
- Microhematocrit centrifuge or centrifuge with microhematocrit reading
- Microhematocrit reader
- Rigid biohazardous container
- Patient's medical record
- Laboratory logbook

STANDARDS: Complete the procedure within _____ minutes and achieve a minimum score of _____%.

Time began _____   Time ended _____

Steps	Possible Points	First Attempt	Second Attempt
1. Sanitize hands.	5		
2. Verify the order, and assemble equipment and supplies.	5		
3. Greet and identify the patient, escort the patient to the examination room or laboratory, and explain the procedure to the patient.	5		
4. Put on gloves and PPE as indicated.	5		
Collecting the Specimen			
5. Perform a capillary puncture and dispose of the lancet in a ridged biohazardous container.	10		
6. Wipe away the first drop of blood with a gauze pad.	5		
7. After the samples have been collected, hand the patient a clean gauze square and instruct to apply direct pressure to the puncture site.	5		
8. Seal the dry end of the capillary tubes with sealing clay.	10		
9. Leave the capillary tubes embedded in the sealing clay to prevent damage.	10		
10. Check the puncture site.	5		
11. Remove gloves, and sanitize hands.	10		

Steps	Possible Points	First Attempt	Second Attempt
Testing the Specimen			
12. Place the specimen in the centrifuge after donning gloves. Be sure to keep centrifuge balanced. The sealed end should be placed toward the outer edge. Record placement to prevent errors in identifying specimens.	10		
13. Secure the locking top by placing it over the threaded bolt on the centrifuge head and turning the fastener until tight.	5		
14. Spin for 5 minutes at 2500 rpm or use the high setting. If required by centrifuge being used, lock the high speed.	10		
15. When the centrifuge comes to a complete stop, unlatch the lid, and remove the locking top if appropriate.	10		
16. Position one of the tubes in the microhematocrit reader and adjust as necessary for reading the results.	10		
17. Determine the results of spun microhematocrit.	15		
18. Record the microhematocrit results.	10		
19. Discard the capillary tube in a rigid biohazardous container.	5		
20. Repeat the reading for the second capillary tube.	10		
21. Average the two results, and record the average value as the reading for the patient.	15		
22. Disinfect the work area with 10% bleach solution.	10		
23. Remove gloves and sanitize hands.	5		
24. Document the results in the patient's medical record.	10		
Total Points Possible	200		

Comments: Total Points Earned _____   Instructor's Signature _____

Student Name _____   Date _____

CHECKLIST: DETERMINE A HEMOGLOBIN MEASUREMENT USING A HEMOCUE

TASK: Accurately measure the hemoglobin using a HemoCue analyzer.

CONDITIONS: Given the proper equipment and supplies, the student will determine a hemoglobin measurement using a HemoCue analyzer.

EQUIPMENT AND SUPPLIES
- Nonsterile disposable gloves
- Personal protective equipment (PPE)
- Alcohol wipes
- Sterile disposable microlancet
- Sterile 2 × 2-inch gauze squares
- HemoCue Analyzer
- Control cuvette—normal and abnormal
- Microcuvettes
- 10% bleach solution
- Sharps container
- Biohazardous waste container
- Patient's medical record
- Laboratory quality control logsheet

STANDARDS: Complete the procedure within _____ minutes and achieve a minimum score of _____%.

Time began _____   Time ended _____

Steps	Possible Points	First Attempt	Second Attempt
1. Sanitize hands.	5		
2. Verify the order, and assemble equipment and supplies.	5		
3. Perform the quality control test as recommended by the manufacturer and document in the laboratory quality control logsheet if first test of the day or new container of microcassettes.	10		
4. Prepare the HemoCue analyzers for testing.	5		
5. Place the control cuvette into the holder and push into the photometer to validate the control values. Perform testing using controls and read and record results.	10		
6. Greet and identify the patient, and escort the patient to the examination room.	10		
7. Explain the procedure to the patient.	5		
8. Sanitize the hands and apply gloves and PPE as indicated.	10		
9. Perform capillary puncture and dispose of the lancet in a sharps container. Wipe away the first drop of blood with a gauze pad.	10		
10. Collect the specimen.	15		

Steps	Possible Points	First Attempt	Second Attempt
11. Wipe away excess blood from the tip of the cuvette.	10		
12. Place the cuvette in its holder and push into the photometer.	10		
13. Read and record the hemoglobin value from LED screen.	10		
14. Discard the cuvette into the rigid biohazardous container.	5		
15. Turn the equipment "off" as appropriate. Clean the equipment with a mild soap and water solution.	10		
16. Disinfect the work area with 10% bleach solution.	10		
17. Remove gloves and sanitize the hands.	5		
18. Document the results in the patient's medical record and the laboratory logbook.	5		
Total Points Possible	150		

Comments: Total Points Earned _____   Instructor's Signature _____

Student Name _____   Date _____

CHECKLIST: PERFORM GLUCOSE TESTING

TASK: Collect and process a blood specimen for glucose testing using AccuCheck.

CONDITIONS: Given the proper equipment and supplies, the student will perform a glucose test.

EQUIPMENT AND SUPPLIES
- Nonsterile disposable gloves
- Personal protection equipments (PPE), as indicated
- Supplies for capillary puncture
- Glucose testing equipment (AccuCheck)
- AccuCheck supplies
- Control test solution
- 10% bleach solution
- Sharps container
- Biohazardous waste container
- Patient's medical records
- Laboratory quality control logsheet
- Laboratory logbook

STANDARDS: Complete the procedure within _____ minutes and achieve a minimum score of _____%.

Time began _____   Time ended _____

Steps	Possible Points	First Attempt	Second Attempt
1. Sanitize hands.	5		
2. Verify the order, and assemble equipment and supplies.	5		
3. Prepare the analyzer according to the manufacturer's instructions.	5		
4. Perform a quality control test as recommended by the manufacturer, and document in the laboratory quality control logsheet.	10		
5. Greet and identify the patient, and escort the patient to the examination room or laboratory. Explain the procedure to the patient. Determine when last food was ingested.	10		
6. Perform a capillary puncture.	10		
7. Insert a test strip into the test strip slot.	10		
8. Apply a rounded drop of blood from the capillary puncture to the test strip. Start the timer for testing.	10		
9. Discard the test strip into the biohazardous container.	5		
10. Turn off the glucometer and wipe it with a damp cloth	10		
11. Disinfect the work area using 10% bleach solution.	5		

Steps	Possible Points	First Attempt	Second Attempt
12. Remove gloves and sanitize the hands.	5		
13. Document the results in the patient's medical record and the laboratory logbook.	10		
Total Points Possible	100		

Comments: Total Points Earned _____   Instructor's Signature _____

Student Name _____   Date _____

CHECKLIST: OBTAIN A BACTERIAL SMEAR FROM A WOUND SPECIMEN

TASK: Collect a sample of wound exudates, using sterile collection supplies, and prepare the specimen for transport to laboratory.

CONDITIONS: Given the proper equipment and supplies, the student will role-play obtaining a bacterial smear from a wound specimen.

EQUIPMENT AND SUPPLIES
- Nonsterile disposable gloves
- Personal protective equipment (PPE), as indicated
- Laboratory requisition form
- Plastic-backed small drape
- Sterile gauze (4 × 4 inch)
- Bottle of 10% antiseptic solution
- Surgical tape
- Bandage roll
- Marking pen
- Agar-gel transport system (sterile tube with sterile swab and semisolid solution in the bottom)
- 10% bleach solution
- Biohazardous waste container
- Patient's medical record

STANDARDS: Complete the procedure within _____ minutes and achieve a minimum score of _____%.

Time began _____   Time ended _____

Steps	Possible Points	First Attempt	Second Attempt
1. Sanitize hands.	5		
2. Verify the order. Assemble equipment and supplies.	5		
3. Prepare a laboratory requisition form for microbiology department.	5		
4. Greet and identify the patient and escort the patient to the examination room.	5		
5. Explain the procedure to the patient.	5		
6. Apply gloves and PPE as indicated.	5		
7. Position the patient for easy access to the area for specimen collection.	5		
8. Remove dressing and dispose in a biohazardous waste container. Inspect wound for odor, color, amount of drainage, and depth.	15		
9. Open transport system and obtain sterile swab, being careful to prevent contamination when removing from kit.	10		
10. Change gloves.	5		

Steps	Possible Points	First Attempt	Second Attempt
11. Obtain the specimen from area with greatest amount of exudates by moving the swab from side to side.	10		
12. Carefully return the swab to the tube, taking care to prevent contamination by extraneous microorganisms.	10		
13. Label the specimen.	10		
14. Place the agar-gel transport tube in a biohazard transport bag and seal the bag.	10		
15. Cleanse the wound using medical aseptic technique.	10		
16. Apply a clean bandage to the wound site using sterile technique.	5		
17. Dispose of all waste material appropriately, and disinfect the work area using 10% bleach solution.	5		
18. Remove gloves and sanitize the hands.	5		
19. Complete the laboratory requisition form and transport the specimen to lab as soon as possible.	10		
20. Document the procedure.	10		
Total Points Possible	150		

Comments: Total Points Earned _____   Instructor's Signature _____

Page numbers followed by f indicate figures; t, tables; b, boxes.